3/50

CONCEPT CLARIFICATION IN NURSING

Edited by
Catherine M. Norris, R.N., Ed.D.
Professor of Nursing
School of Nursing
University of Minnesota

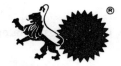

AN ASPEN PUBLICATION®
Aspen Systems Corporation
Rockville, Maryland
London
1982

Library of Congress Cataloging in Publication Data

Main entry under title:
Concept clarification in nursing.

Includes index.
1. Nursing—Philosophy. 2. Symptomatology.
I. Norris, Catherine M. [DNLM: 1. Nursing care. WY 100
C743]
RT84.5.C66 1982   610.73   81-83859
ISBN: 0-89443-825-5

Publisher: John Marozsan
Editorial Director: Darlene Como
Managing Editor: Margot Raphael
Editorial Services: M. Eileen Higgins
Printing and Manufacturing: Debbie Collins

Library of Congress Catalog Card Number: 81-83859
ISBN: 0-89443-825-5

Printed in the United States of America

1   2   3   4   5

To *Hildegard E. Peplau*, nurse, scholar, and teacher, who introduced a generation of nurses to concept clarification as a way to nursing knowledge

Table of Contents

        Karma Castleberry and Frances Seither

        "I Never Felt That Way. If You Feel like That, You
            Must Be Crazy!" 309
        Common Attitudes and Experiences 310
        Nursing and the Concept of Disorientation 312
        Predisposing Factors 313
        Associated Factors 314
        Manifestations 316
        Patient Adaptation 317

Chapter 19—Nipple Confusion in Neonates **325**
        June Kroh Kershner

        Defining Nipple Confusion and Describing Its
            Properties 325
        Suggested Causal Relationships 326
        Physiological, Cultural, and Behavioral Theories Related
            to Nipple Confusion 328
        Explanation of Beginning Conceptual Model 331

Chapter 20—Immobilization in Adolescents **333**
        Audrey J. Kalafatich

        The Literature on Immobility 333
        Immobility and Adolescence 336
        Conclusion 339

Chapter 21—Immobilization: Psychosocial Aspects **341**
        Becky Jane Christian

        Introduction 341
        What the Words Tell Us 341
        Immobilization: Points of View 342
        Relationship Between Age and Onset of Immobility 343
        Onset, Duration, Intensity, and Severity of
            Immobilization 344
        Spatial Relationships and Immobility 344
        Life-Style and Immobility 344
        Emotional Life and Immobility 345
        Other Considerations 346

Foreword

Over the course of her career, Catherine M. Norris has consistently presented ideas that were timely, provocative, and intellectually challenging. This book is squarely in that tradition. Dr. Norris deals with the difficult issues involved in developing a knowledge base for a practice discipline, one of the most critically important and difficult undertakings with which nursing is presently concerned.

The effort in nursing to identify the knowledge on which nursing practice is based is a long-standing one. Attempts to develop that knowledge through scientific investigation of clinical problems are becoming increasingly sophisticated, reflecting two major trends over the past 20 years: (1) increased variety and strength of academic programs preparing nurses as investigators and (2) serious attention to the need for nurses to be expert clinicians. These two interrelated thrusts have given rise in recent years to rapid expansion in the number of doctoral programs in nursing, which should further hasten the development of a sound practice base for nursing.

The serious attention being given by nurses to research and the revolution in science that has been occurring in the past two decades should make for an unprecedented richness in theoretical and methodological approaches to the construction of nursing knowledge. It is time for creativity to combine with the broader and more sophisticated understanding of scientific methods to produce a rich and useful practice base. The work of Catherine M. Norris and the contributors to her book will add greatly to this effort.

Dr. Norris asserts that if nursing indeed has a holistic emphasis, then more attention must be given by nurse clinicians and scholars to developing approaches to patient care that reflect not only psychosocial but also biological bases of human behavior. While not denying the need for nurses to understand the psychosocial dimensions of behavior, Dr. Norris emphasizes an area that she believes has been relatively neglected in recent years: physiological aspects of behavior. In focusing on lower-level physiological needs, she is trying to address the imbalance that has characterized much of nursing literature in recent years.

Another kind of imbalance that has characterized the development of nursing knowledge, according to Dr. Norris, is the overreliance on theories and conceptual frameworks from other disciplines. Dr. Norris argues for more use of essentially inductive approaches to the development of concepts. Again, not denying the need for deduction and interaction between deductive and inductive processes in developing concepts and theories, she focuses on the use of induction in clarifying concepts relevant to nursing practice and urges the use of multiple methods for clarifying the concepts of the profession. Dr. Norris describes Carnap's classical approach to concept formation, but she also examines and gives examples of numerous other approaches, including phenomenological and ethnoscience methods. Above all, she encourages nurse scholars and clinicians to "pursue the unlikely, the ridiculous and incongruous as well as the fantasies, dreams, nightmares, and hunches."

Choosing 15 concepts, 10 of which she and the contributing authors clarify in some detail and 5 others that are briefly identified, Dr. Norris develops the overall umbrella concept of "protection." Suggesting that this concept is broad enough to organize all of the other concepts under it, she develops a beginning theory of physiological protective phenomena. Her discussion of criteria to use in setting priorities for promoting and attending to the protective mechanisms will serve as a useful guide for nurse researchers and clinicians in choosing problems of significance for study.

This book and the ideas presented in it more than fulfill the promise of a fine practitioner, scholar, and educator. *Concept Clarification in Nursing* will serve as a basis for countless serious deliberations by nurse clinicians and scholars concerned with the practice base of their discipline.

—*Ada Jacox, R.N., Ph.D.*
Professor of Nursing
University of Maryland

Preface

One of the goals of *Concept Clarification in Nursing* is to foster the development of increasingly meaningful descriptions of nursing phenomena. Out of these descriptions will come critical questions and hypotheses which nurses will need to explore. Out of these descriptions, nurses will ultimately build the base for a substantive body of knowledge for the discipline called nursing.

The nursing phenomena selected have been studied from a variety of points of view. The concepts represented by these phenomena have been clarified to a great extent so that they can be useful in helping nurses at all levels to better understand the phenomena with which they work and to recognize one kind of knowledge that they need to seek in order to do their job well. The overall goal is to involve more nurses in the sometimes fascinating, often frustrating, frequently messy, and once in a while exciting work of clarifying the concepts of nursing.

Concept Clarification in Nursing is not a nursing text, though treatment of material does reflect recent work and recent thinking. It was developed to illustrate one approach to developing nursing knowledge. It was written for clinicians, especially, so that they could have a clearer perception of the role all nurses have in studying the phenomena involved in their practice. It was developed for students so that they could move ahead in developing and refining the methodology of concept clarification. It was developed for faculty who are concerned with inductive as well as deductive methods in introducing students to the study of nursing. And it was written for a new group of researchers in nursing—descriptive researchers who will contribute substantially to the discipline of nursing.

When nursing first began to strive for professional status, one of its greatest deterrents was lack of prepared researchers. To develop a corps of researchers, nurses were trained in a variety of scientific disciplines. For a profession in a hurry this was faster than having large numbers of nurses spending years doing descriptive work and developing methodologies for studying clinical nursing phenomena. But the greatest advantage of having nurses prepared for research in the social, behavioral, and biological sciences was that the methodologies of these sciences gave nursing a research armamentarium at a time when it was urgently needed.

As it happened, these pioneer nurse researchers were trained essentially in the psychosocial disciplines, a situation related to the fact that baccalaureate nursing graduates met admission requirements for the psychosocial doctoral programs but had insufficient science and mathematics preparation for admission to physiology and biochemistry majors. Graduates of these programs came back to nursing bringing research methodologies and substantive content from the social sciences to bear upon nursing problems. Research methodologies were often modified to conform to the aims, purposes, or framework of nursing, but they had not been created for use with nursing's client-patient universe, nor were they created for use within the contexts in which nursing is done.

It is much easier to operate out of a discipline whose concepts and theories have been all worked out. While many studies based on these orientations have been useful in improving practice, questions are becoming more frequent and urgent about the application of findings and assignment of meaning from these studies to the population with which nursing is concerned. Borrowed experimental approaches from the sciences need to be monitored to prevent nurse doctoral programs from providing misapplied, misused research training. We need to approach the whole area of research in nursing with the awareness that when nurse researchers have expertise in a body of knowledge—say anthropology, psychology, or sociology—they must relate the conceptual framework of the discipline to a conceptual foundation for nursing. This volume attempts to analyze concepts in light of the purposes and values of nursing.

Above and beyond the ambiguities, vagueness, and fragmentation of nursing conceptual frameworks for research is a more critical question: How do nursing researchers know they are studying the basic problems of nursing or even that they are studying nursing problems at all? One could presumably all one's life study trivia that would never have systematic impact (potential for explanation, predictive ability, or potential for becoming an integral part of theory). Research generated from social science and physiology concepts can bypass the experience nurses have with patient-client problems. Also, in these sciences, researchers live with the materials they work with and know what they will do in the laboratory. When nurse researchers do not go into clinical settings, that is, use two laboratories, one to collect data and check out results and the other to analyze data, they do not address the real world of nursing or the crucial nursing problems that exist. Progress may be made at levels not meaningful in nursing care, even though the findings might be meaningful to members of the discipline from which the methodology was derived.

With the proliferation of doctoral programs in nursing, it could be that nursing researchers trained in other disciplines who are the teachers of doctoral students in nursing are going to provide these students with a cross-discipline orientation to research and research methodology. Despite any benefits of this approach, there could be further delay to the development of a substantive body of nursing knowledge and the creation of methodologies to study nursing phenomena. If nursing is to advance its professional status, if it is to become more than a psychosocial discipline and regard people in a holistic way, it must do its descriptive work. That, in essence, is the mission of this volume.

Many phenomena commonly confronting nurses have not been studied using descriptive techniques by any clinical health profession. These phenomena remain at the level of folklore for the average professional. The nursing care in these cases is at the level of empiricism. While physiologists may have done considerable study related to these phenomena, their findings have not been picked up by either clinical workers or health care scientists for study. Nursing needs to do its descriptive work on these and other nursing concepts, and to telescope the work so that it does not take centuries to get accurate, comprehensive data about clients-patients and about nursing practices. This means that nurses need to monitor and describe the work of nursing. In one sense, such an approach represents a backward step from the rigorous research stance of the last two decades. In another sense, however, contributing to the development of sound conceptual frameworks for nursing will ultimately be a step ahead.

The concepts chosen for clarification in this volume are concerned with common human problems classified at lower levels in hierarchies of needs. They were chosen because of frequency of occurrence and because nurses are expected to do something about their existence if nurses are present when they occur. Each chapter represents substantive knowledge more than a methodology for developing a conceptual foundation for nursing. Rather than rework existing abstract nursing concepts, a different, more concrete level of concept was selected.

Concepts chosen were examined so as to eliminate medical phenomena as much as possible. For example, the understanding of myocardial infarct is necessary to medicine. It is interesting to nurses, but nurses do not work with it. Concepts necessary to nursing in this context might be dyspnea, restlessness, and nausea. Physicians are interested in these behaviors, but their real focus is on the treatment of the infarction.

Which concepts were to be explored was determined by the nurses willing to work on them. Nurses volunteered or were located to clarify the concepts of nausea, vomiting, thirst, hunger, fatigue, immobility, insomnia, pressure sores, itching, disorientation, and chilling. No nurse was found willing to clarify diarrhea, constipation, impaction, incontinence, frequency, dribbling, retention, flatulence, anorexia, weakness, perspiration, hiccoughs, or dyspnea. Gastrointestinal tract phenomena, especially those of the lower tract, do not seem to be interesting to nurses. Many of these patient problems that daily confront nurses and the healthy population are the kinds of experiences nurses would like to forget about. They do not want to talk about them or report them at scientific meetings. One exception is Barbara Hansen, who developed a typology of stools on which she reported at the American Nurses' Association Convention in Hawaii in 1978. Such resistance may relate to the role of women in ancient societies. "Those who do demeaning work—who clean up the messes of others—are treated with little respect" (S. Smoyak in Norma Chaska, *The Nursing Profession,* New York, McGraw-Hill, 1978, p. 324).

It is easier to move from the empirical world into areas of abstraction with concepts like role or anxiety than it is with nausea, itching, and flatulence. Since successful coping with primitive physiological processes is required to provide the base for higher-level needs to move into ascendancy (H. Peplau, *Interpersonal Relations in Nursing,* New York, Putnam, 1951, p. 182), it is somewhat difficult to understand nurses' reluctance to deal with lower-level needs. If they are not dealt with, we may create a strange discipline where, in addition to emphasis on the psychosocial dimension, we deal only with the upper half of the human body. This leaves the lower half to some emerging discipline (or to the devil, who proverbially takes the hindmost). Let us hope that ignoring many of the phenomena of nursing is inadvertent rather than a denial that they are our concerns while we look for higher-level concepts that would appear to put us on equal footing with other disciplines in the upper levels of the scientific ether.

At this early stage in describing the specified phenomena, contributors were not asked to conform to a particular method of concept clarification or to do formal concept construction. They were not asked to review the clinical, theoretical, or research literature. They were not asked to do any clinical study or to control their work with patients or clients. It was understood that they would each develop a methodology using authorities in the field or original ideas of their own. This is particularly evident in the instances where the same concept was developed by different people, as in the work on fatigue, nausea, vomiting, and immobility. Some concepts have more hypothesis-producing power related to developing substantive knowledge than others, and others generate hypotheses that are related to nursing process. Differences in approach may be determined by the amount of research and clarification already done. Some concepts have had almost no work, while others have been developed both in nursing and by other disciplines. Differences in level of sophistication of various chapters demonstrates that nurses at all levels can begin to do concept clarification.

Concept Clarification in Nursing attempts then to get at the scope of concept clarification for the phenomena studied and provides the reader with ideas about the possibilities for identifying various aspects of the concepts, since these concepts, on the whole, are so complex that they will very likely become theories as their components are named and operationalized. One problem nurses have in clarifying concepts is the need to devise, invent, or otherwise elucidate nursing care for the phenomenon they clarify, almost as if producing questions for study and hypotheses was not an acceptable way to conclude a piece of nursing research work. Some contributors to this volume demonstrate this need for immediate application of new insights.

In the future, nurses will study or use only that piece of the total concept that relates to the work at hand. For example, if a nurse is studying "morning sickness" in pregnancy, only this aspect of the total concept of nausea and vomiting would be tapped. Or if fatigue in multiple sclerosis is being considered, only those aspects of fatigue related to neuromuscular disease would be selected in building the conceptual basis for study.

It is my wish to acknowledge the contribution of many people to my thinking and to take full responsibility for how the contributions of these people are developed here. First, there are hundreds of students who argued, debated, and complained, thus helping to refocus my thinking on the primary thesis of the book. Dr. Anna M. Voda provided contact with graduate students who were working on concepts. In addition, Dr. Voda read most of the manuscript and made invaluable suggestions. Dr. Ada K. Jacox continues her long years of support for my work. It is especially appreciated because I know how many reservations she has about the route I take. Drs. Jan Beckstrand, Karma Castleberry, Beth Gedan, Frances Seither, and Marilyn Sime read the chapter on itching and made helpful suggestions for refining this material. Mary L. Morris read many chapters and provided detailed suggestions that were useful in rewriting, editing, and organizing the volume. Dr. Dorothy Bloch read the manuscript when it was to be only a periodical article. Her suggestions changed the course of the work. To all of these people I am grateful. The contributors were patient with rewrites, editing, and the long wait while I labored over my chapters. They never lost faith about this as one approach to nursing knowledge. They are a very special group of people to me. Dr. Suzanne Smith Coletta and Debra Osnowitz of Nursing Resources gave freely of their expertise and their support. They too made an invaluable contribution to getting the book in print.

Catherine M. Norris
September 1982

Contributors

JUNE ABBEY, R.N., PH.D.
Professor of Nursing
School of Nursing
University of Pittsburgh
Pittsburgh, Pennsylvania

JACQUELINE ANDERSON, R.N.,
M.S.
2541 East Blacklidge
Tucson, Arizona

KARMA S. CASTLEBERRY, R.N.,
PH.D.
Assistant Professor of Nursing
Radford University
Radford, Virginia

BECKY JANE CHRISTIAN, R.N.,
M.S.
Instructor in Family-Child
Nursing
School of Nursing
University of Missouri
Columbia, Missouri

MILDRED I. FREEL, R.N., M.ED.
Associate Professor
College of Nursing
University of Iowa
Iowa City, Iowa

LAURA K. HART, R.N., PH.D.
Associate Professor
College of Nursing
University of Iowa
Iowa City, Iowa

AUDREY J. KALAFATICH, R.N.,
ED.D.
Clinical Specialist, Nursing of
Adolescents
St. Louis Children's Hospital
St. Louis, Missouri

JANE KROH KERSHNER, B.S.N.,
C.P.N.P.
Pediatric Nurse Practitioner
College of Medicine
University of Arizona Health
Sciences Center
Tucson, Arizona

SUSAN G. MINOW, R.N., M.S.
Critical Care Education
Coordinator
Idaho Falls Consolidated
Hospitals
Idaho Falls, Idaho

MARY L. MORRIS, R.N., ED.D.
Professor of Medical-Surgical
Nursing
College of Nursing
The University of Tennessee
Center for the Health Sciences
Memphis, Tennessee

CATHERINE M. NORRIS, R.N.,
ED.D.
Professor of Nursing
School of Nursing
University of Minnesota
Minneapolis, Minnesota

GUADALUPE S. OLIVAS, R.N.,
M.S.
Doctoral Candidate
College of Nursing
University of Arizona
Tucson, Arizona

MARY PROKOP, R.N., B.S.
Staff Nurse, ICU/CCU
United Health Services
Endicott, New York

MARY PAT RANDALL, R.N., M.S.
142 Manor Drive
Beckley, Virginia

DEBRA RHOTEN, R.N., M.S.
929 Louisiana S.E.
Albuquerque, New Mexico

MARY ANN SCHROEDER, R.N.,
PH.D.
Assistant Professor of Research
School of Nursing
University of Pittsburgh
Pittsburgh, Pennsylvania

FRANCES G. SEITHER, R.N., PH.D.
Professor of Nursing
Radford University
Radford, Virginia

MARY L. SHANNON, R.N., ED.D.
Professor of Medical-Surgical
Nursing
Medical-Surgical Nursing
Graduate Program
University of Tennessee Center
for the Health Sciences
Memphis, Tennessee

ANN M. VODA, R.N., PH.D.
Professor of Nursing
School of Nursing
University of Utah
Salt Lake City, Utah

Part I

Foundations of Concept Clarification in Nursing

This brief review of concept clarification in nursing highlights three directions for refining concept work—deepening understanding, perfecting existing concepts and developing new methodologies, and providing effective synthesis.

This section lays the foundation for developing exploratory and descriptive methods to build nursing knowledge by using clinical observation as a starting point. Chapter 1 presents an overview of the history of concept clarification. Chapter 2 categorizes concept clarification as a scientific activity and specifies how to identify this as *nursing* activity. Further, we learn what the outcomes of concept clarification contribute to nursing knowledge.

Chapter 3 provides material to orient nurses to the work of concept clarification. *Collegial support* is seen as one possible solution to dealing with frustrations in this work. Communication among colleagues also contributes through consensual validation, intellectual stimulation, and criticism. Biases of prospective concept workers are discussed from the points of view of concept selection, values, and role of nursing. Safeguarding the nursing perspective as well as identifying expectations about outcomes of the work are also explored. The communication base required by concept workers is emphasized. Finally, a brief introduction to the area of categorization and a statement about the limitations of concept clarification are given.

Chapter 4 describes the methodological structure of qualitative research and briefly introduces 10 potential methods that have emerged from the social sciences and from nursing. Half of the methods represent nursing innovations and the others have been modified to relate to nursing.

Chapter 1

History of Concept Clarification in Nursing

Catherine M. Norris

Physicians have already spent 400 years clarifying the phenomena of medicine and continue to do descriptive work. Nursing has, by contrast, a 25- or 30-year history of descriptive work. Preliminary descriptive research in medicine has provided the volume and type of data from which both predictive and intervention models can be constructed. These models are used in developing programs that compute diagnoses, treatment options (including risks for each option), and prognoses. Models are also constructed and applied to project health risks for people 5, and even 10, years in the future. Predictive and intervention models exemplify the phenomena being studied as well as representing abstractions of great masses of data. Mathematical models, such as those being developed in the field of medicine, embody considerable scientific achievement.

THEORY CONSTRUCTION PROBLEMS

Projecting, diagnosing, and intervening in illness is possible even though the conceptual framework of the discipline of medicine limits full perception of patients' problems. Specifically, physicians have been unable to build a *holistic model* of the human being. Descriptive work has been and is being done within the psyche–soma dualistic model. This restrictive model has resulted in a separate theory for each disease or syndrome studied by medicine. For some diseases there are several—often competing—theories. The inability to abstract and synthesize these theories has trapped medicine in a simplistic chief-complaint framework that makes complex behavioral data incomprehensible. Further, medicine's long association with physiology, engendering increasing reliance on cellular- and subcellular-level data, has fostered reductionism with resulting devaluation of human life. Increasing public pressure to reduce costs of medical care forces physicians to make more cost-effective use of their time. This in turn reinforces simplistic approaches to people and unicausal theories of behavior as well as the mind–body dichotomy.

3

The young and as-yet-unsophisticated field of nursing has so far avoided the theory-construction problems of medicine and, it is hoped, can do descriptive work within the holistic frameworks developed for the discipline. Ideally, nursing will do sufficient descriptive work before putting its practice theories and models in final form. Nurses are only beginning to build nursing knowledge formally, and only this will permit the evolution of the discipline.

COMPILING KNOWLEDGE

About 25 years ago, a few teachers of nursing started clarifying nursing concepts and publishing their results. Their first attempts were aimed not toward creating a nursing discipline but, instead, toward compiling professional-level knowledge that could be transmitted to students and used in developing clinical nursing skills. Nursing as a profession could not be limited to procedures and nursing activities, especially since an ever-increasing and competitive corps of technical nurses was emerging to challenge whether the practice of the professional nurse was different from technical practice in kind or in level of sophistication.

Practice as a Source of Knowledge

In addition to lacking differentiation between the discipline of nursing and a body of nursing-practice knowledge, the first concepts clarified for nursing were essentially developed without consideration of method. Most nurses focused on patient problems with the aim of discovering nursing knowledge. "Anxiety—A Factor in Nursing Care" (Gregg 1952), "Reassurance" (Gregg 1955), "The Nurse and the Dying Patient" (Norris 1955), "Loneliness" (Peplau 1955), and "The Nurse and the Crying Patient" (Norris 1957), were among the early concepts developed. Tudor (1952), in what has become a classic study in nursing, took the concept of mutual withdrawal beyond earlier studies by demonstrating how clinical data can be used in clarifying a concept.

Shortly thereafter, nursing routines were scrutinized for knowledge that would guide practice beyond dependence on policy, "should systems," and techniques. Works that looked at nursing practice as a source of nursing knowledge include "When a Student Dislikes a Patient" (Highley and Norris 1957) and "Feeding: A Therapeutic Routine in Nursing" (Norris, Shea, and Eller 1963).

CONCEPT-BUILDING IN THE SPECIALTIES

Much of the early work of clarifying nursing concepts was done with psychiatric concepts (Burd and Marshall 1963). Fortunately, psychiatric nurses avoided diagnostic categories. Using symptoms and patient problems, they were able to relate their own work to the uniqueness of nursing. Psychiatric nursing appears to have been in the avant-garde in concept clarification. This is due, at least in part, to the fact that psychiatric nursing had federal support through the National Institute of Mental Health beginning in 1945—almost 20 years before other nursing specialty areas received federal funding under the Nurse Training Act. Psychiatric nurses also benefited from a dynamic teacher and leader, Hildegard Peplau. She convinced hundreds of nurses that documentation of practice and constantly refined conceptualization of that practice were keys to effective professional practice. Peplau identified how theories of nursing would evolve out of this work (Peplau 1969, 1970).

Under the auspices of the Western Interstate Commission for Higher Education, three groups of nursing faculty representing maternal–child nursing, medical–surgical nursing, and psychiatric nursing developed graduate programs in their respective areas. One approach used was the delineation, selection, and clarification of concepts for nursing. The work of these groups and their published reports (Ford, Cobb, and Taylor 1967; Fujiki, et al. 1967; Highley, et al. 1967; Lewis, et al. 1967) contributed to raising standards for graduate nursing education in the West, to delineating nursing content, and to highlighting the need for an intensive research effort.

Through exceptional vision Esther A. Garrison of the National Institute of Mental Health encouraged the Southern Regional Education Board and the School of Nursing at the University of California, Los Angeles to apply for funds to develop psychiatric–mental health nursing concepts. The applications were subsequently funded and, by the mid-1960s, many nurses became involved in clarifying concepts to improve nursing practice and teaching (Zderad and Belcher 1968; Carlson 1970).

Between 1965 and 1981, several books on concepts were written by nonpsychiatric nurses (Byrne and Thompson 1978; Jason and Trygstad 1979; Kintzel 1971; Meltzer 1969; Mitchell 1973; Murray and Zentner 1979; and Roberts 1978). A variety of theoretical approaches—systems theory, adaptation, basic human needs, and growth and development—were used to provide philosophical orientation, consistency and organization for the concepts selected. Concept readers, containing work formerly scattered throughout the literature, were also compiled (Kintzel 1971).

METHODOLOGY

Methodology for concept development has not been explicit, and work done thus far varies in focus, method, depth, scope, organization, logic and relevance for nursing. Some is, in fact, little more than a review of the literature. Even though ideas about concept clarification have been misused, nursing scholars should be acknowledged for identifying how different nursing is from medicine, for redefining nursing's independent functions, and for maintaining a humanistic, holistic approach to individuals and communities when other health professionals succumbed to the medical model.

By 1965, some nursing scholars became concerned about the lack of knowledge of concept clarification—knowledge prerequisite to the research process. Berthold (1964), in a paper still pertinent to nursing's concern with descriptive research, deals in depth with both empirical and theoretical clarification of concepts. The Western Interstate Commission for Higher Education in Nursing received federal support to conduct summer workshops so faculty could identify the core concepts of nursing appropriate to the various levels of nursing programs. During this ferment, Kramer (1970) suggested that explicating concepts using inductive-research methodologies would have the greatest payoff in the identification of specialized concepts in nursing.

Observers of nursing during the period 1950–1975 saw a concerted drive for a body of nursing knowledge by nursing scholars untrained in the methods of concept clarification, theory development, and descriptive methods of research. The occasional nurse who used the podium or the literature to support a descriptive route to knowledge was a "voice crying in the wilderness" as far as the average clinician, teacher, or even researcher in nursing was concerned. The immediate need for a body of knowledge has already been identified as a deterrent to research; further roadblocks came from the area of nursing research itself. In a desperate attempt to move the profession ahead and enter the competitive scientific world, nursing, along with other emerging disciplines, attempted to bypass the task of describing its phenomena. Instead, the profession touted experimental research as the best route to go. While the lack of description did not create problems for some researchers, others were and continue to be hampered by the lack of operational definitions, the ambiguous and multiple definitions, definitions developed for other disciplines, and the lack of conceptual models from which testable hypothesis could be formulated.

Descriptive Work

Nursing now seems to be taking a step back by doing descriptive work. But there appears to be a growing recognition that if we are to move knowledge from the level of folklore to science and theory and move intervention from the empirical to the scientific mode, our knowledge base depends upon clarifying nursing phenomena to make them fully researchable. Batey (1977) identified the greatest limiting factor in published nursing research as problems with the conceptual phase of the nursing process. She highlights how limited a study is when the investigator uses an ambiguous concept. The Frances Payne Bolton School of Nursing's 1967 Symposium on Theory (Berthold 1968; Dickoff and James 1968; Johnson 1968; and Rubin 1968), The University of Kansas Conferences on Nursing Theory (Norris [Ed.] 1969, 1970; Jacox 1974) provided great impetus to concept clarification and theory development.

1. Concept clarification became more formalized, organized, and complex.
2. Nurses became conversant with theories and theory building.
3. Nursing education programs began to include courses in theory construction, theory analysis, and comparative theories.
4. The number of nurse theorists increased.
5. Graduates of nurse-scientist programs were able to contribute substantially to theory despite the fact that their training was in another discipline.

Nursing Perspective in Research

Donaldson and Crowley (1978) refocused nursing's attention on nursing: they reiterated the requirement of a nursing perspective for nursing research. More important, they stressed that "Disciplines reflect true distinctions between bodies of knowledge per se. . . ." The discipline of nursing, then, is unique. While nurses may draw upon many other disciplines, nursing itself provides the focus, orientation, and values that guide practice, teaching, and research. Also, these scholars distinguished the "discipline as a body of knowledge that is separate from the activities of practitioners. . . ." These three points—nursing perspective, essential uniqueness of a nursing body of knowledge, and separation of the discipline from the practice—help nurses zero in on nursing phenomena and support nurses to free themselves to work on aspects of the substantive body of knowledge without having to identify what it means for either practical knowledge or the body of professional knowledge. The nursing care study may be a useful tool in learning nursing but we can now dispense with it as a means to develop a body of nursing knowledge. Donaldson and Crowley have pinpointed what constitutes basic research in nursing: concept clarification in the future must meet the criteria for basic research.

Barnett (1972), in her work on the concepts of touch, illustrates more formal methodology than those clarified earlier. Gregg (1973) demonstrated how the concept of aggression could be simplified and how doctoral-level research studies might evolve out of particular kinds of work on a concept. Weiss' (1979) work on the concept of touch, Francis' (1976) work on loneliness, and Norris' (1978) work on restlessness illustrate systematic approaches to definition and clarification in concept work. In their studies on the concept of empathy, Mansfield (1973) and Forsyth (1979) used organized methods of study, as did Kim (1980) in her work on pain and Rawnsley (1980) in studying privacy. Ryden (1977) used categorization to develop a hierarchy related to a concept of energy. Wilson (1977) turned to qualitative comparative analysis methods to study the social-process concept *limiting intrusion* within a framework of social control in an experimental treatment community for schizophrenics. These emerging methodologies are discussed in a later chapter.

Historically, nursing concepts have been studied generally. If, for example, hope was the concept, a report on its clarification would be a summary of a literature review and a summary of the investigator's observations. Future studies of hope might be general but might also have a specific focus on one aspect of hope—such as initiation, maintenance, the end of hope, or hope under specific clinical conditions (e.g., in parents of infants with Down's syndrome or in terminal cancer patients). Differences in hope might also be compared among different kinds of family and social support systems.

The literature of concept clarification in nursing reports few studies of nursing concepts that involved a study design. We now know that, to be systematic in our work of building substantive nursing knowledge, we need to refine existing methods and develop new ones that allow us to explicate the empirical concepts about which we need knowledge.

Our past work, for the most part, represents satisfaction with analysis and summary of study findings. Descriptive work was adequate for a time in which teachers were searching for knowledge for an emerging professional discipline. Now that the crisis this search represented has passed, those who are clarifying concepts in nursing need to be experts in relationships, whether from logic or philosophy of science. It is out of this knowledge that valid syntheses will come, syntheses that will be understandable to all students of nursing because they can study the synthetic statements or arguments and do not have to guess how investigators related phenomena—concept to behavior, for example—or how they got from A to C. This is not to say that synthesis is not often a very creative experience. Rather, however synthesis is carried out it needs to be reported within a logical framework if we are to move toward explanation.

FUTURE TRENDS

Examination of our history in concept clarification has shed some light on future directions. Three major concerns emerge: (1) Concepts explored generally in the past need to be studied to clarify their components and their roles in specific clinical situations; (2) Current methodologies for concept clarification need to be refined, and new methodologies need to be developed; and (3) Nurses need to be familiar with modes of synthesis.

REFERENCES

Barnett, K. A theoretical construct of the concepts of touch as they relate to nursing. *Nurs. Res.* 21:102–110, Mar.–Apr. 1972.

Batey, M.V. Conceptualization: Knowledge and logic guiding empirical research. *Nurs. Res.* 26:324–329, Sept.–Oct. 1977.

Berthold, J.S. Theoretical and empirical clarification of concepts. *Nurs. Sci.* 2:406–422, Oct. 1964.

Berthold, J.S. Prologue. *Nurs. Res.* 17:196–197, May–June 1968.

Burd, S., and Marshall, M. *Some Clinical Approaches to Psychiatric Nursing.* New York: Macmillan, 1963.

Byrne, M.L., and Thompson, L.F. *Key Concepts for the Study and Practice of Nursing.* St. Louis: Mosby, 1978.

Carlson, C.E. (Ed.). *Behavioral Concepts and Nursing Intervention.* Philadelphia: Lippincott, 1970.

Carlson, C.E., and Blackwell, B. (Eds.). *Behavioral Concepts and Nursing Intervention* (2nd ed.). Philadelphia: Lippincott, 1978.

Dickoff, J., and James, P. A theory of theories: A position paper. *Nurs. Res.* 17:197–203, May–June 1968.

Dickoff, J., and James, P. Researching research's role in theory development. *Nurs. Res.* 17:204–206, May–June 1968.

Donaldson, S.K., and Crowley, D.M. The discipline of nursing. *Nurs. Outlook* 26:113–120, Feb. 1978.

Ford, L.C., Cobb, M., and Taylor, M. *Defining Clinical Content: Graduate Nursing Programs: Community-Health Nursing.* Boulder, Col.: Western Interstate Commission for Higher Education, 1967.

Forsyth, G.L. Exploration of empathy in nurse–client interaction. *Adv. Nurs. Sci.* 1:53–61, Jan. 1979.

Francis, G.M. Loneliness: Measuring the abstract. *Int. J. Nurs. Stud.* 13:153–160, 1976.

Fujiki, S., Clayton, B.C., Estes, N.J., Kalkman, M., and White, O.H. *Defining Clinical Content: Graduate Nursing Programs: Psychiatric Nursing.* Boulder, Col.: Western Interstate Commission for Higher Education, 1967.

Gregg, D.E. Anxiety—A factor in nursing care. *Am. J. Nurs.* 52:1363–1365, Nov. 1952.

Gregg, D.E. Reassurance. *Am. J. Nurs.* 55:171–174, Feb. 1955.

Gregg, D.E. Proposing two approaches to doctoral education in nursing. In E.A. Garrison (Ed.), *Doctoral Education for Nurses.* San Francisco: University of California, 1973.

Hames, C.C., and Joseph, D.H. *Basic Concepts of Helping.* New York: Appleton-Century-Crofts, 1980.

Highley, B.L., Berlinger, M., Hillard, P., Lonnstrom, B.T., and Murray, B.L. *Defining Clinical Content: Graduate Nursing Programs: Maternal Child Health Nursing.* Boulder, Col.: Western Interstate Commission for Higher Education, 1967.

Highley, B.L., and Norris, C.M. When a student dislikes a patient. *Am. J. Nurs.* 57:1163–1166, Sept. 1957.

Jacox, A.K. Theory construction in nursing: An overview. *Nurs. Res.* 23:6–8, Jan.–Feb. 1974.

Jason, S., and Trygstad, L.N. *Behavioral Concepts and the Nursing Process.* St. Louis: Mosby, 1979.

Johnson, D.E. Theory in nursing: Borrower and unique. *Nurs. Res.* 17:206–209, May–June 1968.

Kim, S. Pain theory: Research and nursing practice. *Adv. Nurs. Sci.* 2:43–59, Jan. 1980.

Kintzel, K.C. *Advanced Concepts in Clinical Nursing*. Philadelphia: Lippincott, 1971.

Kramer, M. Concept Formation. In M.V. Batey, *Communicating Nursing Research*. Boulder, Col.: Western Interstate Commission for Higher Education, 1970. Pp. 246–266.

Lewis, L., Carozza, V., Carroll, M., Darragh, R., Patrick, M., and Schadt, E. *Defining Clinical Content: Graduate Nursing Programs: Medical–Surgical Nursing*. Boulder, Col.: Western Interstate Commission for Higher Education, 1967.

Mansfield, E. Empathy: Concept or identified psychiatric behavior. *Nurs. Res.* 22:525–529, Nov.–Dec. 1973.

Meltzer, L.E., Abdella, F.G., and Kitchell, R. (Eds.). *Concepts and Practices of Intensive Care for Nurse Specialists*. Philadelphia: Charles, 1969.

Mitchell, P.H. *Concepts Basic to Nursing*. New York: McGraw-Hill, 1973.

Murray, R.B., and Zentner, J.P. *Nursing Concepts for Health Promotion*. Englewood Cliffs, N.J.: Prentice-Hall, 1979.

Norris, C.M. The nurse and the dying patient. *Am. J. Nurs.* 55:1214–1217, 1955.

Norris, C.M. The nurse and the crying patient. *Am. J. Nurs.* 57:323–327, 1957.

Norris, C.M., Shea, F.J., and Eller, F. Feeding as a therapeutic routine. Parts I & II. *Perspect. Psychiatr. Care* 1:33–39, Mar.–Apr. 1963, 1:13–27, May–July 1963.

Norris, C.M. Toward a science of nursing. *Nurs. Forum* 3:10–45, 1964.

Norris, C.M. (Ed.). *Proceedings Nursing Theory Conference*. Kansas City: University of Kansas, Department of Nursing Education, 1969–1970.

Norris, C.M. Restlessness. In C.E. Carlson and B. Blackwell (Eds.), *Behavioral Concepts and Nursing Intervention*. Philadelphia: Lippincott, 1978.

Peplau, H.E. Loneliness. *Am. J. Nurs.* 55:1476, Dec. 1955.

Peplau, H.E. Theory: The professional dimension. In C.M. Norris (Ed.), *Proceedings First Nursing Theory Conference*. Kansas City: University of Kansas, Department of Nursing Education, 1969.

Peplau, H.E. In L.T. Zderad and H.C. Belcher, *Developing Behavioral Concepts in Nursing*. Atlanta, Ga.: Southern Regional Education Board, 1968. Pp. 12–15.

Peplau, H.E. In C.E. Carlson, C.M. Norris, S. Lange, B. Blackwell, and D. Moses, *Identification of Basic Mental Health Content in Nursing*. Boulder, Col.: Western Interstate Commission for Higher Education, 1970.

Putnam, P.A. A conceptual approach to nursing theory. *Nurs. Sci.* 3:430–442, Dec. 1965.

Rawnsley, M.M. The concept of privacy. *Adv. Nurs. Sci.* 2:25–31, Jan. 1980.

Roberts, S.L. *Behavioral Concepts and Nursing Throughout the Life Span*. Englewood Cliffs, N.J.: Prentice-Hall, 1978.

Rubin, R. A theory of clinical nursing. *Nurs. Res.* 17:210–212, May–June 1968.

Ryden, M.B. Energy: A crucial consideration in the nursing process. *Nurs. Forum* 16:71–82, 1977.

Smith, J.A. The idea of health: A philosophical inquiry. *Adv. Nurs. Sci.* 3:43–50, April 1981.

Tudor, G.E. A sociopsychiatric approach to intervention in a problem of mutual withdrawal on a mental-hospital ward. *Psychiatry* 5:193–217, May 1952.

Weiss, S.J. The language of touch. *Nurs. Res.* 28:76–79, March–Apr. 1979.

Wilson, H.S. Limiting intrusion—social control of outsiders in a healing community. *Nurs. Res.* 26:103–111, March–Apr. 1977.

Zderad, L.T., and Belcher, H.C. *Developing Behavioral Concepts in Nursing*. Atlanta, Ga.: Southern Regional Education Board, 1968.

Chapter 2

Concept Clarification: An Overview

Catherine M. Norris

CONCEPT CLARIFICATION AND SCIENCE

The groundwork for all advances in science requires clarifying the basic ideas involved. These basic ideas are called *concepts,* and they are the analytic tools· of the discipline. Concepts are also the only means of connecting an empirical science to the "real world." The work of clarifying and relating the basic ideas is called *concept clarification.* Concept clarification needs to be done within the framework of exploratory and descriptive research, which is hypothesis- and theory-generating in contrast to deductive research, which tests hypotheses and theories. Concept clarification and deductive research together permit continuous growth of a body of knowledge. Concept clarification without experimental research is ineffective in that it cannot by itself fulfill the requirements of knowing. Experimental research without concept clarification is meaningless. If a concept is not clear, subsequent research may be based on false assumptions, false premises, and hypotheses that have no relevance to the real world.

Concepts are abstractions of concrete events. They represent ways of perceiving phenomena. Concepts are generalizations about particulars such as cause–effect, duration, dimension, attributes, and continua of phenomena or objects. Concepts have many degrees of abstraction—from symbolizing something very concrete to taking in a whole species, all living things, the world, or even the universe.

An example of a readily understood concept in nursing is that of vomiting: here, the concept is the *word symbol,* not the act itself. On another level, vomiting might be categorized as a symptom of gastrointestinal upset or as a protective mechanism of the body. At yet another level, it might be perceived as one of the most primitive protective body responses of carnivores. One might, in fact, suggest that vomiting is one of the most primitive body responses of all vertebrates. This last statement would indicate, however, that we have gone beyond empirical reality. With each new level of abstraction, the symbolic concepts must relate and include the concrete phenomena from which one started abstracting. Being able to do this is prerequisite to working with concepts.

Concept Clarification and Research Design

Experimental research design requires thorough explication of the concept or concepts involved, including an operational definition. Also, a model of the concept including its components and the stated relationships among them allows an investigator to examine the adequacy of the hypothesis to be tested and to effectively identify dependent and independent variables. A concept model that clarifies the placement or relationship of the concept to existing theory provides a frame of reference within which experimental research can be carried out. For example, to attempt experimental research on some aspect of sleep or fatigue or nausea requires thorough, organized, and systematized knowledge of the concepts, with awareness of relationships among their parts and to the theories to which they belong. Without such an organized body of knowledge, an investigation is unrelated to the real world, unrelated to the perspective of nursing, and without known boundaries. If, on the other hand, findings of experimental research completed on some aspect of sleep or fatigue or nausea are not incorporated into the concepts and the concepts revised in view of this new knowledge, the concepts then become meaningless for guiding practice or developing the discipline. The crucial hypotheses and critical experiments that move an empirical science forward depend on dynamic interactive relationships between descriptive and experimental research. It is understood that neither experimental research nor concept clarification demands or waits for complete definition. Yet every discipline must explicate its basic ideas so that they can acquire more meaning. Analysis and clarification are powerful tools in dealing with knowledge.

CONCEPT CLARIFICATION AND NURSING

In that nursing seeks to describe, clarify, predict, and control certain aspects of the world in which nurses work, it can be classified as an *empirical*, rather than a nonempirical, science. All advances in science require clarifying and relating the basic ideas involved. Specifically, advances in nursing science require clarifying the basic ideas in nursing and relating them to nursing's unique purposes, perspectives, and universe of discourse. Donaldson and Crowley (1978) abstracted from the nursing literature three general themes that express the core and scope of nursing.

1. Concern with the principles and laws that govern the life processes, well-being, and optimum functioning of human beings—sick or well.

2. Concern with the patterning of human behavior in interaction with the environment in critical life situations.
3. Concern with the processes by which positive changes in health status are affected.

Using these items in lieu of a definition of nursing allows identification of basic concepts of nursing. Because nursing is a profession, two kinds of basic concepts are required: one type relates to abstract knowledge and knowing; the other type is process-oriented and answers questions about how knowledge is useful in solving nursing problems. Another way of stating this is to say that descriptive research, including concept clarification, revolves around ways of knowing and represents one area of basic research in nursing. Process-oriented concepts, while requiring clarification, must ultimately be tested and proven successful or discarded as unsuccessful applications of knowledge.

Concepts discussed in this text are concerned with building substantive knowledge in nursing. The concepts selected can be subsumed under the basic ideas in the previously mentioned themes one and two identified by Donaldson and Crowley (1978). They relate to phenomena that confront nurses regularly in working with people, sick or well. They are all related to basic human needs and represent lower-level physiological needs. No application to practice is represented in this text except insofar as hypotheses and models raise questions or postulate relationships to practice. This is a departure from nursing's approach to concept clarification wherein recommendations for practice were inferred directly from substantive knowledge.

When concepts are clarified precisely, their influence is powerful. This is called the *power of naming*. The sources of this power include the depths to which conceptual thinking explicates meaning and value and the general applicability of the concept to many specific instances.

CONCEPT CLARIFICATION AND NURSING RESEARCH

Only recently have nurse researchers suggested that (1) nursing needs to do much more extensive research and (2) scientists in nursing need to evolve descriptive research methods to examine nursing phenomena fully. The pace of the movement using research methods other than experimental methodologies is urged by several nursing scholars and heightened by the dire need to make a body of nursing knowledge explicit. But some forces within the profession tend to slow the development of descriptive research as a discipline. Teaching and research nurses have been highly trained in disciplines whose descriptive work has long been completed; these disciplines thus give training in descriptive methods low priority. (Note, however, that descriptive methods for academic disciplines might not be useful in delineating a professional discipline.)

Also, descriptive research depends heavily upon both clinicians and researchers. Historic and existing elitism surrounding researchers has alienated the two groups. New patterns of relationships being explored will foster greater cooperative and collaborative study.

Early nursing identity with liberal arts colleges, which often sponsored nursing education in academia, made rigorous research the road to respectability. It is still common for members of academic disciplines to classify nursing as a semi- or paraprofessional discipline. But nurses are beginning to make decisions about themselves as members of a discipline.

Identification of physiological functioning and malfunctioning as lower levels in hierarchies of needs may account for the lethargy in making commitments to describe these concepts for nursing. The topic of pain, however, has had considerable attention from nurse researchers. Therefore, it may be aversion to odors, noise, and other so-called repulsive aspects of behavior that are usually handled privately. Nursing is now, it is hoped, ready to give greater emphasis to descriptive research and to develop more effective methodologies for accomplishing descriptive research tasks. Backed by the profession, more clinicians and researchers can be expected to make personal commitments.

CONCEPT CLARIFICATION AND THEORY BUILDING IN NURSING

Theory can be derived inductively and/or deductively; Stevens (1978) describes the methods as "by reason" and "by assertion." Historically, theory generation in nursing has employed concepts from academic disciplines that were used to explain nursing situations and to guide nursing practice. Aspects of human behavior and interaction situations used in this way include stress, coping, adaptation, healthy environment, growth, holistic functioning, and anxiety. Concepts selected were explicitly related to predicting or explaining human behavior. Often, concepts were defined in terms of the two disciplines, theoretically in the discipline from which the concept was selected using empirical indicators derived from knowledge of nursing. Thus, elements of theory from other disciplines may have been modified from their "pure" form in the original discipline for use as guiding principles in nursing. But, as seen in the original or as modified for nursing, the work of most nurse theorists has not been tested in empirical situations or even systematically observed in these clinical contexts.

Grand Theory

Theory essentially developed by assertion is often called *grand theory*. Grand theories are useful, even when untested, because they give direction to the discipline, identify major and recurring concepts and concerns of the discipline, and give focus and provide a framework for practice and, possibly, research. The grand theory situation is typical, however, of a prevailing problem in all behavioral sciences, including nursing: that is, a gap exists between theories and empirical research based on these theories. The higher the level of abstraction used in theory construction, the higher or more general the level of concept definition. The more abstract the concept definition, the harder it is to define it operationally to ensure its reliability. Guidance for research or practice using this model of theory development is limited even though the theory may ultimately prove useful and valid. We might observe that this approach to theory in nursing has produced conceptual frameworks rather than theory: that is, the level of generality is so abstract that the "theory" cannot be used as theory, since, by definition, one should be able to generate testable hypotheses from theory.

Inductive Approach

The inductive approach to theory construction is based at the empirical level which, in nursing, is in the clinical situation with patients and clients. It is concerned with the behavioral phenomena with which these people confront nurses or which nurses can anticipate. The phenomena involved are those related to human health, illness, and comfort—fundamentals with which nurses are expected to deal in relation to social prerogatives and mandates allowed or given to them. In the inductive approach, theory is generated from observations that are analyzed and used to construct concepts that explain the observed phenomena and that can be used to understand multiple instances of the phenomena in the future. No concepts are borrowed, modified, or reconstructed from other disciplines. The goal is to collect empirical data and analyze it in ways that build increasing levels of abstraction, which include increasingly more of the phenomena being studied. Highly abstract theories of human behavior in health and illness may ultimately be constructed. Because inductive inference often begins with specific cases and moves toward generality, it is more likely that at some point the inductive model will fit into one or more deductively constructed theories. The more the professional membership agrees about its mission and common ideas, the more likely inductive and deductive work on theory construction will articulate each other. It seems pointless for nurses to argue about the better way to develop theory; rather, it is better to recognize that both are necessary. The real challenge may be to find ways to increase mutual complementarity.

SPECIFIC GOALS OF CONCEPT CLARIFICATION

First, by observing and describing nursing phenomena repeatedly and by studying the phenomena from the viewpoints of various disciplines—that is, cogitating and reflecting about possible meanings, possible relationships, possible sequences or order, and possible causes and effects—we hope to *describe, explain, and give meaning to human behavior*. For example, nurses have studied the healing effects of insulin on decubiti; they wonder why insulin promotes the healing of these bedsores (Van Ort and Gerber 1976). Then a nurse physiologist points out that zinc is required for the action of tissue-growth hormone and asks whether it is not the zinc in the protamine zinc insulin used that is the active agent in healing. Such an elucidation spawns needed research for ways to use other zinc compounds to heal decubiti or for a study replicating the original bedsore study, substituting regular insulin for protamine zinc insulin.

Second, we hope to *systematize observations and descriptions*. In studying fatigue, nurses might want to know the specific behaviors along a continuum that ranges from tired, over-tired, fatigued, to exhausted. Systematization (i.e., establishing categories, continua, hierarchies, and the like) might tell nurses something about temporal sequence and seriousness, as well as about relationships to other events or environments. For example, in a sequence of vomiting that ranges from descriptions of nonfunctional vomiting (motion sickness) to "spitting up," simple vomiting and vomiting under pressure to projectile vomiting to complicated vomiting to emergency vomiting, nurses could identify priorities for care. In systematizing restlessness, we see that restlessness occurs first as small-muscle activity, proceeds to gross-muscle activity and then to total-body involvement and that each successive stage expresses greater discomfort (Norris 1978). If the accuracy of this system is proved, nurses eventually could assess and intervene in its earliest stages before considerable discomfort develops.

A third goal of concept clarification is an *operational definition of the concept under study*. An operational definition is required to answer at least one question, "How will I know this concept when (in the broadest sense) I see it in operation?" Imprecision in the use of terms, lack of clarification of nursing phenomena, and lack of discriminatory skills make operational definitions difficult. Most people trained in science are more skilled in analysis—the principal mode of the scientist—and less skilled in synthesis—the principal mode of the practitioner. Perhaps we need to teach nurses to operate more effectively in the mode of synthesis if we are to have operational definitions of nursing concepts as a basis for our research. Still, imprecision in the terms we elect will cause us problems. For the concept of disorientation, terms like "confusion," "psychosis," and "chronic brain syndrome" hamper an operational definition of the expression from a nursing perspective. If this quandary is not resolved we might speculate whether disorientation needs to be replaced by a new, precise term. The question here is whether we should eliminate "confusion" in favor of "disorientation" or whether nurses, by working on both concepts, can identify the imprecisions and correct them. Presently, "disorientation" belongs to a hodgepodge of imprecise terms.

Fourth, the work of concept clarification should produce a *model*. Models are intellectual inventions that may take several forms, ranging from those using spoken language only, to those which use only mathematical or statistical terms. The common sense language-descriptive model is the most difficult to understand because of the ambiguity of language. In other descriptive models, terms used are defined which increases precision and improves the communication value of the model.

Construction of a model requires a sophisticated level of synthesis. Synthesis is done after the data is collected in inductive work while, in deductive theory construction, it precedes data collection. All of the data collected is moved to a level of abstraction where large volumes of data can be represented graphically. In developing the model, the task of categorization needs to be completed or reexamined to move the concrete data to more advanced levels of abstraction, that is, increasing generalization about the data. This task provides the worker with a smaller and more manageable number of elements. For example, we could not easily work with the 100 or more signs and symptoms of nausea and vomiting. If these symptoms can be grouped into 6 categories, however, they become manageable intellectually, in their organization, in the meanings they give the data, and in communication with others.

Another task in model construction is distinguishing the relationships among the various kinds of categories of data in some communicable way. While causal relationships may be the most commonly sought, many others may be required for clarification of nursing phenomena. Other common relationships include independence–dependence, concomitance, concurrence, sequence, seriousness, temporal relationships, speed or rate relationships, damping, and outcome.

All of the investigation data is represented in an abstract descriptive, pictorial, or mathematical form. This does not imply simplicity. On the contrary, understanding models may require long study. All hypotheses emerge from a model—explicit or not—and they are stimulated by questions the model creates, inconsistencies observed, and inadequacies or "holes" in the schematic representation. Thus, the model is the ultimate test of the researcher's comprehension of the data and ability to synthesize it into an integrated whole that others can study and raise questions about. One danger for the worker is in collecting vast amounts of data, including many variables, and trying to explore every relationship yet never determining how it all fits together.

At this point in nursing research, many models will be constructed for the same concept, whereas in the future these may be integrated into a single, comprehensive model. For example, a model for a general concept of nausea and vomiting is now quite different from a model of "morning sickness," and these two are removed from nausea with myocardial infarct and nausea and vomiting of oncology patients undergoing radiation therapy or chemotherapy. Each of these aspects would also vary if different nurses did the work because of diversified perceptions, approaches to synthesis, and errors in interpretation of data and synthesis. As more nurses investigate nausea and vomiting under similar and varied circumstances, they will create new models and correct errors in old ones. All of these models deserve exploration, for they are needed to formulate a thorough explication of nausea and vomiting. Models for the many aspects of nursing phenomena presage the day when more inclusive models of phenomena can be constructed and specify the questions to be answered in developing nursing's unique knowledge.

A single concept is not enough in any discipline; each concept needs to be related to, combined with, or integrated into other concepts, a construct, existing theory, a new theory fostered by clarifying the concept, or new relationships among existing theories. A concept represents a fragment of knowledge about one behavioral phenomenon. Its full meaning rests in its relationship to the holism represented by key elements of the discipline or to one of the grand theories that permits organizing the knowledge of nursing. Relationships between the single concept and the larger body of knowledge need to be stated explicitly; such relationships or the logic involved in inferring them is usually not accomplished readily. Insights noted during concept clarification work are helpful in defining relations, but testing the logic of relationships and examining the fit of concepts within larger constructs takes months.

The fifth, and final aspect of concept clarification, is *hypothesis formulation.* In scientific inquiry using exploratory and descriptive methods, data are analyzed and, through a kind of synthesis often referred to as *inductive inference,* general principles or even empirical laws are formulated. But in almost all instances, a hypothesis states some probable, directional relationship between two or more variables. Such a hypothesis may prove useful as a pro tempore principle for guiding practice. Testing the hypothesis moves the work into the experimental mode, where conclusions are stated with more certainty—that is, one learns whether the hypothesis was or was not supported by the results. This does not mean that a conclusion is absolute, but only that it is relevant for situations tested.

Hypotheses emerge from a variety of activities. Hypothesis formulation requires skill in synthesis, that is, relating two or more variables in specified ways. In studying vomiting, for instance, workers found that herbivorous animals do not vomit. This produced a line of reasoning that might propose this. People who are ovo-lacto-vegetarians vomit more than omnivorous eaters and more than strict vegetarians. People on a vegetarian diet for a period before surgery vomit less than those who remained omnivorous right up to surgery. (Is this what people mean when they talk about purifying the body as they return to a vegetarian diet after a period of being carnivorous?) Morning sickness of pregnancy would be less on a vegetarian diet than on an omnivorous diet. These hypotheses are far out, but in view of the discomforts of nausea and vomiting and the serious side effects of many antiemetics, they may be worth pursuing.

The work of concept clarification relates to theory at rudimentary levels—factor isolation, description and systematization and prediction (hypothesis formulation). Prescriptions inferred need to be considered as either hypothetical or empirical in nature. It is through systematization, especially, that relationships among highly diverse data emerge. Systematization activities include observing, discovering, common sense thinking, engaging in logical deduction and induction, searching for meaning, developing insights, testing out ways to organize, and speculating about types of relationships. The basic ideas in nursing to which nurses must respond are phenomena presented by patients and clients or confronted by nurses in work situations.

SUMMARY

Common sense analysis of concepts is not enough, but common sense is the source for all science. Common sense data require analysis, refinement, amendment, and even contradiction, but this is where all sciences begin; it is the point at which we begin to explain behavior. Common sense explanations are the referents for understanding empirical reality.

Clarifying concepts is descriptive work. It is rarely possible to leap from an event to theory without describing the event or phenomenon. As specialists within the profession, nurse clinicians may need fewer descriptive elements, such as criterion attributes or even different perspectives of the various elements (Benner 1981), in order to name the concept and relate it to theory. Our aim as scholars is to make this true for nurses in all areas of practice.

REFERENCES

Benner, P. Characteristics of novice and expert performance: Implications for teaching the experienced nurse. In K.L. Jako (Ed.), *Proceedings: Researching Second-Step Education*. San Francisco, Calif.: Sonoma State University, Department of Nursing, 1981.

Donaldson, S.K., and Crowley, D.M. The discipline of nursing. *Nurs. Outlook* 26:113–120, Feb. 1978.

Norris, C.M. Restlessness. In C.E. Carlson and E. Blackwell, *Behavioral Concepts and Nursing Intervention*. Philadelphia: Lippincott, 1978.

Stevens, B.J. *Nursing theory: Analysis, application, evaluation*. Boston: Little, Brown, 1979.

Van Ort, S.R., and Gerber, R.M. Topical application of insulin in the treatment of decubitus ulcers: A pilot study. *Nurs. Res.* 25:9–12, Feb. 1976.

Chapter 3

Concept Clarification: Approaches and Preliminaries

Catherine M. Norris

INTRODUCTION

Nursing is still in the early stages of exploratory and descriptive research: methodologies developed by nurses and relevant methodologies from other disciplines are often not well developed. Instrumentation is also lacking. Primitive methodology in untested form, without consensual validation or rejection from the profession, does not facilitate concept clarification. Despite its deficiencies, we believe that concept clarification is a key in building the substantive—as opposed to the practice, knowledge, and theory—aspect of the discipline.

Most individual nurses, like the profession in general, are still novices in concept clarification. But there is evidence in the literature of a positive momentum for explicating new methodologies (Forsyth 1980; Francis 1976; Gregg 1973; Hansen 1981; Kim 1980; Mansfield 1973; Norris 1975; Rawnsley 1980; and Weiss 1979).

Many nurses have contributed to revitalizing the methodology of this aspect of nursing scholarship, and there has been support for basic nursing research (Donaldson and Crowley 1978; Crawford, Dufault, and Rudy 1979). Clarifying the concepts of the discipline could surely be subsumed under the rubric of basic research. Benoliel (1977) stressed that identifying categories of concepts used in practice is essential. Several nurse scholars (McKay 1977; Schlofeldt 1977; and Silva 1977) have stressed the need to develop methods explicating nursing phenomena.

Beginning graduate students have difficulties with still-nebulous methodologies and their plea is always, "Tell me how!" At a certain level, one can describe concept clarification as complex, creative, inventive, imaginative, intellectual activity. It can also be described as slow, frustrating, messy, lonely, and sometimes unproductive. Such abstractions only set the stage for confronting the job or making an initial commitment to the work; it does not address the "how" question. It is tempting to provide formulas for research, but one should keep in mind that guidelines can often have an inhibiting or misleading effect on neophyte researchers. Guidelines may stifle imagination and constrict the world view of nurses who are beginning the work of building the nursing knowledge. Guidelines may foster premature closure and possibly the false assumption that the work is done or complete.

Whatever methodologies are taught and however sophisticated nurses become in applying them, learners must freely pursue their own hunches and develop their own methods. Intellectual ventures into unfamiliar territory may be critical to building nursing knowledge. Students of nursing must pursue the unlikely, the ridiculous, and the incongruous as well as their own fantasies and hunches. Capitalizing on their own styles of exploration, analysis, and synthesis nurses can refine their skills as they work.

The remainder of this chapter is devoted to a description of my work in easing the transition from concept development to concept clarification.

COLLEGIAL SUPPORT

Nurses involved in concept clarification are, in a sense, pioneers and as such face all of the concomitant challenges and risks of the role. Pioneers become totally involved in their work and are often lonely because no one else is as interested in or as knowledgeable about the work underway. Often the data are intuitively experienced, and intuitions are difficult to process and to formulate in concrete terms. Sometimes the data consist of vague and ambiguous cues that are difficult to pursue and to formulate conceptually.

Almost all concept workers experience one or more of these common problems. They make errors in relating one aspect of the data to another; they spend long periods of time tracking down data that are of minimal or no consequence to the concept being studied; they go too far in extrapolating results of animal research to human phenomena; they cannot identify when the period of maximum payoff in data collection has been reached; they can hardly believe breakthroughs coming out of their own reflection upon the data or the discoveries coming out of their own creativity; they hesitate to depart from conventional modes of thinking as they work with concepts. In addition, pioneers may have many highs and many lows of mood as they correct their errors, rework their formulations, and discard materials that represent weeks of nonproductive effort.

The nature of scientific work requires collegial support. Colleagues are essential for the optimism and progress they foster as well as for the support they offer. They also raise questions in ongoing intellectual debates and help refine methods. Excitement expressed among colleagues is contagious and self-affirming. Thus, contracting with a colleague or paid research associate is critical for the researcher.

SOME SOURCES OF BIAS

Concept Selection

A possible source of bias is in selecting a concept that has personal significance or is based in a personal problem—whether it be severe trauma, present or past health problems, feelings about competence and worth, or feelings about deficiencies or unmet needs. Concept research is measured in years; emotional involvement may complicate the task. Biased research workers may experience added frustration and fatigue when concept elements are undefined; elements may be left selectively unexamined if they heighten anxiety. Meaning and process can be distorted when observations or relationships do not conform to the researcher's expectations or are too painful to contemplate. If a concept of personal significance is selected for study, the researcher must then decipher his or her motivation before pursuing the investigation. On the other hand, the nurse scholar must have a real interest and commitment to the concept selected since the researcher–subject relationship may endure for years.

Values

Another possible origin of bias is the value system of the researcher. Everyone's cultural, socioeconomic, professional, and personal value systems affect whatever work they do. In concept clarification work, as with any intellectual pursuit, one must monitor the values one brings to the study. For example, in working on nausea and vomiting, if the main value dealt with is disgust, the analytic work may be weighted toward repulsive aspects; emotional components will possibly be overemphasized in the operational definition and model. If a nurse sees nausea and vomiting as symptoms of illness, clarification will give weight to the illness aspects. Time spent developing these behaviors as illness, much as the medical model, may block examination of protective functions of these phenomena, which would be important to nurses.

Role

A third source of bias is in the interpersonal role required in some techniques used in exploratory and descriptive research. In many interview and observation situations, for example, the researcher is a variable: that is, the subject affects the nurse, and the nurse affects subject. One research role that takes into account the impact of the researcher on the interpersonal field being studied is that of participant–observer. Even though this role makes situations more complex than the "objective" observation, it allows the nurse to pursue and collect more relevant data than would be available to a nonparticipant observer. The researcher is thus freed of inhibitions, especially in the area of feelings and values, inherent in objective observation.

Reducing bias depends on the researcher's awareness of reactions to subjects and the impact of role, approach, and charisma upon them. It also rests on the researcher's ability to assess how his or her reactions and those of study subjects can affect the interpersonal field. During phenomenological aspects of the work, the researcher must identify how he or she knows that it is the subject's experience of the event that is reported as opposed to the researcher's subjective feelings. While most nurses learn some skill in participant observation during their basic nursing education, additional skill is required to gain objectivity in analyzing research data. Reducing biases stemming from roles in descriptive research is difficult and challenges the nurse scholar.

ORIENTING CONCEPTS

Investigators of nursing phenomena, even those who attempt a tabula rasa approach, enter empirical fields where phenomena occur with implicit or explicit conceptual frameworks, values, and needs that affect the identification of the data, or kinds of data, they will seek. Since the concepts comprising one's orientation guide work and affect the total research enterprise, they should be rendered explicit.

Purposes and Perspective of Nursing

Concepts need to be clarified within clearly stated goals and purposes of nursing. Such a statement must be in conceptual, as opposed to action or concrete, terms. The level of abstraction must provide scope and depth but not be so general that it encompasses everything in the health care and socioeconomic system. Concepts refined using a nursing perspective become uniquely useful to nurses. They have limited meaning for other disciplines. For example, fatigue has been clarified as a concept for both industry and physical education. The purpose of concept clarification in industry is to increase worker productivity. In physical education, the purpose of the work is to increase physical stamina and energy for athletic competition. In aero–outerspace research, the goal is to prevent errors and reduce astronauts' irritability.

The specific purpose of clarifying the concept of fatigue for nursing might be its relation to the healing process, pain reduction, and relaxation. Or, it might be clarified from the standpoint of a physiological protective mechanism in health maintenance. There are other perspectives in clarifying fatigue for nursing; each purpose will change the focus of the work, the definition of function, and the kinds of hypotheses generated. If the purpose of studying fatigue is energy conservation for patients, the focus might not be upon healing or health, but upon those activities that dissipate patients' energies in a purely physical sense. If healing is the focus, physiological catabolic processes might be studied. If health maintenance is the purpose of the work, physiological anabolic processes might be examined. Again, this means that concepts clarified for nursing may not necessarily translate to other disciplines. If goals and purposes are conceived too narrowly, however, the number of concepts is limited and their development for nursing might be fragmented, superficial, and constricted (or limited) in scope.

Our Medical Orientation

When is sickness not sickness? Using a pathophysiological approach to concept clarification, the worker proceeds from the presenting phenomenon into pathology until a relationship to some disease appears relevant or until a correlation with symptoms of illness is found. Since symptoms are to be relieved and diseases are to be cured, the phenomenon under study could never be correlated with a healthy function such as protection. One is not free to examine whether the phenomenon has different functions at different times at different points along a continuum. If medicine has not found the particular phenomenon interesting, there may be no existing continuum—temporal, acuteness, or sequence—and fine discriminations among concept variables may not have been made. From this medical perspective, nurses could not arrive at a course of action that allowed the phenomenon to continue unabated or an intervention that supported the phenomenon to continue or initiated the occurrence of the phenomenon. If a phenomenon such as vomiting is protective, it needs to be studied in terms of the circumstances under which it should be supported, allowed to continue, or even initiated. This view will not be found in the medical literature where most of the discussion on vomiting appears. Vomiting, as far as medicine is concerned, is a symptom to be terminated as expeditiously as possible, usually with drugs whose side effects may be dangerous or even life-threatening (e.g., prochlorperazine, Compazine).

Occasionally, when an overdose of a drug has been taken or poison ingested orally, vomiting is induced by an emetic. This is done only when the toxic substance is not corrosive and there is no danger of inducing or increasing gastric bleeding. But even in these instances, for a number of real and contrived reasons (neatness, orderliness, esthetic factors, and subconscious needs to punish, etc.), evacuating and washing the stomach using large gastric tubes is usually preferred to initiating the normal protective response of vomiting. There are phenomena which, because they are not symptoms, are not studied by medicine. Mobility and restlessness are two such phenomena and are not even indexed in the *Cumulative Index Medicus*. Nurses can thus study these phenomena without becoming enmeshed in the literature of symptomatology and cure.

In clarifying the normal health protective functions of behavioral phenomena nurses confront every day, many questions must be answered before concepts can be introduced into nursing practice. Once the concept is clarified, questions about the extent to which phenomena are protective will arise (e.g., fatigue, thirst, and disorientation). Questions about modes of support and initiation of the phenomena also have to be studied. Criteria for identifying when behavior is no longer protective or has failed in its protective function, such as occurs in vomiting or thirst, have to be developed through research. This kind of assessment would be critical for nurses since it could change the course of nursing action for many human behavioral phenomena.

Work Orientation

Descriptive research is concerned with generating ideas and hypotheses as opposed to testing hypotheses, the modus operandi of experimental research. All goals of concept clarification are *generative,* the ultimate of which is hypothesis formulation. Clearly, the search for meaning, explanation, is the basic goal. It is almost impossible to study any concept in all its meanings.

> It is essential to be consciously aware of the choices made in regard to the aspects or meaning included, the explicit limitations imposed and the interpretation of the results in accordance with the choices (Berthold, 1964).

For example, in the study of nausea and vomiting, anorexia nervosa and bulimarexia are left untouched. Taste alteration, which is sometimes confused with nausea, was deleted from the study as well as all the specific diseases of which nausea and vomiting are symptoms.

As is true of all science, findings are not necessarily true. Rather, they are always open to modification and reformulation even though when using evaluation criteria they prove useful and powerful. Concept clarification is one way to create new knowledge for the discipline at a critical period in its development; therein lies the satisfaction in this work.

Replication of exploratory and descriptive studies is neither possible nor desirable. Instead, further exploratory and descriptive studies of the phenomenon might be useful, since new study might modify scope, range, regularities, and tendencies found in previous study. Results of descriptive studies are used to structure experimental studies and to construct theory.

CONSIDERATION OF LANGUAGE

Everyday language is not an adequate tool for exploratory and descriptive research. Nursing's disadvantage in both clinical practice and research is lack of consensus concerning concept definitions. Habit makes it difficult to examine critically concept usage in everyday language. Terms like *hunger, thirst,* and *fatigue* are hard to define precisely for use in scientific work. Constant use of such terms in both social and professional contexts makes it difficult to do the ongoing monitoring that ensures exactness. Nurses who use common-sense definitions without elevating them to a scientific level face two problems: (1) The concept may be so widely used and so broadly defined that it eludes definition. (2) Each person trying to cope with broad definitions uses his or her personal experience to give it meaning. Every common-sense concept ends up having subjective connotations as well as imprecise, general meanings. This traps the nurse, including the researcher, into the same position as the layperson.

Not only do words lack the refinement in definition required but many terms imply a nonexistent conceptual scheme or system. Concrete descriptions, regardless of accuracy, detail, and delineation of relationships among events, do not provide conceptual means for either description or prediction. Ordinary language lacks elements of a system (i.e., categories, taxonomies, rules) necessary for a scientific discipline; this is true regardless of the skills of the researcher. Even numbers are relative and lack precise values, especially when considered simply; take, for example, the number 2. Is it the distance between 1 and 2, 2 and 3, 1.5 and 2.5? For example, Gordon (1981) reports this incident:

> One of his (Fuller Albright's) favorite stories was about his visit to Shohl in New York, then the expert in mineral metabolism. Fuller described his arrival just as Shohl was about to show some students how to use the slide rule (*Note:* the slide rule is a crude analog portable calculator lacking circuits, transistors, or batteries and worked by hand!). Together, Albright and Shohl went into a lecture room dominated by an enormous slide rule, and Shohl explained that the slide rule was based on the simple principle that adding logarithms is multiplication. According to Fuller, Shohl marked off 2 on the D scale, explained that the scale represented the logarithm of 2, then added 2 on the C scale and concluded, "2 × 2 = 3.99." Fuller always savored this story because it depicted his view of the inexactness of mathematics in clinical investigation.

Consider the number 2 again. Is it a single point in some unspecified order, or what? In concept clarification, it may be necessary to invent new language or to develop methods of quantification. While mathematical or other symbol quantification may be an ultimate goal in scientific research, finding ways to systematize data may fulfill some of the same purposes and provide similar relative values.

Qualitative and Quantitative Language

Nurse researchers under pressure to quantify the phenomena of nursing could easily come to the same conclusion as have many philosophers: "that there are two kinds of features in nature, the qualitative and the quantitative (Carnap 1966)." Carnap (1966, pp. 58–59) makes several excellent points in speaking to this issue:

> . . . we must emphasize that the difference between qualitative and quantitative is not a difference in nature but a difference in our conceptual system . . . in our language. . . . We have the language of physics, the language of anthropology, the language of set theory, and so on. In this sense, a language is constituted by rules for a vocabulary, rules for building sentences, rules for logical deduction from those sentences, and other rules. The kinds of concepts that occur in a scientific language are extremely important. What I want to make clear is that the difference between qualitative and quantitative is a difference in languages.

The qualitative language is restricted to predicates, while the quantitative language introduces what are called *functor symbols,* that is, symbols for functions that have numerical values.

Definition

Workers approach concept clarification with the expectation that many of the elements or components composing the concept, in addition to the concept itself, require definition modification to improve the communication value. While the *common-sense,* or reportorial, *meaning* may be left unchanged, there are two major ways of redefining units of language. One method is to make an arbitrary definition and say, "For the purposes of this research or this theory, this word (term or phrase) will mean such-and-such."

This is called a *stipulated definition*. The researcher may hope that this kind of definition will come into general use like the terms *sensory overload* and *sensory deprivation* or that it will facilitate comparison with other concepts. At the very least, meaning in the research concerned will be precise and understandable as a result of such definitions. The stipulated definition is useful when there are many ambiguities or tangential elements that cannot be resolved as part of the work itself. It is bound to be replaced at some point by what Martin (1972) calls *rational reconstruction*. In rational reconstruction there is an effort to improve usage for scientific purposes through logic, refinement, and establishing coherence with existing knowledge (Martin 1972).

My work on nausea and vomiting in this text exemplifies both stipulated and rational reconstruction definitions. I stipulated that spitting up is vomiting and that regurgitation and gagging are nausea. Because of the many differences between spitting up and vomiting, spitting up may eventually be rationally reconstructed based on parameters other than the ejection of stomach contents through the mouth. These other parameters might include the immature nervous structures in infancy or differences in muscle contraction in the spitting up of infants. In defining nausea, I logically developed mutually exclusive categories of the phases of nausea, and from these, constructed a taxonomy of nausea that includes many variables not included in the reportorial or dictionary definitions. This rational reconstruction task also included more precisely aligning the definition to existing knowledge about nausea.

Hempel (1966) uses three terms, *analytical* (description), *extensional* (application), and *stipulative* (specified) *definitions* to express the relationship of the word to be defined (definiendum) and the definition (definiens) as demonstrated in the three basic types of definitions just discussed. If the definiens is used to analyze the sense or connotation of the definiendum or the researcher's stipulated sense of the definiendum, the definition is an *analytical* one. Definitions where extension or application of the definiendum are identified are called *extensional* definitions. Using this particular definitional system gives greater specificity to the definitions—analytical, stipulative, extensional, stipulative analytical, stipulative extensional, analytical extensional—to nurses doing descriptive research. Again, an operational definition is one goal of concept clarification. (See Chapter 2.)

Phonetics, Morphology, and Syntax

Both the scientific and the common-sense terms for behavioral phenomena need to be examined from the framework of linguistics. Language sounds have positive and negative, or both, values. Some sounds are more highly positively or negatively charged than others. Sounds and the way they are vocalized in the language provide clues to the way behaviors are viewed and valued. Language is essential in explicating experience and defining the quality of experience.

Similar words and phrases need to be analyzed in terms of whether they reflect synonymous experiences. For example, in common-sense language, fatigue and tiredness may appear to be almost synonymous. But many people experience tiredness as positive, especially if it follows a satisfying activity. Fatigue may be experienced negatively as overtiredness. Some people cannot be discriminating about their experience even when words have different common-sense meanings. People have reported, for example, that they could not discriminate between their nausea or hunger, for example. If the nurse's orientation to language is not finely honed, differences in meanings of the same words, similar words, and unrelated words may not be discovered until a great deal of the work of synthesis has been done. This would involve the researcher retracing his or her steps.

It is useful to note certain words or terms that keep coming up when your concept is discussed. For example, the word *boredom* recurs when people describe their fatigue. When this happens, discriminating between the two words during data analysis is important and relating the two in the process of synthesis is indicated. Boredom may be on a continuum with fatigue or it may have a causal relation to fatigue. The difference between the two may be in varied degree of feeling. In analysis, a worker might ascertain the circumstances under which they occur and whether they occur together or in sequence. They could be studied from the perspective of differences in energy available as well as accompanying degree of optimism. Nurses need to differentiate concepts from contexts of use and purposes served in other disciplines—industry, physical education, medicine, psychiatry, psychology, and so forth.

Adequacy of language. It is often assumed by casual observers that all languages have all the words, concepts, and structures required by the people using the language. However, there are many cross-cultural differences in language relating to concrete objects and abstractions. Some languages have, for example, several words to describe aspects of pain, grief, and love. Some societies, like the Navajo, have no words to describe internal bodily organs and their functioning. Some languages have no words for finely discriminating nuances of color, weight, or temperature. And some primitive cultures have language for concrete thinking about objects and events yet have limited language for conveying generalizations or abstractions. The demands of sustaining life for primitive peoples are focused on concrete realities; abstract language is not needed and thus none has developed. In different ways, every language places restrictions upon what can be communicated.

Another important orienting idea is the need for continuous assessment of the adequacy of language of the research subjects selected, especially those belonging to another culture or those for whom English is not a first language.

> Language is one of the most important instruments of adaptation . . . [It] is more than its vocabulary, grammar, sound structures, etc. It is also the repository of the modes of thought, the notions of causation and the conceptual and cognitive categories of the culture (Hymes 1968).

If language is an instrument of adaptation, one would expect language coping patterns to emerge in the face of all new challenges. When coping does not result in modifications of language, we can expect silence, apathy or denial— defenses concerned with inability to modify language, with giving stereotype responses, or with refusal to use language (i.e., unwillingness to talk about the challenge). Different cultures have various coping mechanisms for dealing with death. Death is a challenge in every culture, but even though the English language has words for expressing grief and comfort, many people do not use the language, but cope with death symbolically (e.g., by sending flowers or food instead of interacting). Coping with social change has resulted in language modification in Western society during the last fifteen years, particularly as sexual function in life and sexual practices have evolved. The effect on research methods has been revolutionized as well. Thus we see that coping strategies related to language and cognitive style permitted by language operate in all human functioning. A classic example of the astute descriptive researcher identifying some of these strategies may be found in *Awareness of Dying* (Glaser and Strauss 1965).

Significance of Categories

Certain ideas about how data will be analyzed and synthesized may be useful in selecting data-collection methods. First, categorization involves classifying the various aspects, components, or elements of a concept based on similarities and differences. Identifying and describing concept attributes promotes explanation and prediction. For example, if aversion to the concept of vomiting recurs with patients and health personnel, a next step might be to pinpoint a class of behaviors as producing aversion. Such a list might include nausea, gagging, retching, belching, and the like. Or, we might want to count the number of times aversion is observed and then term it aversion. A second advantage of categorization is that some methods of qualitative research require both immediate categorization of observations and ongoing hypothesis generation. These two activities can go on simultaneously with observation for the duration of observations.

Third, no nurse researcher enters a clinical area (empirical situation) without preconceptions about the kind of data to be found there. If a conceptual frame of reference is used to guide study, it will influence both what is observed and the kinds of categories constructed; what is observed and what categories are assigned may conflict with the conceptual frame of reference. Neither of these phenomena are counter-productive as long as biases are identified and corrections made. When working materials—observations, categorizations, and hypothesis generation—conflict with theory, theory must give way to modification or to new theory formulation.

One method of classification, *nominal scaling,* involves grouping all similar attributes or like data into mutually exclusive categories. The only evaluative criteria are that whatever variables are grouped together are the same, similar, or have at least one shared property and that they can be defined as different and identifiable from the variables found in any other group. For example, if vomiting is placed in a category or class named "human protective behaviors," it must be clear how the attributes of variables in this category differ from variables in any other category. Note that nominal scaling provides no other information. In the vomiting instance, we do not learn whether vomiting is more or less protective than any other protective mechanism; we are not told that vomiting is often preceded by nausea or whether it occurs more frequently than another protective mechanism, for example, elevated body temperature. Nominal scaling does not specify whether vomiting is more or less uncomfortable than fatigue or thirst; it just provides unidimensional data.

Categories may be assigned on the basis of properties, including size, width, mass, bulk, weight, color, capacity, location, and context in which the phenomenon occurs as well as temperature, time, frequency, duration, type, form, intensity, or seriousness. What the experience is phenomenologically for those subjected to it also may be classified.

Another approach to categorization is to search for ways to make comparable categories. This involves organizing existing categories according to some shared relationship. Once data are moved into the realm of comparability, they provide much more information than nominal scaling and facilitate much stronger statements. For example, one might say that NPO patients lost weight in a 24-hour period; this is a simple nominal classification of NPO patients. We can make two other classifications and demonstrate how they help us to compare. Of NPO patients, 20 percent lose more than 2 percent of their body weight in 24 hours; 80 percent do not lose more than 2 percent of their body weight. Most of the NPO patients who lose more than 2 percent of their body weight in 24 hours are 65 years of age or older; fewer than 49 percent are 65 years of age or under. Weight loss of 2 percent in 24 hours with patients who are NPO indicates early dehydration. So more than half of NPO patients 65 years of age or older who were studied are in a state of early dehydration at the end of 24 hours (Voda 1978). Comparative categories provide nurses with increased, stronger information than do simple nominal scaling statements. Also, philosophy of science accepts both of these comparative statements as statistical statements. Having both comparative and statistical qualities makes these statements more effective in that they are more productive of information and more predictive of future NPO patients. This is particularly important with qualitative concepts since one function of both comparative and statistical categories is to quantify. They are further important to a professional discipline because they form the base upon which clinical decisions may be made when more certain statements or laws are lacking. The examples that follow illustrate some of the thinking that goes into categorization.

Cultural value. The value of the phenomenon in our society and other cultures may be important. For example, a culture in which there is usually not enough to eat may value vomiting because it signifies more than enough to eat. Another society may attach negative value to it because it represents gluttony—an immoral act or sin—and still another may devalue it because the act is perceived as disgusting. Values may vary between health care disciplines: for example, in medicine, vomiting is a good chief complaint whereas in nursing, it may have protective value and in social work it may have no significance at all.

Population. Which populations are affected by the phenomenon and how does the phenomenon become operational in these populations? How do these populations explain the phenomenon and its function and sequelae? And, how similar or how different are the perceptions of the affected population from the explanations of scientists and professionals? The history and impact of many experiential phenomena differ depending on whose point of view—patient–client or professional—is under observation. Only recently has medicine evaluated old wives' tales and folk medicine for treatments that might be useful in scientific medicine; for example, rauwolfia has been discovered to be useful in the treatment of hypertension. The delay in recognizing the value of culturally evolved care is related to the scientist's trust in science and distrust of the pragmatic. Nurses working in concept clarification need to be open in observing affected and associated populations.

Impact on society. Importance of phenomena to the society relates to the extent to which they affect people (e.g., degree of misery they cause—whether this is discomfort, pain, loss of status, loss of personal appearance or personal values because of bad odor, deformity, or other devalued state). How subjects of the phenomenon influence the productivity and the economics of the social system is an important observation in terms of looking at priorities for coping and solving the particular problem. How the phenomenon affects the family and kinship system provides another measure of social impact.

Function. The function of the phenomenon is critical to understanding its occurrence and its resolution if indicated. It may be that under certain circumstances, no function can be found. In the study discussed earlier, this was the case in nausea and vomiting due to motion such as occurs in seasickness.

Cause and effect. Actually, this is a false category because it is almost impossible to verify that A causes B. Scientists do not look for causes; they search for relationships. A scientist might say, "if A, then B" or "A and B." This establishes an associational relationship but the claim of cause-and-effect is not made. Postulating relevant relationships usually comes late in the process of concept clarification, after the greater mass of data about the phenomenon has been collected. This may be a difficult phase of the work because of the knowledge required to build logical, clear "connectives" or relationships between the phenomenon under study and concomitant or sequential processes or events. Knowledge of physiology, pathophysiology, psychology, or social sciences may be necessary to synthesize complex relationships in terms of the holism of individuals. When working with complex concepts, it is difficult to know what questions to ask of a resource person. It may be even more difficult to understand the answers. We need to be able to learn from scientists, including philosophers, who are not nurses. Expecting any one to deal with a mass of data is exploitative, however. The nurse researcher needs to go as far as possible in independently systematizing the data and identifying the critical questions.

SETTING IT UP TO SEE WHAT IS THERE

It is difficult to be sensitive to all of the aspects, phases, or variations of nursing phenomena. The careful observer has to go beyond subject data (e.g., the person saying, "I am nauseated; this is how I feel"). The observer might ask, "Are there observations I can make about degree of nausea? Are there observations I can make that predict whether this person will vomit? Can I make observations that provide clues to intervention?" Or, if the researcher is observing the redness of the skin around a decubitus ulcer, he or she may be unaware that there are many shades of red that appear differently in various qualities and levels of light. If the observer is not aware that redness must be calculated using a color scale under standardized lighting at a known candlepower, observation of one patient is not accurately comparable with any other patient. Descriptions obtained under such uncontrolled conditions are not reliable; no matter how many observations are made, no generalization is possible.

Requirements for clarifying concepts include that nurses discriminate between similar and dissimilar events. Because nurses are educated within the framework of individual uniqueness and individual differences, there is a tendency for them to look for differences; other disciplines focus on the identification of similarities. Another requirement is that methods of construction quantify without minimizing qualitative or value-laden materials. Values may concern seriousness of impact, traditional approaches, or possibly, what has been most meaningful to the common-sense orientation. The existence of value is one of the basic reasons why concept clarification is necessary in nursing. Quantification of information may provide a different value system for a profession like nursing, or it may create a new perspective from which to view nursing. In other words, concepts may have more than one value depending upon the groups using them. As stated previously, to medicine vomiting is considered a significant chief complaint, valued because it is a "good" symptom of illness; in nursing, vomiting is seen as the protective first line of defense against noxious agents entering the body. Frequency of occurrence creates another value because of the amount of physician time required or the amount of money required to treat it.

LIMITATIONS OF CONCEPT CLARIFICATION

The main danger of abstracted empiricism or the inductive method used in this particular way is in allowing the work to become mired in tangential trivia or concepts. These trivial, usually low-level concepts (e.g., concrete observations) could be studied rigorously for years without ever accomplishing the formulation of nursing concepts. This is the opposite of the dangers of grand theory, in which the basic ideas may be stated so broadly that no one cannot identify the specific statements that delineate professional nursing. If the major ideas cannot be identified, hypothesis generation is impossible.

A further limitation of the inductive mode of clarifying concepts is that they deal with empirical reality, thus ruling out any conceptualization of the ideal. Especially in a profession, developing statements of ideal types, ideal performance, and ideal interventions may be important for transmission of knowledge to the learners and students of the discipline. Grand theory as developed by nursing may better serve this function.

Concept clarification is but one of many ways to develop knowledge. The role of research is paramount in confirming or refuting whether categories are valid, whether elements of a phenomenon belong in categories assigned and, whether causal, coexistence, or sequential relationships exist.

REFERENCES

Benoliel, J.Q. The interaction between theory and research. *Nurs. Outlook* 25:108–113, Feb. 1977.

Berthold, J.S. Theoretical and empirical clarification of concepts. *Nurs. Sci.* 2:406–422, Oct. 1964.

Carnap, R. In M. Gardiner (Ed.), *An Introduction to the Philosophy of Science.* New York: Basic Books, 1966. Pp. 58–59, 108.

Crawford, G., Dufault, K., and Rudy, E. Evolving issues in theory development. *Nurs. Outlook* 27:346–351, May 1979.

Donaldson, S.K., and Crowley, D.M. The discipline of nursing. *Nurs. Outlook* 26:113–119, Feb. 1978.

Forsyth, G.L. Analysis of the concept of empathy: Illustration of one approach. *Adv. Nurs. Sci.* 2:33–42, Jan. 1980.

Francis, G.M. Loneliness: Measuring the abstract. *Int. J. Nurs. Stud.* 13:153–160, 1976.

Glaser, B.B., and Strauss, A.L. *Awareness of Dying.* Chicago: Aldine, 1965.

Gordon, G.S. Fuller Albright and postmenopausal osteoporosis: A personal appreciation. *Perspect. Biol. Med.* 24:547–560, Summer, 1981.

Gregg, D.E. Proposing Two Approaches to Doctoral Education in Nursing. In E.A. Garrison (Ed.), *Doctoral Preparation for Nurses.* San Francisco: University of California, 1973.

Hansen, B.W. In *CURN Project,* Reducing Diarrhea in Tube-fed Patients, Vol. 2. New York: Grune & Stratton, 1981.

Hempel, C.G. *Philosophy of Natural Science*. Englewood Cliffs, N.J.: Prentice-Hall, 1966. Pp. 86–87, 101–105.

Hymes, D.H. Functions of Speech: An Evolutionary Approach. In Y.A. Cohen (Ed.), *Man in Adaption*. Chicago: Aldine, 1968.

Mansfield, E. Empathy: Concept and identified psychiatric nursing behavior. *Nurs. Res.* 22:525–530, Nov.–Dec. 1973.

Martin, M. *Concepts of Science Education*. Glenview, Ill.: Scott, Foresman, 1972. Pp. 75–102.

McKay, R.P. Discussion: Discipline of nursing-syntactical structure and relation with other disciplines and the profession of nursing. In M.V. Batey (Ed.), *Communicating Nursing Research: Optimizing Environments for Health: Nursing's Unique Perspective*. Boulder, Col.: Western Interstate Commission for Higher Education, 10:23–30, 1977.

Norris, C.M. Restlessness: A nursing phenomenon in search of meaning. *Nurs. Outlook* 23:103–107, Feb. 1975.

Rawnsley, M.M. The concept of privacy. *Adv. Nurs. Sci.* 2:25–31, Jan. 1980.

Schlotfeldt, R.M. Nursing research: Reflection of values. *Nurs. Res.* 26:4–9, Jan.–Feb. 1977.

Silva, M.C. Philosophy, science, theory: Interrelationships and implications for nursing research. *Image* 9:59–63, Oct. 1977.

Voda, A.M. Preoperative Water Loss. In E. Bauwens (Ed.), *Clinical Nursing Research: Its Strategies and Findings*. Indianapolis, Ind.: Sigma Theta Tau, 1978.

Weiss, S.J. The language of touch. *Nurs. Res.* 28:76–80, Mar.–Apr. 1979.

Chapter 4

Concept Clarification: Evolving Methods in Nursing

Catherine M. Norris

If concepts are "gateways to the world of nursing," methods for clarifying the concepts need to be made explicit. Many methods are promising for doing effective concept clarification, but a limited number of formal methodologies are described in the literature. There is comparatively copious literature related to two or three conventional methods but newer methods, briefly described in this chapter, were abstracted from reports of concept clarification.

To editorialize about "the state of the art" and to ensure the survival of the nursing profession, we need to clarify our concepts. This requires at least two types of value changes.

1. Nurse scientists educated in methodological rigor need to investigate and develop other tools of science that can contribute to creation of the substance of nursing.
2. All methods of study need to be considered.

Exploratory and descriptive research have been assigned low priority by nurse researchers, so these methods are often rejected out of hand. Thus many attempts at concept clarification are misguided. But with adequate study and feedback from colleagues, work that shows promise or needs modification can be refined to meet the requirements of research. Nurses have the opportunity to develop a large, respectable armamentarium of exploratory and descriptive methodologies for adding to the substantive body of nursing knowledge. The power of these methods for developing operational definitions, typologies and taxonomies, models, hypotheses, and theory needs recognition as scientific work. The publication of *Advances in Nursing Science* represents one very positive step in this direction.

This chapter will present a brief description of a limited number of methods for concept clarification. Other methods, such as one-person studies and pilot studies, are covered in almost all beginning research texts. Inclusion here does not imply that these methods are better than others or that one method stands out. Rather, the choice to include several varied methodologies demonstrates our need to experiment with existing methods and develop new ones from nurses' and others' perspectives. While the methods of other disciplines are possibly applicable to nursing, these other groups usually develop their own or tailor existing methods to meet their needs, as nurses have done with so-called grounded theory (Glaser and Strauss 1967).

QUALITATIVE METHODS

Qualitative methods are often called *inductive methods* of study and include both exploratory and descriptive methodologies, even though it is recognized that there is no theory free research.

Until recently, social and behavioral scientists conformed to the experimental research model of the physical and natural sciences. *Qualitative research* was identified as exploratory and preliminary to experimental research. Since this approach was reassuring to the scientific community and to the social and behavioral scientists themselves, nothing was done to disturb the uneasy truce between "hard" and "soft" scientists for half a century. Only in the last 20 years have scientists in the sociopsychological and professional disciplines asserted that qualitative research has an important place in scientific work.

Exploratory and descriptive methods were once the route through which a discipline gained entry into the unknown and discovered enough about concepts involved to permit generation of hypotheses relevant for experimental research. But there is increasing evidence that qualitative methods are often the most efficient or sole manner of studying an empirical situation. Sometimes these methods are more adequate than experimental methods in extracting the kind of information contained in a situation. Qualitative research may be related to the final goal (i.e., not as a prelude to experimental research) as in studying the inner perspective of people's experience. It may have the goal of theory generation or it may include the best method for studying empirical phenomena. Qualitative research is also called *first-level inquiry* by some researchers.

STRUCTURE IN QUALITATIVE RESEARCH

Because nursing concepts may be undefined or poorly defined and because relationships between concepts are often not explicit, the theoretical framework may be little more than a written statement of the nursing perspective out of which one operates; there is never a hypothesis stated. If we can state a hypothesis, we have enough knowledge about the concept or concepts to test it out using experimental methods. A "what" question is asked at this first level of inquiry; the less known about the concept, the more direct and concrete the question. If little is known, the researcher might ask questions such as, "What is restlessness?" or "What is taste alteration?" If more is known about a concept, we might ask a more complicated question like, "What does postmyocardial infarct nausea mean in the rehabilitation trajectory?"

The methodologies will be simply structured, semistructured, or unstructured, and at least one method is structured by the nature of the data to be collected. This general nature of qualitative methodologies already assures that these studies cannot be replicated; nor would we want to replicate them. If the studies have generated a model from which testable hypotheses evolve, we do not as yet need more concept clarification. If no model is forthcoming, other descriptive approaches to study of the phenomenon might be appropriate. Data would be analyzed conceptually and arithmetically in exploratory research with findings expressed as categories, typologies, operational definitions, models, percentages, means, and frequencies. In descriptive research, simple (descriptive) statistics as well as conceptual analysis and synthesis would be used to analyze the data. Findings would be expressed as correlations, variance, and hypotheses.

METHODS

The remainder of this chapter consists of brief descriptions of in-use and potential methods that may have relevance for concept clarification. These include

Criterion attributes
Phenomenological techniques
Discovery or idea testing
General systems theory
Ethnoscience
Wilson's technique or model
Dimensions and attributes
Cross-sectional survey
Theory, research, practice analysis, and reconceptualization
Philosophy of science tools.

OVERVIEW OF MORE COMMON METHODS

Criterion Attributes

Because nursing concepts are distressingly vague, they often do not clearly discriminate their empirical instances. Methods developed around the discrimination, specification, description, and weighting of a concept's attributes could prove extremely useful to the nurse researcher. This method is commonly called the *criterion attribute method*.

Phenomenology

While the phenomenological approach to concept clarification is not in accord with scientific empiricism, it appears to be an approach that has potential for nursing. This is especially relevant since participant observation, a technique for collecting phenomenological data, is already in use by nurses in their work with patients. Davis (1973) succinctly characterized the approach; "The phenomenological movement is an attempt to understand empirical matters from the perspective of those being studied." There has been steadfast unwillingness among health care professionals and scientists about having patients or subjects wittingly supply the data or solve research problems. But the major reason for lack of acceptance of this approach concerns the problem of reliability, which is problematic for all qualitative research.

Reliability was formerly, in the discipline of sociology and, to some degree, psychology, the science climber's most favored step on the ladder to scientific respectability. This stance often resulted in neglected validity problems. Preoccupation with reliability prevented clarification of why we seek knowledge and ignored phenomena about which we need knowledge. While researchers using qualitative methods are interested in reliability and have developed procedures for intersubject and transubject understanding of data, many researchers continue their work—not waiting for solution of the issue of reliability.

Workers unconstrained by the reliability debate believe that qualitative methods are legitimate for arriving at personal knowledge and subjective understanding as well as for identifying relations between symbolic data. They believe that to refuse to tap this knowledge would hamper development of truthful definition of the nature of people. One basic assumption of the scientist who uses qualitative methods is that reliable knowledge can be found in ways other than by sensory observation and reason. Intuition may be a case in point. Traditional science has essentially not attempted to identify the processes of intuition, to put it in a framework of data-collecting instrumentation, or to even recognize it as a legitimate source of knowledge.

Nurses, most of whom are women, can offer a great deal to the development of reliable qualitative methods if they were allowed autonomy and if the value of these methods were recognized. Mead (1978) notes that women

> show marked differences in the way they tackle problems. . . . Most men doing any kind of work that involves human beings and animals think they themselves are some kind of animal. They try to understand

animals by identification. . . . Women, on the other hand, have been taught to look at animals, or babies, as different from themselves. This is an exceedingly important dimension of research.

Scientific method as it exists today was developed by men; this is not stated to default current method in any way. Rather, it prefaces the question about how women, were they free, would develop methodologies that would provide meaningful descriptions about the nature of the world, of health, and our existence. Consider whether traditional scientists using "The Scientific Method" would ask questions like "How does it feel to be dying?" "What does it mean to a woman to lose a breast and how [does she go about] coming to terms with such a change in physical appearance?" (Quint 1962) "How do different senders and receivers of touch perceive their interaction?" (Weiss 1979) "How does it feel to be raped?" (Ipema 1979) "What color is your pain?" (Stewart 1977) "Does your hot flash have an odor?" (Voda 1981).

Discovery or Idea Testing

The methodology of discovery using "comparative analysis methods as an inductive, hypothesis-seeking strategy for generating plausible 'middle range' substantive and formal theory" (Wilson 1977) has become the method of choice in nursing. This method, also called *idea testing*, was first developed as grounded theory methodology (Glaser and Strauss 1967) for use in sociology.

Replacing the sociological framework with a nursing structure, this method proves useful not only for the discovery of substantive theory but also for the clarification of theoretical building blocks, or nursing concepts. In the discovery method, the investigator identifies a phenomenon for study and places him- or herself in situations where the phenomenon occurs. We may start by observing everything or only the particular phenomenon under consideration. Soon the investigator starts to hypothesize and seeks to confirm or invalidate the hypotheses. Multiple hypotheses are studied simultaneously; careful field notes produce even more hypotheses. As hypotheses are verified, they are set aside and attention diverted to emerging hypotheses. In time, hypotheses are organized into categories or a central framework; the framework then guides data collection and the work becomes much more analytical. When investigators believe that work is completed, they withdraw to reflect upon the data and its analysis, to check out findings with colleagues, and to study the literature.

General System Theory

General system theory operates within a holistic paradigm, and developments in the theory may make it useful in concept clarification. First there are changes in some of the basic concepts of science ". . . we see old concepts of energy, force and causality being replaced by concepts of probability, information and organization in all fields of science (Battista 1977)." When Bertalanffy (1968) developed the theory, it was essentially descriptive, but recent contributions resulting from synthesis of information theory and cybernetics as well as the addition and integration of structuralism now permit the theory to be explanatory. Battista (1977) notes that purposive behavior can be accounted for "by conceptualizing all interactions to occur as information processing feedback loops or as servomechanisms. This has . . . allowed system theorists to shed new light on such behaviors as drinking, eating and mating."

Ethnoscience

Ethnoscience methods were developed by anthropologists and evolved out of "a profound realization: the people we . . . seek to help have a way of life, a culture of their own (Spradley 1979)." Such methods constitute a systematized way of entering the separate realities of others and making those realities comprehensible to us. Ethnoscience relies heavily on the interview and participant–observation used in some ways that are different from both discovery method and phenomenological methods. "Field work" or the data-collecting phase "involves the disciplined study of what the world is like to people who have learned to see, hear, speak, think, and act in ways that are different." The goal is to learn from people—to put the subjects in teacher roles. Investigative skills required include knowing how to collect cultural data, knowing how to analyze cultural data, and formulating ethnoscientific hypotheses. There are many similarities in methods of grounded theory and ethnoscience: for example, simultaneous hypothesis formulation and data collection.

Wilson's Technique

The process of concept analysis using the techniques described by Wilson (1969) in *Thinking with Concepts* was the first step of Forsyth's work in clarifying the concept of empathy. These techniques include:

1. Description and analysis of model cases, or analysis of empirical events that can be said by most observers to represent an instance or occurrence of the abstract concept
2. Description and analysis of alternative cases that represent the occurrence of the contrary
3. Review of existing literature to extract explicit or implicit meanings
4. Extraction of provisional criteria that may be used in naming the occurrence of the phenomenon

5. Examination of such factors as social contexts, underlying anxieties, and application of varying means in different social situations.

"The techniques are not necessarily used in step-by-step fashion; rather they tend to emerge simultaneously once the initial steps of analysis have been undertaken (Forsyth 1980)." Forsyth's analysis of model and alternative empathic events in nursing situations revealed the following conditions or provisional criteria: consciousness, temporality, relationship, validation, accuracy, and intensity.

The next step in this study was identifying and differentiating related concepts of sympathy, pity, and compassion from empathy. This highlighted the following two provisional criteria for empathy: objectivity and freedom of evaluation. At that point, the eight provisional criteria were envisioned as necessary conditions for the existence of an instance of empathy.

Dimensions Examined Using Specified Attributes

In studying the concept of privacy, Rawnsley (1980) identified three dimensions of the concept as follows: privacy as a legal right, privacy as a social privilege, and privacy as a psychological need. The concept was then explored in terms of the three dimensions in an attempt to define privacy, to identify its population, to speculate about its functions, to trace its historical development, to identify questions that need to be answered, and to project research questions. This methodology contains some elements of the criterion-attribute method in terms of the variables to be examined under the three identified dimensions. While the methodology appears simple and useful for the beginner, the clarification of privacy rests more heavily on the investigator's knowledge of the concept and ability to critically analyze.

Cross-Sectional Survey

Francis (1976) studied secondary loneliness experimentally and descriptively using cross-sectional survey methodology. This research "provided a logically defined variable (loneliness) and a system of concepts (cathectic investment and significantly associated variables such as gender, age, and race) in which the concepts fit logically." While relationships among concepts could not be explained, the theoretical significance of the research lies in the finding of a new concept, *cathectic investment,* to integrate into a potential theory of loneliness. Knowledge-extending methods like cross-sectional survey require careful deliberation.

Theory, Research, Practice Analysis, and Reconceptualization

Kim (1980) approached the concept of pain by critically analyzing pain theory, pain research, and nonresearch-oriented professional nursing literature on pain. She applied her research results to create categories of pain-relieving nursing activities, to identify clinical implications of pain research for nursing, and to identify areas in which nursing practice likely originates from either theory or research or both as well as areas in which theory and research are not related to practice. Finally, she recommended directions for future research and proposed the utilization of both research and practice findings for modifying theory.

The gate control theory of pain was identified as having evolved to the point where it "provides a more comprehensive understanding of the pain mechanism which reflects both physiological and psychological dimensions (Kim 1980)." After describing the theory, Kim (1980) evaluated it using the criteria of operational and empirical adequacy, contribution to understanding, and pragmatic adequacy. Pain research was then (reviewed and) evaluated by means of reliability and validity criteria. Finally, nursing practice was analyzed in terms of what nurses are doing for patients in pain; out of this analysis came the seven categories of pain-relieving nursing activities. The analysis of nursing practice was carried out using both theory and research findings to identify areas of fragmentation and to pave the way for the creation of a pain-care theory and improved pain-care practice.

The descriptive-level study previously discussed was feasible because of the extensive literature available in theory, research, and practice. The investigator's intellectual familiarity and facility in the areas of practice, theory, and experimental research allowed her to pursue such a study effectively. Any investigator attempting an endeavor such as the study outlined must also be able to understand statistics to the level of multivariate analysis in order to comprehend and analyze the research reports on, in this instance, pain. Theory, research, practice analysis, and reconceptualization, then, is not a method for the concept-clarification novice.

Philosophy of Science Tools

Several nurse scholars (McKay 1977; Schlotfeldt 1977; and Silva 1977) have suggested that nurses might look to philosophy as one source of methodology for developing a substantive body of nursing knowledge (see Chapter 5, Long-Term Itching). Philosophy of science deals with the logical analysis of concepts, statements, and theories of science. "Science begins with direct observations of single facts (Carnap 1966)." In nursing, one set of facts is, for example, observations of the client–patient population; once these facts are in hand, the first step in treating them is searching for patterns, repetition, and regularities. Then we process the facts—that is, that which is observable—and elevate them to an abstract level.

One kind of abstraction that specifies regularities and patterns in observed phenomena is a statement called a *law*; a law is always a relational statement (e.g., sequence of events, causal factors, associational relationships). The simplest abstraction of this type is an *empirical law*. Empirical laws generalize direct observations nurses make in collecting their data. Another kind of abstraction, a *theoretical law*, generalizes nonobservable aspects of the concept being studied and goes beyond empirical laws. Nurses use the abstractions, or laws, both informally and in formal, structured ways to explain and predict nursing phenomena. The quality of subsequent steps in the methodology process depends on the initial veracity of the law: in other words, the better the law, the better the explanation, and the better the explanation, the greater the predictive power.

APPLYING LEARNED METHODS

In addition to method, in-depth knowledge of nursing's perspective and scope as well as depth insight into the study subject influence both choice of questions and quality of data obtained. Expertise in some other area such as philosophy, physiology, psychology, or anthropology allows the investigator to pursue a concept to its fullest extent. The researcher's own conceptual ability and ability to cope with abstractions dealing with varying kinds of relationships also has a profound influence on the ultimate outcome.

In summary, nursing needs a qualitative-research armamentarium for use in clarifying the phenomena of nursing. Further, nurses need to perceive themselves as scientists as they develop expertise in applying these developing research tools.

REFERENCES

Agar, M. *Ripping and Running: A Formal Ethnography of Urban Heroin Addicts.* New York: Seminar Press, 1973.

Battista, J. The holistic paradigm and general system theory. *Gen. Systems* 22:65–71, 1977.

Berger, P.L., and Luckman, T. *The Social Construction of Reality.* Garden City, N.Y.: Anchor–Doubleday, 1966.

Bertalanffy, L.V. *General System Theory.* New York: Braziller, 1968.

Berthold, J. Theoretical and empirical clarification of concepts. *Nurs. Sci.* 2:406–422, Oct. 1964.

Blumer, H. *Symbolic Interactionism.* Englewood Cliffs, N.J.: Prentice–Hall, 1969.

Blumer, H. The problem of the concept in social psychology. *Am. J. Sociol.* 46:707–719, 1940.

Blumer, H. What is wrong with social theory? In W.J. Filstead (Ed.), *Qualitative Methodology.* Chicago: Markham, 1970.

Bogdan, R., and Taylor, S. *Introduction to Qualitative Research Methods: A Phenomenological Approach to the Social Sciences*. New York: Wiley–Interscience, 1975.

Brunner, J.S., Goodnow, J.J., and Austin, G.A. *A Study of Thinking*. New York: Wiley, 1956.

Carini, P.F. *Observation and Description: An Alternative Methodology for the Investigation of Human Phenomena*. Grand Forks, N.D.: University of North Dakota Press, 1975.

Carnap, R. *An Introduction to Philosophy of Science*. New York: Basic Books, 1966.

Davis, A.J. The Phenomenological Approach to Nursing Research. In E.A. Garrison (Ed.), *Doctoral Preparation for Nurses . . . with Emphasis on the Psychiatric Field*. San Francisco: University of California, 1973.

DeGroot, A. *Methodology: Foundations of Inference and Research in the Behavioral Sciences*. Hawthorne, N.J.: Mouton, 1969.

Ennis, R.H. Operational definitions. *Am. Educ. Res. J.* 1:183–201, May 1964.

Fawcett, J. The relationship between theory and research: A double helix. *Adv. Nurs. Sci.* 1:49–62, Oct. 1978.

Forsyth, G.L. Analysis of the concept of empathy: Illustration of one approach. *Adv. Nurs. Sci.* 2:33–42, Jan. 1980.

Forsyth, G.L. Exploration of empathy in nursing client interaction. *Adv. Nurs. Sci.* 1:53–61, Jan. 1979.

Francis, G.M. Loneliness: Measuring the abstract. *Int. J. Nurs. Stud.* 13:153–160, 1976.

Glaser, B.G., and Strauss, A.L. *The Discovery of Grounded Theory: Strategies for Qualitative Research*. Chicago: Aldine, 1967.

Glaser, B.G. *Theoretical Sensitivity*. San Francisco: University of California Press, 1978.

Gordon, M., and Sweeney, M.A. Methodological problems and issues in identifying and standardizing nursing diagnoses. *Adv. Nurs. Sci.* 2:3–15, Oct. 1979.

Gordon, R. *Interviewing Strategies: Techniques and Tactics*. Homewood, Ill.: Dorsey, 1969.

Graham, K.R. *Controlled Interpersonal Interaction*. New York: Brooks–Cole, 1977.

Gurvitch, G., Scheler, M., and Vierkrandt, A. The Essentials of the Phenomenological Method. In H. Spiegelberg (Ed.), *The Phenomenological Movement* (2nd ed.), Vol. 2. Boston: Kluwer, 1976.

Homans, G.C. *The Nature of Social Science*. New York: Harcourt Brace Jovanovich, 1967.

Husserl, E. *Ideas: General Introduction to Pure Phenomenology*. New York: Collier Paperback, 1962.

Ipema, D.K. Rape: The process of recovery. *Nurs. Res.* 28:272–275, Sept.–Oct. 1979.

Jacox, A. Issues in Construction of Nursing Theory. In C. Norris (Ed.), *Proceedings: First Nursing Theory Conference*. Kansas City, Ks.: University of Kansas Medical Center, Department of Nursing Education, March 20–21, 1969.

Kim, S. Pain theory: Research and nursing practice. *Adv. Nurs. Sci.* 2:43–59, Jan. 1980.

Kockelmans, J., and Kisiel, J. (Comps). *Phenomenology and the Natural Sciences, Essays and Translations*. Evanston, Ill.: Northwestern University Press, 1970.

Kwant, R.C. *The Phenomenological Philosophy of Merleau-Ponty*. Pittsburgh: Duquesne University Press, 1963.

McFarlane, J.K. The role of research and the development of nursing theory. *J. Adv. Nurs.* 1:443–451, 1976.

McKay, R.P. Discussion: Discipline of Nursing-Syntactical Structure and Relation with Other Disciplines and the Profession of Nursing. In M.V. Batey (Ed.), *Communicating Nursing Research: Optimizing Environments for Health; Nursing's Unique Perspective*. Boulder, Col.: Western Interstate Commission for Higher Education, 1977.

Mead, M. Women and Men in the Natural and Social Sciences. In National Science Foundation, *Increasing the Participation of Women in Scientific Research: Summary of Conference Proceedings, October 1977*. Washington, D.C.: National Science Foundation, 1978.

Mehan, H., and Wood, H. *The Reality of Ethnomethodology*. New York: Wiley, 1975.

Newman, M. *Theory Development in Nursing*. Philadelphia: Davis, 1980.

Peplau, H.E. Theory: The Professional Dimension. In C. Norris (Ed.), *Proceedings First Nursing Theory Conference*. Kansas City, Ks.: University of Kansas Medical Center, Department of Nursing Education, March 20–21, 1969.

Quint, J.C. Delineation of qualitative aspects of nursing care. *Nurs. Res.* 12:204–206, Fall 1962.

Quint, J.C. Research—how will nursing define it? The case for theories generated from empirical data. *Nurs. Res.* 16:109–114, Spring 1967.

Rawnsley, M.M. The concept of privacy. *Adv. Nurs. Sci.* 2:25–31, Jan. 1980.

Reilly, D.E. Why a conceptual framework? *Nurs. Outlook* 23:566–569, Sept. 1975.

Scholtfeldt, R.M. Nursing research: Reflection of values. *Nurs. Res.* 26:4–9, Jan.–Feb. 1977.

Silva, M.C. Philosophy, science, theory: Interrelationships and implications for nursing research. *Image* 9:59–63, Oct. 1977.

Smith, R.B., and Manning, P. (Eds.). *Qualitative Methods*. New York: Irvington, 1979.

Spradley, J.P., and McCurdy, D.W. *Anthropology: The Cultural Perspective*. New York: Wiley, 1975. Chap. 3.

Spradley, J.P. *The Ethnographic Interview*. New York: Holt, Rinehart & Winston, 1979.

Spradley, J.B. *Participant Observation*. New York: Holt, Rinehart & Winston, 1980.

Spradley, J.B., and Mann, B.J. *The Cocktail Waitress: Women's Work in a Man's World*. New York: Wiley, 1975.

Stewart, M.L. Measurement of Clinical Pain. In A.K. Jacox (Ed.), *Pain: A Source Book for Nurses*. Boston: Little, Brown, 1977.

Straus, E.W. *Phenomenology: Pure and Applied*. Pittsburgh: Duquesne University Press, 1964.

Voda, A.M. Climacteric hot flash. *Maturitas* 1:1–21, Jan.–Feb. 1981.

Weiss, S.J. The language of touch. *Nurs. Res.* 28:76–80, Mar.–Apr. 1979.

Wilson, H.S. Limiting intrusion—Social control of outsiders in a healing community. *Nurs. Res.* 26:103–111, Mar.–Apr. 1977.

Wilson, J. *Thinking with Concepts*. London: Cambridge University Press, 1969.

Zaner, R.M. *The Way of Phenomenology*. New York: Pegasus, 1970.

Zderad, L.T. Empathy—From Cliche to Construct. In C. Norris (Ed.), *Proceedings: Third Nursing Theory Conference*. Kansas City, Ks.: University of Kansas Medical Center, Department of Nursing, 1970.

Part II

A Sampling of Concepts Clarified for Nursing

In this section, 18 chapters of clarification work representing 10 nursing concepts are reported by 19 nurse investigators. In Chapter 5, Long-term Itching, I attempt to clarify a concept using the tools of philosophy of science. While problems persist in methodology of assigning meaning to verbalizations at the figurative and symbolic levels and concerns about the depth of philosophy of science knowledge required endure, this work may catalyze another method for clarifying concepts.

In Chapter 6, clarification of nausea and vomiting is from the standpoint of a discovery methodology. Ultimately focusing on the occasional self-induced vomiter as compared to the ill vomiter a formulation was developed that proposes the basic function of nausea and vomiting is *protective*. The definitions, taxonomy, and model developed may be useful in further, more rigorous study of the concepts.

In pursuing her interest in the meaning of nausea in the illness trajectory of patients with MI Minow (Chapter 7) first reviewed the literature related to post-MI complications. She conducted further literature search for the anatomical and physiological links between nausea and MI. A convenience sample of 10 patients was studied. Nausea was related to time of diagnosis, chest pain, vomiting, a variety of autonomic nervous system changes, and subjective complaints. Severity and frequency were also studied. Finally, complications of MI were related to complaints of nausea. Findings are synthesized in a model and hypotheses for further study are offered.

Voda and Randall (Chapter 8) conceptualize morning nausea of pregnancy out of a woman-centered wellness perspective. Using a semistructured interview methodology, they conducted a pilot study to explore the morning-sickness phenomenon from the perspectives of the experience, circumstances related to the experience, and variations of the experience. Using this empirically generated data and review of the literature, they developed a physiological model within a framework of normal function to explain morning sickness. Out of the model, they identify 10 questions to be answered about the phenomenon.

Olivas used discovery methods to study the problem of thirst (Chapter 9) in a convenience sample of a particular group of patients on fluid restriction. She summarizes her observations in terms of behavioral problems and patterns and poses questions nurses need to answer. Her examination of the literature on thirst and relating the phenomenon to the clinician and clinical practice highlight the need for nurses to study current practices. The literature review also clearly differentiates "true thirst" from "false thirst" and provides the base for a model depicting the effects of fluid restriction on thirst and drinking behavior. All of this sets the stage for Olivas' reconceptualization of the thirst phenomenon for nursing practice. In Chapter 10, Olivas provides the reader with the contrast between concept clarification through empirical study and concept clarification through deductive methods. Using Gibb's paradigm, Olivas masterfully creates a theoretical model of thirst.

Using a loosely formulated discovery methodology, Anderson (Chapter 11) studied NPO patients, nurses' notes on these patients, and nurses in clinical settings to learn more about patients' expressions of hunger, nursing perceptions, and nursing interventions in hunger. She identifies three categories of hunger experience as well as associated behavioral changes. Next, she compared her findings about clinical hunger to those reported in the literature, examined various coping capacities for dealing with hunger, and related them to nursing. Anderson developed three models based on her work: the hunger continuum, behavior in hunger, and intervention in hunger.

Chapters 12 and 13 offer another kind of contrast. Abbey, who has worked with the concept of shivering and surface cooling for more than a decade, deals with the concept in a general sense. Schroeder, on the other hand, zeros in on a specific instance of shivering—shivering of postpartum women. Abbey's work stands apart because it consisted partly of experimental research; she integrated her findings into her conceptualization of shivering. Abbey presents a model of normothermic regulation. Schroeder offers a typology for shivering during the childbearing process and a set of propositions generated from exploratory informal survey data.

Three chapters discuss fatigue. In an extensive, critical literature review Hart and Freel (Chapter 14) essentially use the medical model for analyzing the concept of fatigue. When these investigators project nursing functions, they make an elegant statement of four health-promoting life-style modifications relative to fatigue and postulate one fatigue-preventing function. In Chapter 15, Morris adopts a third-person posture to report on her own fatigue during a long-term health problem. She relates the data from this one-person study to research findings and other fatigue variables reported in the literature, but is not inhibited in describing the full scope of her experience. Rhoten's work (Chapter 16) differs from the other two chapters on fatigue in that she focuses on the fatigue of one specific group, postsurgical patients. From reviewed literature she developed the

"Rhoten Fatigue Scale" and an "Observation Check List." Using these instruments with a semistructured interview, Rhoten did a pilot study with a convenience sample of five postoperative patients. Her findings generated a hypothesis about which postoperative patients might be at high risk for fatigue; attributes were identified that have potential use in building an assessment tool to determine level of fatigue. The three studies of fatigue contrast levels of knowledge at which concept work can be done. They point out that most nurses, beginning where they are, can do concept clarification.

Prokop, in her work on insomnia (Chapter 17), applied her observations as a night nurse to conceptualize insomnia as a protective response of the organism to potential danger.

Disorientation is more complicated than its traditional dictionary definition, Seither and Castleberry (Chapter 18) indicate. Of particular interest in their report is the recognition that transitory disorientation is a universal phenomenon in functional states like boredom and preoccupation. A beginning typology of disorientation and a mode of adaptive function of disorientation evolved out of their work. Kersher (Chapter 19) deals with one small aspect of disorientation of the infant to nurturer—human or mechanical. Her observations were used with findings and suggestions reported in the literature to reconceptualize the phenomenon and create a conceptual model of nipple confusion in the neonate.

The chapters on immobility each clarify a specific aspect of the concept. Kalafatich (Chapter 20) uses a pilot study of adolescent girls under treatment for scoliosis to observe responses to threatened and actual immobilization. She compares her findings with the findings of other studies reported in the literature. In Chapter 21, Christian uses a one-patient method to delineate the psychosocial aspects of immobilization for study. Out of her study, Christian develops a classification of immobilization by type of limitation, identification of criterion attributes related to immobilization, a classification of psychosocial reactions to immobilization, an assessment model of immobilization, and a model of the concept of immobilization.

Shannon's scholarly review of the literature on pressure sores (Chapter 22) is in line with the medical model that is used when investigating a physiological failure. The etiological causal model emerging from her work could be tested to see whether it would identify people at high risk for pressure sores. Shannon also created a descriptive model for future nursing research.

Most of the contributors in Part II mentioned one or more relationships between their concept and other existing concepts; this aspect of the work will be discussed in Chapter 23. Different levels of sophistication in approaching concept clarification are represented in the following chapters. This is purposeful because it supports the view that clinicians at all levels have a contribution to make. Scholars in nursing can contribute their special knowledge in more sophisticated conceptual clarification work.

Chapter 5

Long-term Itching

Catherine M. Norris

Several nurse scholars (Jacox 1974; McKay 1977; Schlotfeldt 1977; and Silva 1977) have suggested that nurses might look to the discipline of philosophy as one source of methodology for developing a substantive body of knowledge. The tools of philosophy of science may hold some promise for this task. Until recently, philosophers of science have essentially subscribed to logical positivism. This traditional approach could never include a body of professional knowledge as a science. Recent challenges to logical positivism (Feyerabend 1978; Kuhn 1970; Laudan 1977; Popper 1979; and Suppe 1974) may foster development of knowledge in the professions that meet reconceptualized criteria for being named sciences as opposed to older restrictive views of science that include only basic disciplines like mathematics, physics, or chemistry.

The purpose of this chapter is twofold. First, selected tools used by philosophers of science as they examine a science are briefly described. Second, exploratory work using these tools in clarifying the phenomenon of long-term itching is presented. This work is only a beginning. It is intended to stimulate other professional nurses to explore these or similar ideas as routes to building a body of nursing knowledge.

TOOLS OF PHILOSOPHY OF SCIENCE

A cursory examination of some of the tools used by philosophers of science is presented to enrich understanding of this manner of treating empirical observation. The reader is encouraged to refer to books in the reference list (particularly Carnap 1966; Feyerabend 1978; Laudan 1977; Popper 1979; and Suppe 1974) for further study (particularly in relation to forms of logical statements as well as the truth table and explanatory arguments). Also, the reader is encouraged to project other ways these tools could be used since this chapter is intended to point a direction rather than present a well-formulated method for explicating nursing phenomena.

The following tools were selected for brief definition and discussion: facts and statements; identification of patterns, repetitions, and regularities; assignment of meaning; and empirical and theoretical laws and formal explanation.

Facts and Statements

There are varied types of statements scientists can make. An *empirical observation* or *factual statement* is one type. A factual statement specifies an observable event that occurred at a specified place within a specified time frame. This specific judgment is about a single event, sequence of events, or activity.

A factual statement is often called a *singular statement*. Factual statements are singular statements, even though all singular statements are not facts. Facts always refer to particulars. All science (i.e., all scientific knowledge) begins or has its source in particular observations of particular events at particular times by particular people and the attempts of these particular people to comprehend observations made. But all observations do not lead to scientific knowledge. Observations require cognitive work that attempts to explain the observations.

All statements that do not specify an observable event are, then, intellectual inventions. For example, a nurse might observe the fact of a patient thrashing around in bed but make the statement that the patient is restless. The term *restless* is an intellectual invention to explain the fact of thrashing around in bed. It is also an intellectual invention that by naming, assigns some kind of meaning understood among nurses about the fact of a patient thrashing around in his or her bed. To the extent that the word *restless* is not just a synonym and nominal definition for thrashing around in bed, but a diagnosis, it is an *inference*. Inferences are not facts, but statements. They are intellectual inventions called *conditional statements* based on numbers of like or similar empirical observations (i.e., inferences express movement from observation of particulars to generalization about those particulars). Inferences are conditional in the sense that they are still subject to testing and verification for the population nursed. But inferences are important types of statements in nursing, for they often form the basis for clinical judgments. In this sense, nurses use inferences almost as laws since they are the closest we can come at a given moment to tested knowledge. For example, if all newly admitted patients thrashed around in bed, and no research reports about the phenomenon could be found, nurses might make the inference that all newly admitted bed-patients become restless. Then, nurses might base a plan for prevention or intervention on this inference. In so doing, they would give their inference the force of law.

Inferences are also important statements in nursing because they are treated as having communication value they may not in reality have. In the case in point, a question could be raised as to whether thrashing around in bed as a single behavioral operation is sufficient for assignment of the name *restless*. Are there operations like repetitiveness of behaviors, urgency to perform the behaviors, limited control of the behaviors or other behavioral operations that are also necessary to meet the conditions for naming *restless*?

It is important for the nurse using tools of the philosopher of science to comprehend the differences between facts and statements. This is difficult because of the frequent use of the cliches like, "It is a fact that . . ." or, "It's a commonly known fact." It is also important to identify the basis of the intellectual inventions on which statements are based.

A further word about statements. "The patient is thrashing around in bed," as has already been noted, is a fact and also a statement. It is a simple statement (i.e., one clause with one subject and one predicate). "The patient is restless" is also a simple statement, but not a fact. Statements are true or false; they cannot be both and they cannot be neither. If a nurse makes the statement, "The patient is thrashing around in bed and thrashing around in bed is restlessness," she has combined two simple statements (using the conjunctive "and") to make a compound statement. If either of the simple statements in the compound statement is not true, the whole statement is false. For example, if operations other than "thrashing around in bed" were required to compose sufficient conditions for naming the behavior *restless,* this would make the statement false even though one operation or condition for inferring the state *restless* is present.

Defining *fact* as an observation of some particular at a particular time, a first task for investigators doing concept clarification when dealing with empirical patient, nurse, and nurse–patient observations would be to identify and list all the facts, separating compound sentences and phrases into simpler ones. As in the example of thrashing around in bed, the kind of facts—thrashing and related behaviors—might be specified as the particular facts to be abstracted from records of empirical observations.

Repetition, Patterns, and Regularities

As a scientist, the nurse studies the facts, as far as they can be known to him or her, to search for repetition of events or behavior. (The term *behavior* as used here includes signs and symptoms.) If the nurse is concerned about thrashing around in bed, all behavior perceived to be thrashing around in bed is described. The facts will include possibly a wide range of behavior interpreted as thrashing around and some count of frequency of the behavior as well as a total count of the behavior for the period of observation. Frequency of occurrence and total number of occurrences provide some indication of importance to the individual or group under study.

Not only are behaviors and events repeated, but they may be repeated in some kind of pattern. Some are preceded by, succeeded by, or accompanied by other phenomena as trauma is always a prelude to physiological or emotional shock. A pattern indicates association of trend, tendency, or even regularity. Regularity indicates the extent to which phenomena occur under the specific circumstances alone or in some type of association. When the pattern or association is regular (i.e., without exception) the statement made about this regularity is referred to as a law, such as "Shock is preceded by trauma."

Associations represent a variety of relationships. It has already been suggested that thrashing around in bed may have a part–whole relationship to restlessness (i.e., in order for a judgment of restlessness to be made, there must be other behaviors present). In part–whole relationships, the part may not substitute for the whole in either structure or function. Thus, a part is dependent on the whole for both structure and function; the part is also necessary to the whole. If, however, restlessness represents a set of behaviors and subsets include thrashing around in bed, tapping fingers on the table, pacing and frequent shifting of sitting position, the characteristics of this kind of association are categorical. Thrashing around in bed in this context is an independent kind of phenomenon in that it has structure and function of its own. It is related to restlessness, however, by one or more common characteristics. These kinds of relationships provide description of phenomena.

As scientists, nurses will want to study repetitions, patterns, and regularities for relationships that go beyond description and advance toward explanation. One kind of compound statement that begins to do this describes the conditional relationship. For example, if the patient is thrashing around in bed, he or she is unable to sleep. This does not make a causal claim but only says that thrashing around in bed is a sufficient condition to prevent someone from sleeping.

In the explanatory phase of scientific activity, the causal relationship is of primary importance. Causal relations attempt to specify what it means to say, "One event caused another." Causal explanations attempt to answer "why" questions. Causal relationships have to do with processes. It is not accurate, for example, to say, "The patient mussed the sheets." It is more accurate to say, "The activity of the patient thrashing around in bed mussed the sheets." Causal relations have to do with all the conditions surrounding events. So to make a causal statement about a newly admitted patient thrashing around in bed, we would have to investigate and analyze all the conditions surrounding the patient— not only admission processes and hospital living but all the other processes that might be pertinent. If a causal relation is found between acting in the role of stranger or facing the unknown and a patient's thrashing around in bed, it must emerge out of the total context of his or her situation. The astute reader is already saying, "A causal relation also means predictability (i.e., if all of the facts and

laws had been known, thrashing around in bed could have been predicted)''
(Carnap 1966, p. 192).

It needs to be clear that the repetitions, patterns, and regularities scientists
look for would stem from the perspectives and purposes of the particular discipline. Nurses are oriented to studying life processes, human well-being, and
high-level human functioning. Nurses are concerned with health-related behavior
in interaction with the environment and are interested in processes that promote
and maintain health. Nurses focus on processes that restore health. Nurses'
purposes include discovery and application of laws and principles that govern
these processes in sickness and health (Donaldson and Crowley 1978).

Assignment of Meaning

Assigning meaning is a critical and challenging task for the concept clarifier.
For example, nurse–patient interactional observation records are often permeated
with slang. How does the nurse scientist assign meaning to these expressions?
These records also typically include three levels of communication: literal, figurative, and symbolic. If a patient talks about someone giving him or her a "pain
in the neck," this figurative statement requires some kind of treatment to put it
into the literal level of communication. In addition to observations of verbal
behavior, gestures and nonverbal vocalizations require meaning assignment if
they are to be understandable.

In observing the nonsensate behavior of people, instruments that measure
behavior indirectly have to be used or developed in order to assign meaning.
For example, in order to observe body temperature, an indirect measuring instrument, called a thermometer, can be used. To assign meaning to the readings
achieved using a thermometer, many readings were made and related to theories
of metabolism, maintenance of body temperature, inflammation, dehydration,
and other theories of human pathology. Nurses may be only at the beginning of
developing an armamentarium of instruments for indirect measurement.

In addition to putting observations into a form where they can be assigned
some form of understandable meaning, the concept clarifier cannot leave his or
her work until it is removed from the state of an isolated bit of knowledge. This
involves relating it to theory or existing knowledge.

When assigning meaning, the nurse as scientist asks how meaning is assigned.
In scientific theory, terms have very precise meanings. Such specificity is required if the statements in the theory are to be verified by testing. Definitions
may use common-sense meaning or other already accepted meanings of words.
One kind of definition is to give the term a special meaning for the time or cases
under consideration (Hempel 1966). This is called a *stipulated definition* and

generally is not as strong because its applicability is circumscribed and time-limited. In the absence of existing scientific theory about a phenomenon, we may use another theory (e.g., interpersonal theory) to assign meaning.

Even though theory used to assign meaning is a qualitative one, it is more adequate for assigning meaning than simple common sense or a dictionary as the terms are accepted and have fairly specific meanings for scientists and practitioners in the behavioral sciences. On the other hand, meaning may be more precise through the use of primitive terms or interpretive sentences (Hempel 1966) that specify a specific test or proof. For example, if frustration is the helpless feeling related to a block in progress toward a goal and aggression is the overt act that functions to reduce helpless feelings, the interpretive sentence might read, "Removing blocks to goal accomplishment reduces feelings of helplessness and aggressive behavior." This pretheoretical statement makes the previous theoretical statement more specific and thus provides a better definition of frustration.

Since use of an inference system for assigning meaning to the symbolic and figurative expressions may not be clear to the reader, an example may prove useful.

An example: assigning meaning to feelings of frustration and aggressive behavior. Frustration–aggression, an important theory within interpersonal theory, will be used to demonstrate assignment of meaning. Since its construction in the thirties (Dollard 1937; Dollard et al. 1939), the theory has been revised by others (Bronson and Desjardins 1971; Eleftheriou and Scott 1971; and Welch and Welch 1971). Dollard and colleagues' (1939) basic postulate was that aggression is always a consequence of frustration and that the existence of frustration always leads to some form of aggression. The theory states that some need is felt and a goal is set. A goal-directed response drive is initiated and at some point short of goal accomplishment, there is interference or blocking to the drive and achievement of the goal cannot occur. This situation constitutes frustration felt, for example, as helplessness or anger and calls forth an aggressive response. The strength of the aggressive response is related to the strength of the need, the timing of the interference in the goal-seeking behavioral sequence, the strength or completeness of the interference and the person's substitutive, sublimative, and compromising capacities in relation to goal achievement.

Recent additions to the theory include the generalization that "any behavior in order to become important, must have survival value (i.e. perform an adaptive function for the individuals involved) (Scott 1971, p. 11)." Scott (1971) further specifies that frustration–aggression is adaptive only where individuals are able to recognize each other as individuals. Indiscriminate attacks would have negative survival value. In summarizing physiological research on frustration–aggression, Eleftheriou and co-workers (1971) postulate "that while the aggressor learns to survive and adapts readily to the fighting process, the vanquished, if he does not die, maintains an existence highlighted by severe and extensive changes in all physiologic systems.'' Scientific research is close to important breakthroughs related to physiological changes related to frustration–aggression. Animal research (Eleftheriou and Scott 1971, pp. 34, 73) has demonstrated that losers in frustration–aggression interaction have lower levels of brain ribonucleic acid. This permits postulating the already common observation that emotional reactions interfere with learning. This method of using a theory to assign meaning could be used with other observed behavioral events.

Laws

One kind of abstraction that specifies repetitions, patterns and regularities is a statement called a *law*. As Carnap (1966, p. 3) writes, "The laws of science are nothing more than statements expressing these regularities [of the phenomena under study] as precisely as possible." Laws specify a uniform relationship between facets of or the whole of different empirical phenomena. Laws are more than assertions; they are not conceptualizations of the accidental relationship in that they are based on evidence that provides for understanding of how and why they are true. Thus, even though hypotheses express regularities between phenomena, they only propose the regularity as possible with the evidence still forthcoming.

If a regularity in relationship exists all of the time, wherever it is observed, the statement is referred to as a *universal law*. Universal laws are stated without reference to time, place, or person. Most universal laws exist in the natural sciences and mathematics. An example of a universal law that nurses use is, "If a solid is dissolved in a liquid, then the boiling point of the liquid is raised." There is not enough nursing knowledge and not even enough evidence about nursing phenomena to use in doing the deductive work required for explanation at the level of universal laws. The functions of laws are to explain facts already known and to predict phenomena that are not known.

Two kinds of laws can be distinguished in science: empirical laws and theoretical laws. The simplest abstraction of regularity that qualifies as a law is an *empirical law*. Empirical laws generalize the relationships between direct observations nurses, for example, make in collecting the data of nursing. In other words, empirical laws are derived from observing the relationship between two kinds of events or variables. These describe the regularities in our experience and we infer that the themes or patterns observed will, given the same circumstances, be duplicated or repeated. "Empirical laws are laws that can be confirmed directly by empirical observations (Carnap 1966, p. 225)." Empirical laws always explain facts.

Theoretical laws are statements expressing invariant relationships between two or more theoretical phenomena. They are used to explain regularities that cannot be directly observed and measured. For example, they include phenomena (e.g., gamma rays, beta rays, personality) that cannot be seen or directly measured but about which we have laws that explain both structure and behavior. Often the things or variables specified in theoretical laws have not been directly or even indirectly observed when they are first conceptualized. As the reality of these phenomena and their invariate relationships are supported through research and testing, however, theoretical laws lose their hypothetical (or proposed) status and take on the force of fact. Theoretical laws do not explain facts. They often explain empirical laws by hypothesizing beyond these laws and the testing of the hypothesis. This testing leads to the second function of theoretical laws, which is the derivation of new empirical laws.

Support of empirical law through observation, and confirmation of theoretical law through testing is never-ending. To the extent that the law is used as a basis for explaining another law, it retains the ascription of theoretical. Sets of theoretical laws (in the second sense of the term), logically related to explain another law, may be called *theory*.

Both empirical and theoretical laws may be deterministic or statistical. *Statistical laws* represent something being true in a percentage of cases, a percentage of the time, or in a certain ratio. Statistical laws maintain that if certain conditions exist, something else will also exist or occur at a specified relative frequency. When repetition, regularity, or patterns occur less than 100 percent of the time, the best statements nurses may be able to make might be, "Insomnia often accompanies emotional stress," "Nausea usually precedes vomiting," "Activity may reduce feelings of hunger," "Projectile vomiting nearly always indicates a crises," or "Hunger is occasionally mistaken for nausea (i.e., experienced as nausea)."

We may use quantifiers like "a few," "rarely," "about half," "sometimes," or "99.99%." Statistical laws may be stated in common-sense language, or they may be carefully defined quantitatively to increase the precision of the statement. Quantifiers like "few," "some," and "rarely," make weak statements. They are usually to be avoided because a law has limited usefulness when a statistical relationship is so weak. Statistical laws are probabilistic in that they state that under certain conditions certain events will probably happen.

Deterministic laws are stated in either quantitative or qualitative terms. The basic difference between a statistical law and a deterministic law is that a deterministic law is a statement about a certainty rather than a probability. At this point in nursing, statistical laws are not only important but necessary if we are to manage and understand the vast number of facts we gather.

In addition to the truth value of laws, it is paramount to recognize that one of the functions of laws is to rule out more and more possibilities, moving from unlimited possibilities to fewer and fewer possibilities with each restatement. All laws are predictive of some relationship or relationships. Empirical laws are more predictive and have limited explanatory power compared to theoretical laws. In nursing we are not in a position to do formal scientific explanation until we identify laws that may be useful in explanation.

Teleological laws need to be mentioned briefly. *Teleological laws* explain something of its purpose (e.g., the purpose of itching is to warn about stress). Teleological laws are weak laws since they do not address "why" questions nor can they ever explain causal relationships.

WAYS OF SCIENTIFIC EXPLANATION

When asked for a scientific explanation, we are past the point of description and are asking for answers to "why" questions. Why does a certain sequence of events occur? Why does something occur part of the time or most of the time and not all of the time? Why do certain events occur together? Scientific explanations must be intellectually constructed; no one can claim to have observed more than a sample of the world of empirical reality. In nursing, moving beyond trial-and-error approaches to intervention requires baseline data derived from scientific description and explanation.

In a scientific explanation, the arguments that go into the explanation must be based on laws.

Scientific Arguments

Several kinds of formal arguments are used in providing scientific explanations. The most common and generally most respected ones among scientists (at least until recently) are deductive–nominological explanations. Deductive–nominological explanations (D–N) (nominological means having to do with laws) argue from universal laws to explain some condition or conditions. Laws used in D–N arguments cannot include specification of time, place, or person. Even a law relative to a particular culture would not be permissible. D–N arguments help to establish laws that hold throughout the universe; these arguments are truth-preserving. As stated previously, we observe facts. We cannot observe laws; we reason them from facts. We construct explanations using laws. The conclusions of D–N arguments do not go beyond the content of the premises and laws contained in the argument (i.e., the content of the explanation or conclusion is contained in the premises). They can be used to predict but only those things that appear within the premises. The premises logically imply the conclusions. If the premises are true, the conclusions must be true.

D–N explanations require a law that is testable, a form of argument, and true premises. Using this type of explanation, the form of structure of the argument is

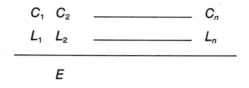

$$\frac{C_1 \ C_2 \ \text{——————} \ C_n}{L_1 \ L_2 \ \text{——————} \ L_n}$$

$$E$$

On this form, C represents the conditions, premises, antecedent conditions, or assertions about facts. The subscripts identify that a number of conditions or premises may be stated with n representing the last number for the premises and laws used in a particular explanation.

The letter L represents the laws or universal generalizations. The subscripts identify that more than one law may be necessary to the explanation. The statements that L and C represent are called the "Explanans."

The single line that divides the premise-type statements and the universal (law) statements from the explanation tells the reader that this is the D–N argument. The single line also says that premises logically lead to the conclusion.

The letter E represents the explanation, or explanandum. This statement fits the phenomenon to be explained into a pattern of uniformities and shows that its occurrence was to be expected (See Carnap 1966; and Hempel 1966).

The following example of a D–N explanation uses assertions about observed facts and a law. All of the facts are connected by the law. This is necessary for the logical development of the explanation.

C_1 Mosquitos, when threatened, withdraw.
C_2 Spiders, when threatened, neutralize the threatening agent.
C_3 Rattlesnakes, when threatened, attempt to destroy the threatening agent.
C_4 Squids, when threatened, create a visually impenetrable environment.
C_5 Hunting dogs, when threatened, become impervious to the full impact of the threat.
C_6 Deer, when threatened, increase their rate of functioning to cope with threat.
C_7 Humans and other vertebrates, when threatened, draw upon stored supplies of energy.
C_8 Stone crabs, when threatened, quickly hide in the sand.
C_9 Chameleons, when threatened, change color to blend with the environment.

C_{10} Wasps and hornets, when threatened, become irritated or hyperirritable.

L All living organisms are capable of protective responses.

E Living organisms respond in a variety of ways to protect themselves when threatened.

This D–N argument is true and fulfills the two D–N functions: preserving truth and predicting that which is in the premises. We cannot disagree with them.

Professionals need conclusions that go beyond the data at hand (i.e., are ampliative) and conclusions that are not universal, since people and their behavior do not conform very often to universal laws and conclusions.

Inductive–Statistical Explanations

Another form of explanation, inductive–statistical (I–S) is used to explain conditions of uncertainty. While not truth-preserving, this form of argument is amplifying. In D–N argument, if the premises are true, the conclusion must be true; in I–S argument, the premises may be true while the conclusion is false. This is so because the explanation is ampliative, meaning that it goes beyond the premises or infers certain probabilities from the premises. The content of the premises is not in the conclusions, as it is in D–N argument, but must be connected to the conclusion. Statistical explanations are important because much of what happens in the universe is not "all or none." All people who touch poison-ivy leaves do not get a rash, but a considerable percentage do. All people who have metastatic cancer do not die, but a very high percentage do.

I–S explanations must meet all the conditions of D–N explanations (i.e., they must contain a testable law), be in proper logical form, and the premises have to be true. But the explanation (inference) may be false. In addition, I–S explanations must meet the requirement of maximal specificity (i.e., all relevant evidence must be presented). The law in I–S explanations will be a testable statistical law. The form or structure of I–S explanations is

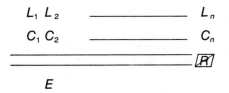

The letter L stands for a statistical law. The letter C is a premise that states an individual case. The subscripts indicate that many premises or laws may be

used, with n representing the last of a series. The double line indicates that the conclusion that follows is a probability. And the boxed r symbolizes the strength of the probability. The example that follows is the kind nurses recognize.

L   Seventy percent of patients who have cardiac-valve replacements develop mental symptomatology.

C   Mr. Jones has had a mitral-valve replacement.

$$\overline{}\; \boxed{strong}$$

E   Mr. Jones will develop mental symptomatology.

This constitutes a brief introduction to some of the tools used in philosophy of science. This kind of opening statement has little utility for nurses if it is not followed up for full comprehension of the complex concepts that underlie these tools.

This chapter also aims to illustrate how philosophy-of-science tools might be used in describing and explaining nursing data. The phenomenon studied was long-term or episodic itching. While the work is only a beginning, it is presented in the hope that it will stimulate others to develop this as a method producing nursing knowledge.

For 30 years, the author has kept notes of interpersonal interaction with patients, recording verbalizations people with chronic itching use to describe themselves and the dynamics of their interpersonal interaction. Data were also collected from nursing notes and student process records when they related to long-term itching problems. For the data of this chapter, a composite nurse–patient interaction was created from these notes.

THE PHENOMENON OF LONG-TERM ITCHING

This interaction is exemplified by the following dialogue, which demonstrates a first encounter between Miss Cubanich, a nurse, and Mrs. Dermis, a new patient:

Miss Cubanich: Mrs. Dermis, I'm Miss Cubanich. I'd like to talk with you about how you feel and what led to your coming here. Can you tell me a little about how you feel?

Mrs. Dermis: Oh, I can tell you about how I feel. I love to talk, but I'm afraid I'll only get under your skin. I've been to lots of doctors, but no one has been able to touch the problem.

Miss Cubanich: I would like to hear what you have been through. Would you tell me about it?

Mrs. Dermis: My problem is this itch. At times it's all over, but usually it's just on the palms of my hands and the soles of my feet. Sometimes I could jump out of my skin with it. A dozen doctors have treated me, and I've consulted a dozen more who wouldn't touch me with a 10-foot pole.

Miss Cubanich: That must be pretty discouraging.

Mrs. Dermis: It sure is. You can't be as thin-skinned as I am and take all that frustration. I just keep my feelers out for new dermatologists and give each one a chance. My husband thinks I change doctors too often, that I'm a soft touch, but I'm the one who suffers. It's no skin off his back. He's so hidebound that he thinks it will just go away if I wait long enough. But I think special folks need special strokes.

Miss Cubanich: Does he complain about the bills?

Mrs. Dermis: He's a skinflint all right, but one complaint from him and I tell him to go scratch himself.

Miss Cubanich: How can the nurses help you best while you are here?

Mrs. Dermis: I always feel like I'm on vacation in the hospital. Even though I smart and tingle all over when I'm admitted, I just soak up all the attention. Of course, some nurses' interest in patients is only skin deep; they rub you the wrong way, and you just itch to smack them one. But I'm learning to be thick-skinned with them.

Miss Cubanich: Do you use a special soap?

Mrs. Dermis: Yes, I use ABD soap. Just the thought of using the same soap these other patients use gives me the willies—makes me prickle, you know. Common soap would skin me alive. I'd feel as though I'd had a hiding at the very best.

Miss Cubanich: Do you have your medications with you?

Mrs. Dermis: Oh, yes. I can't be without those. I'd dry up and blow away.

Miss Cubanich: The doctor wants you to try a few days without medication so we can assess your condition.

Mrs. Dermis: That cuts me to the quick. I don't see how I can do that. That son of an itch! Ha! Ha! That sure is the nitty gritty of being a patient. Well, as far as nursing goes, you won't find me complaining. When I get stung, I'm more apt to take it out of my own hide.

Miss Cubanich: We'll do everything we can to make your stay with us comfortable.

Mrs. Dermis: I'm just tickled to death you dropped in. You seem to have a feel for my problem—a happy touch.

Miss Cubanich: Please feel free to call on us. I'll be in to see you often, too.

Mrs. Dermis: I'll press the flesh on that. Keep in touch!

Miss Cubanich: Note in the Clinical Record: Patient has long history of pruritus from which she experiences considerable discomfort. She needs good basic physical care and emotional support.

Composite treatment of all subjects as a single unit can be a useful first step in clarifying a phenomenon. Even though it resembles a caricature, a composite of this type can explicate the full range of expression and full scope of behaviors encompassed within a phenomenon—in this instance, chronic itching.

The nurse's note that the patient has pruritus is a common conceptual synthesis of an empirical situation. Nurses learn a large physiological and pathological vocabulary that functions as shorthand for long descriptions and takes small space on clinical records and supposedly provides for greater specificity and precision than the vernacular would. It does not take a skilled clinician to recognize that, in this case, the language of science oversimplifies the problem. Feyerabend (1978) succinctly describes one aspect of this problem in discussing scientific education. "It simplifies 'science' by simplifying its participants." In the not-too-recent past, the term "pruritus" would have been accepted as a name identifying this patient's experience. More recently, this would have been questioned in terms of a nurse's ability to deal with psychodynamic data. Even though we have come a long way in developing the nursing processes of assessment, diagnosis, and evaluation of nursing, we still often lack conceptual clarity and regular application of processes that provide precision in naming and explicating nursing phenomenon. Further, we often lack awareness that these two problems exist.

Today, nurses are expected to work with empirical data in such a way that the phenomena they are dealing with are clear. In responding to this expectation, what did the nurse in this situation do? She explains Mrs. Dermis's experience as "pruritus." Mrs. Dermis states that she itches. That she itches, then, is a fact, and to the extent that pruritus is the same thing as itching, the patient's pruritus is also a fact. In this case, the observation is made by Mrs. Dermis, since the fact of her itching cannot be observed by others. The nurse makes a statement, or intellectual intervention, to explain facts or to assign meaning, "The patient has pruritus." To the extent that the word *pruritus* is not just a synonym and nominal definition for itching, but a diagnosis, it is an inference.

The nurse adds the adjective "uncomfortable" to pruritus, which is also inferential rather than factual. Mrs. Dermis's uncomfortable pruritus is really not a fact because Mrs. Dermis did not state she observed it and the nurse does not observe it either. Nor do the terms meet the requirements of a scientific explanation. Even though they are neither fact nor scientific explanation, clinical inferences are expected to clarify. But, in this clinical situation, the definitional inference is too general and provides premature closure by focusing attention on itching while ignoring much of the information contained in the data. The nurse needs to be able to bring *all* possible data together in a conceptual synthesis (inference) in assigning meaning. Miss Cubanich has done a selective synthesis.

Getting the Facts

In the composite empirical situation under consideration, 45 facts were stated representing Mrs. Dermis's perceptions of experience and are factual in that sense.

> I can tell you (Miss Cubanich) how I feel.
> I love to talk.
> I'm afraid I'll get under your skin.
> I've been to lots of doctors.
> No one (doctor) has been able to touch the problem.
> My problem is this itch. At times it's all over, but usually it's just on the palms of my hands and the soles of my feet.
> Sometimes I could jump out of my skin.
> A dozen doctors have treated me.
> A dozen more (doctors) wouldn't touch me with a 10-foot pole.
> It sure is (discouraging).
> I am too thin-skinned to take all the frustration.
> I just keep my feelers out for new dermatologists.
> I give each one (dermatologist) a chance.
> I think my husband thinks I change doctors too often.
> I am the one who suffers (with a change of doctors).
> I think it's no skin off his back (husband's) if I change doctors.
> I think he is so hidebound (husband).

I think he thinks it (itching and dermal oversensitivity) will just go away if I wait long enough.

I am special.

I need special strokes.

He (husband) is a skinflint.

One complaint from him (husband) and I tell him to go scratch himself.

I feel like I'm on a vacation in the hospital.

When I'm admitted, I smart and tingle all over.

I just soak up all the attention.

Some nurses' interest in patients is only skin deep.

They (some nurses) rub you the wrong way.

You (patient) just itch to smack them one.

I'm learning to be thick-skinned with them (nurses with little interest in patients).

I use ABD soap.

The thought of using common soap gives me the willies—makes me prickle.

Common soap would skin me alive.

I'd feel as though I'd had a hiding at the very least (if I used common soap).

I can't be without my medication.

I'd dry up and blow away (without medications).

That cuts me to the quick (doctor's wish to assess her when off medications).

I don't see how I can do that (do without medications).

She refers to the doctor as, "That son of an itch! Ha! Ha!"

That sure is the nitty-gritty of being a patient.

As far as nursing goes, you won't find me complaining.

When I get stung (disappointed, hurt), I'm more apt to take it out of my own hide.

I'm just tickled to death you dropped in.

You seem to have a feel for my problem—a happy touch.

I'll press the flesh on that (agreeing with the nurse to see her often).

She says, "Keep in touch."

Clarifying the Facts

In the 45 factual statements representing Mrs. Dermis's perceptions of experience, there are 28 potentially figurative and slang verbal expressions of feeling. These expressions were translated into literal English, using theory—in this case, interpersonal theory—that deals with symbolization processes to express the reality of experience (Peplau 1951, pp. 294–307) (Table 5-1).

Assigning Meaning to the Facts

Using psychodynamic theories of anxiety, frustration aggression, ego functions, and mental mechanisms, meaning was assigned to the 28 facts that Mrs. Dermis stated in figurative terms.

Repetitions, patterns, and regularity. In reference to the data about relationships, Mrs. Dermis had some experience of every relationship in or through her skin. This includes her husband, doctors, nurses, the environment generally, and the hospital specifically. It might be said that she is using her skin to communicate (relate) self to others.

Mrs. Dermis, in the pertinent feelings statements (empirical observations), expresses what could be interpreted as frustration–aggression eight times, helplessness seven times, anxiety three times, the wish to be cared for three times, uncertainty, anger, discomfort, and pleasure twice, and fear, hurt, avoidance, denial, and vulnerability once. She employs a kind of sardonic humor. The range of feelings expressed encompasses in some degree the scope of human emotions. While uncomfortable feelings are expected with all itching, we cannot generalize from this composite patient situation to other situations. But the identification of regularities provides ideas about the possible shape and range of feeling experienced in chronic itching. This moves the work to assignment of meaning.

Assigning Meaning to the Phenomenon of Long-term Itching

Information about range, scope, and frequency permits a beginning view of the shape of a phenomenon (Figure 5-1). Attempting to show the shape of a phenomenon as one way of assigning meaning involves creating a model. There are risks in model building. One concept of a model is that it is a design of symbols or processes that correspond to a perceptual whole. Stated relationships and position of the various elements in the model can be tested (e.g., it would be possible to ascertain whether, in long-term itching, frustration–aggression is expressed more frequently in interaction with others than are complaints of physical discomfort). Regardless of the discipline, however, the basic data are influenced by the perceptions of the scientist since scientists differ in how they view relationships among data and construct different models to explain the same phenomenon. The three shapes representing long-term itching—the circle, triangle, and ellipse—as illustrated in Figure 5-1 all use the same information but

Table 5-1 Desymbolizing Figurative Communications and Assigning Meaning to Communications

Observations of Skin as a Sensory Organ	Interpretation of Verbalization	Assignment of Meaning
Getting under your skin.	Fear of annoying nurse.	Fear or uncertainty.
No one . . . able to touch the problem.	Doctors cannot help.	Uncertainty, helplessness.
I itch.	My skin is irritated.	Discomfort.
Jumping out of my skin.	I can hardly cope with how I feel.	Anxiety, helplessness.
I am thin-skinned.	Oversensitive to environment.	Helplessness, powerlessness.
My feelers.	I use my skin as antennae in my environment.	Anxiety.
I am a soft touch.	Easily taken in by others.	Helplessness, vulnerability.
No skin off his/her back.	Person does not care.	Denial, anger.
Person is hidebound.	Person not understanding or open.	Frustration, aggression.
I need special strokes.	I am different with different needs in this world.	Wish to be cared for.
Person is a skinflint.	Person is ungiving.	Frustration-aggression.
Person can go scratch.	Power struggle needed to get needs met.	Frustration-aggression.
I smart and tingle.	Uncomfortable with self.	Discomfort.
I soak up attention.	Needs to be given to by others.	Wish to be cared for.
Skin deep.	Some nurses do not relate as needed.	Frustration-aggression.
Rubbing you the wrong way.	Some nurses are irritating.	Frustration-aggression.
Itch to hit.	Would like to punish nurses for their lack of interest.	Frustration-aggression.
Learning to be thick skinned.	Trying to be less sensitive.	Hurt-avoidance.
Thoughts of using same soap gives willies/prickles.	Can suffer just by thinking about it.	Anxiety.
Soap would skin person alive.	Vulnerable to environment.	Helplessness.
Feeling as if with a hiding.	Vulnerable to environment.	Helplessness.
Cut to the quick.	Doctor hurts feelings.	Anger, suffering.
"Son of an itch."	Indirect attack on doctor.	Frustration-aggression.
Getting stung.	Disappointed or hurt by someone.	Frustration-aggression.

Table 5-1 Continued

Observations of Skin as a Sensory Organ	Interpretation of Verbalization	Assignment of Meaning
Taking out of my own hide.	I punish myself.	Guilt, helplessness.
Tickled to death.	I feel pleasure in my skin.	Pleasure.
Having a feel for the problem.	Feels understood by nurse.	Pleasure.
Keeping in touch.	Invites (asks or possibly demands that nurse return).	Need to be cared for.

might alter both focus and perception of information. These alterations would then change the perceived shape of the phenomenon under study. In the elliptical or oval model, the range of emotions might be seen in terms of a health–illness continuum. Clinically, this might have implications for building on or supporting the health of a patient. In the triangular models, frustration–aggression or helplessness could be interpreted as either the overriding or overwhelming aspects of the phenomenon of long-term itching with negative affect involvement. In intervention, we might overlook other feelings expressed.

In the circular models, there might be a tendency to zero in on the "core." There is no data that suggests a core problem, except as frequency might be related.

In addition to looking at shape, naming is another way to assign meaning to a phenomenon. In order to do this, the problems identified must be conceptualized in a more holistic way. This process might be called *synthesizing the concept* or *concept synthesis*. The nurse is obviously working with feelings and relationships. Feelings and relationships are both structures representing parts of a whole that might be called *personality* or *personhood*. One part of personality is named *identity*. Feelings and relationships are two of the parts of identity. The feelings and relationships that Mrs. Dermis expressed omit the basic problem—chronic itching—as the term *pruritus* omitted the feeling and relationship problems. A meaningful whole needs to include recognition that the total person is involved and is responding to itching of long duration. More than this, the total person is responding negatively to itching of long duration. To add to the scope of feelings and relationships, we might finally say, "Mrs. Dermis is involved and responding negatively to a large extent, intrapersonally and interpersonally, to itching of long duration." We cannot say whether her behaviors reflect personality conflict, aberrant physiology, the itching per se, or her response to the approaches and responses of others, but these could be phrased as hypotheses for study. This also does not specify whether Mrs. Dermis's feelings

Figure 5-1 The Shape of Long-Term Itching with Negative Affect

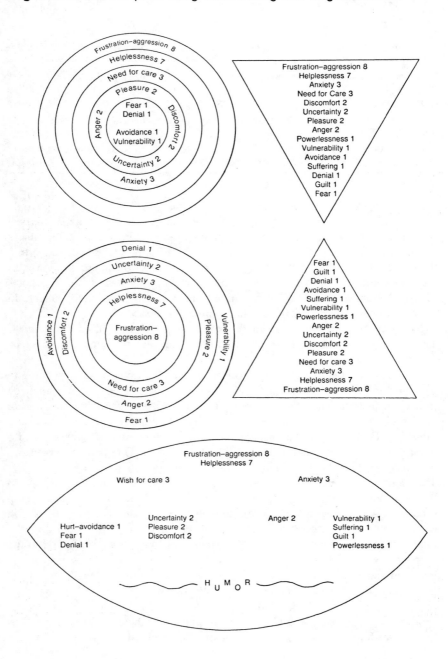

and relationship problems preceded the itching, but suggests a causal relationship (i.e., if long-term itching occurs, then negative feelings arise and relationships change).

The name *pruritus* was discarded because it addresses only one part of the data. Chronic itching, the initial name in this work, addresses only itching and its temporal aspects so it, too, was discarded. Pervasive chronic itching is not precise from a conceptual point of view. The area of pervasiveness is not explicit, and chronic means habitual and constant as much as it means long-term. "Emotionally pervasive long-term itching" might be a possibility since the word *emotionally* would include both intrapersonal and interpersonal spheres. This name omits negative emotions involved in the phenomenon, although this could be stipulated in the meaning of emotion when used in this particular condition. We could assume that the term *emotionally* includes the meaning of pervasive and use the name "emotionally distressing long-term itching." *Emotionally distressing* is such a general term that another name such as "long-term itching with negative affect involvement" seemed more precise. Putting long-term itching first specifies the basic consideration or condition; the word *affect* specifies feeling and the term *negative,* the kind of feeling. The term *involvement* specifies negative affect as an accompanying condition of long-term itching in causative relationship. Other names may be equally precise but the point here is the need to name or specify with precision the empirical phenomenon under study.

LAWS

For the data at hand, five statements in the nature of empirical laws operating in or basic to the phenomenon were identified. In chronic itching with negative affect involvement, the following statements apply:

1. Skin and skin-related terms occur repetitively in conversation.
2. The skin and skin-related terms are used to structure interaction.
3. Interpreting the behavior of others in skin and skin-related terms is a pattern in interpersonal interaction.
4. The skin becomes increasingly sensitive to the environment.
5. There is a pattern of negative feelings.

These laws are based on the regularities noted in observations of people with chronic itching with negative affect. The observations treated as premises can be used in arguing that whenever chronic itching again is observed the same regularities and patterns will also occur (i.e., that regularity in the past makes probable this occurrence in the future). This is the beginning of scientific concept formulation, description, and explanation (Hempel 1966).

Empirical laws, while having power in relation to their predictability, have limited explanatory power (e.g., the five empirical laws identified earlier). Therefore, we are not in a position to do any formal scientific explanation until theoretical laws are identified. Since skin is one basic concept underlying the phenomenon of chronic itching, it seems appropriate to look at laws related to human skin in terms of whether they might have power in explaining chronic itching with negative affect involvement. Some of the empirical laws concerning the nature of the skin are

1. Skin covers the body of all humans. This empirical law can be subsumed under the more general empirical law that all living protoplasm—plant or animal—is contained within some form of membranous structure. All laws related to human skin can be subsumed under more general laws. Also, most of the laws can be related to physical and chemical laws. Some laws related to the skin can be mathematically quantified.
2. Humans have both outer and inner skins.
3. Both outer and inner skins are closely associated with one another.
4. The primary functions of the intact skin are protective.
   a) The intact skin holds the fluids within the body.
   b) The sebaceous glands of the skin keep the surface of the body lubricated (i.e., soft and supple).
   c) Skin sweat glands excrete some body wastes.
   d) Sweat glands in the skin secrete an aqueous solution of salts.
   e) Sweat glands excrete this aqueous solution, which disappears over time on the surface of the skin.
   f) Skin sweat glands secrete bacteriostatic substances.
   g) The intact skin prevents bacteria from entering subcutaneous tissues.
   h) When the arrectores pilorum muscles of the skin are contracted, heat is lost more slowly from the surface of the body.
   i) The skin is a major sensory organ of the body, perceiving touch, pain, pressure, itching, tickling.

Some of the theoretical laws concerning the nature of the skin are:

5. Skin is a medium through which sensations are felt that represent the outer experience of a situation.
6. Only man can differentiate the several sensory experiences of the skin associated with aversive circumstances—tickling, itching, and creeping (Perl 1959).

7. Itching results from weak activation of the same sensory apparatus responsible for pain (Rothman 1943; and Shelby and Arthur 1959).

8. Itching is more protopathic (pain-like in character) than is tickling (Torebjork 1978).

9. Only low-threshold nerve endings respond to itching; high threshold mechanoreceptors do not (Szolcsanye 1978).

10. Itching is a situation in which there is a conditioned reflex mediated in the vegetative nervous system accompanied by changes in the system of endocrine glands (Dunbar 1946).

11. Itching functions as a protective mechanism (Norris 1981).

12. If the skin is to perceive itching as a warning, people must recognize itching as a necessary condition for becoming alerted (Norris 1981).

13. Increased skin sensitivity accompanying chronic itching makes the skin more vulnerable to external environmental stressors.

14. People respond holistically to experience.
    a) If people respond holistically, the most holistic response is the conditioned reflex (Dunbar 1955).
    b) If the conditioned reflex is a holistic response, it contains aspects of both physiology and personality (Shilder 1929).
    c) If physiological and personality aspects of humans are contained in the conditioned reflex, the problems of physiology and personality are also represented (Shilder 1929).
    d) If the conditioned reflex represents personality, then it encompasses emotions that contain a living situation—whether perceived, imagined, real or represented, fully conscious or systematically unconscious as well as the attitude toward this living situation (Dunbar 1955).
    e) If emotion includes an attitude toward a living situation, this attitude is evidenced by feelings and represents inner experience of the situation (Dunbar 1946).
    f) If feelings represent inner experience of a situation, unresolved feelings arising from an inner conflict situation (different strivings) lead to physical manifestations (Dunbar 1955).
    g) If there are inner conflicts expressed through the physical manifestations of the skin, some of the most common psychosomatic aspects of these relationships are expressed by blushing, gooseflesh, hives, perspiration, chilling, itching, crawling, tickling, and prickling.
    h) If there are psychosomatic expressions of relationships expressed by the skin, some (e.g., scratching, itching, or tickling) are pleasurable as in sex play, play of a breeze upon the skin, or relaxation upon removing a girdle or other clothing.

i) If psychosomatic expressions of relationships expressed by the skin are pleasurable, they are only pleasurable up to a point.

j) If psychosomatic expressions of relationships expressed by the skin are pleasurable, anticipation of scratching an itch or tickle is also pleasurable.

k) If psychosomatic expressions of relationships expressed by the skin become unpleasurable (e.g., itching, tickling, or prickling) they can be relieved (stopped or obliterated) by (1) pressure with the hand to release endorphins (opiate polypeptides), (2) scratching that causes nerve-ending destruction lasting about 20 minutes, (3) scratching that causes endorphin release, (4) application of drugs, like carbolic acid solutions, that deaden nerve endings, or (5) neutralization or removal of stressor.

15. People respond holistically to experience. Even though the skin may be the stressed body part, the body responds as a whole to the stress (e.g., allergy to strawberries, allergy to soap, or inability to resolve conflicts).

a) Emotional tension creates disturbances in both skins—sometimes simultaneously, sometimes alternately (Dunbar 1955).

b) Outer skin separates humans from their surroundings but at the same time is the medium of first learned communication with significant others (Dunbar 1955).

c) Skin of infants is more sensitive to communication than is the skin of adults (Dunbar 1955).

d) Flaws or errors in early sensory communication that become themes in infant–parent dynamics prevent learning trust, tenderness, and worthiness of care (Dunbar 1955).

e) One manifestation of unresolved conflict between different strivings is chronic itching (Dunbar 1955).

f) The skin then can function as a target organ for stress to which the organism is subjected (Dunbar 1955).

g) Selection of target organs for stress, while not clearly understood, is related to genetic factors, teaching–learning of behaviors, and personal experience of and with an organ.

h) All humans have one or more target organs for stress.

i) Physical manifestations, of which chronic itching is one example, are initiated from within and without the body.

j) People whose skin is a target organ for stress bring it into much of their communication.

k) Chronic itching structures much of the activity and thinking of those subject to it.

l) Preoccupation with one's skin extends and distorts the protective function of the skin (Norris 1980).

m) Psyche–soma integration in chronic itching operates in such a way that the environment is increasingly experienced and relationships to the environment are increasingly made through the use of the skin.

n) Once a pattern of itching behavior is established, it is replicated by suggestion or through evoking the life situation that recreates the emotion associated with the situation (Dunbar 1955).

o) Typical sufferers from chronic itching have the unresolved conflict between desire for affection and fear of being hurt if they seek it (i.e., touch me, don't touch me) (Dunbar 1955).

p) Compensation for chronic itching (i.e., application of ointments, bathing, rubbing, and sympathy) make resolution difficult (Dunbar 1955).

16. People can help each other through problem-solving interaction.

a) People cannot report objective events; they can only report their inner perception of it.

b) Unfolding experience leading up to present difficulties can help in developing new perspectives.

c) People can support each other in unfolding painful inner experiences.

d) New perspectives allow identification of new coping strategies: (1) New perspectives for Mrs. Dermis would be identification and movement toward the real goal, and (2) learning more healthy aggressive strategies.

e) People can support others in identifying new coping strategies.

f) Resolution is slow due to strength of interpersonal habituation practices, pleasurable compensation for the symptom, ribonucleic acid deficiencies in selective brain tissues, and the fact that the victim is both a loser and an aggressor.

Some of the laws cited above might fall in the category of teleological law. Teleological laws explain something of purpose (e.g., the purpose of itching is to warn about stress). As previously noted, teleological laws are weak since they address, but do not explain, causal relationships. Law 4a and the other laws under "4" are teleological as well as empirical in character. Law 11, which states that itching functions as a protective mechanism, is also teleological.

A law such as "Emotional tension creates disturbances in both skins" (15a) and other laws under "15" are really hypothetical laws. This means they are hypotheses about the mechanism of itching. No one has seen the psyche or soma (theoretical constructs) attacking an organ or putting the ego (another theoretical construct) in conflict so the target organ is put under stress. We cannot see how preoccupation with one's skin extends and distorts the function of the skin. But on the basis of observations, we can invent an explanation. It should be obvious to the reader by now that when one uses laws to clarify a phenomenon, the final set of statements will be large.

EXPLANATIONS

Examples of possible explanations for chronic itching with negative affect involvement were conceptualized from the facts identified in this chapter and from many other experiences with patients who experienced stress through the skin. An inductive explanation using an empirical law to explain (predict) a fact is as follows:

L   People who have long-term itching with negative affect involvement use the skin as a target organ for stress.

C   Mrs. Dermis has long-term itching with negative affect involvement.

_____ /Strong/

E   Mrs. Dermis uses her skin as a target organ for stress.

An I–S argument explaining why a person is identified as having long-term itching with negative affect involvement is based on this law: If a person's skin is a target organ for stress, then this stress is expressed in all modes of a person's behavior. Therefore, if a person has long-term itching and

Premise 1   Skin and skin-related terms occur repetitively in conversation.

Premise 2   The skin and skin-related terms are used to structure interpersonal interaction.

Premise 3   The person often interprets the behavior of others in skin and skin-related terms.

Premise 4   The skin becomes increasingly sensitive to the environment.

Premise 5   The person often expresses negative feelings.

_____ /Strong/

Conclusion   A person may be said to have long-term itching with negative affect involvement.

An I–S argument using clinical data to explain how we can identify the skin as a target organ is as follows:

C_1 Infants who have allergy (stressor) often develop chronic eczema characterized by itching.

C_2 Adults who have allergy (stressor) often develop a rash called hives characterized by itching.

C_3 Children or adults, when they get too hot (stressor), may develop a heat rash characterized by itching.

C_4 Many people who are "nervous" (high-anxiety level) have a chronic rash characterized by itching.

C_5 Excitement (stressor) may create an itchy feeling followed by scratching.

C_6 Use of soap (stressor) may cause skin irritation accompanied by itching.

C_7 Once the skin is sensitized to one allergen (stressor), it may become more easily sensitized to others.

C_8 Certain fabric softeners (stressor) cause itching.

C_9 Thinking about certain stressors (e.g., bed bugs) can cause chronic itching.

C_{10} Certain kinds of clothing like wool (stressor) may cause chronic itching.

L_1 One way stress is manifested in the skin is by itching.

L_2 A target organ is one that is a frequent receptor for the stress mediated response.

E If the skin frequently itches, it may be said to be a target organ for stress.

Description, the first function of a science, is important to nursing at this time. Tools useful in description may be those of philosophy of science. Before nurses can move effectively into formal explanation of the inductive–statistical type, we need greater consensus about the meaning and greater precision in defining the concepts basic to the discipline. We also need to name the phenomena of nursing and to operationalize that which is included in the phenomena. We need descriptive statistical information. This is basic to prediction associated with the descriptive function of science.

The work done in this chapter on long-term itching used an approach that was heavily weighted by assumptions from psychosomatic theory. But emphasis on the nature of facts, assignment of meaning, categorization of facts, search for repetition, patterns and regularities, and the use of laws to explain represent only one way of describing a concept. Progress in explanation in using the explanatory tools of philosophy of science depends upon a much greater data base.

REFERENCES

Bronson, F.H., and Desjardins, C. Steroid hormones and aggressive behavior in mammals. In B.E. Eleftheriou and J.P. Scott, *The Physiology of Aggression and Defeat.* New York: Plenum, 1971.

Carnap, R. *An Introduction to the Philosophy of Science.* New York: Basic Books, 1966.

Dollard, J., Miller, N.E., Doob, L.W., Moweer, O.H., and Sears, R.R. *Frustration and Aggression.* New Haven: Yale University Press, 1939.

Dollard, J. *Caste and Class in a Southern Town.* New Haven: Yale University Press, 1937.

Donaldson, S., and Crowley, D. The discipline of nursing. *Nurs. Outlook* 26:113–120, Feb. 1978.

Dunbar, F. *Emotions and Bodily Changes* (3rd ed.). New York: Columbia University Press, 1946.

Dunbar, F. *Mind and Body: Psychosomatic Medicine.* New York: Random House, 1955.

Eleftheriou, B.E., and Scott, J.P. *The Physiology of Aggression and Defeat.* New York: Plenum, 1971.

Feyerabend, P. *Against Method.* London: Verso, 1975. P. 19.

Hempel, C.G. *The Philosophy of Natural Science.* Englewood Cliffs, N.J.: Prentice-Hall, 1966.

Jacox, A.K. Theory construction in nursing: An overview. *Nurs. Res.* 23:4–13, Jan.–Feb. 1974.

Kuhn, T.S. *The Structure of Scientific Revolutions* (2nd ed.). Vol. 2, No. 2. Chicago: University of Chicago, 1970.

Laudan, L. *Progress and Its Problems.* Berkeley, Calif.: University of California, 1977.

McKay, R.P. Discussion: Discipline of nursing–syntactical structure and relation with other disciplines and the profession of nursing. In M.V. Batey (Ed.), *Communicating Nursing Research: Optimizing environments for health; nursing's unique perspective.* Boulder, Col.: Western Interstate Commission for Higher Education. 10:23–30, 1977.

Peplau, H.E. *Interpersonal Relations in Nursing.* New York: Putnam, 1951.

Perl, E.P. In D.R. Kenshalo (Ed.), *Sensory Functions of the Skin of Humans.* New York: Plenum, 1978.

Popper, K.R. *Objective Knowledge* (2nd ed.). Oxford: Clarendon, 1979.

Reynolds, P.D. *A Primer in Theory Construction.* New York: Bobbs-Merrill, 1971.

Rothman, S. The nature of itching. *Research Publication.* Association for Research in Nervous and Mental Diseases. 23:110–122, 1943.

Scholtfeldt, R.M. Nursing research: Reflection of values. *Nurs. Res.* 26:4–9, Jan.–Feb. 1977.

Scott, J.P. Theoretical issues concerning the origin and causes of fighting. In B.E. Eleftheriou and J.P. Scott, *The Physiology of Aggression and Defeat.* New York: Plenum, 1971.

Shelly, W.B., and Arthur, R.P. The peripheral mechanism of itch in man. In G.E.W. Wolston Holme and M. O'Connor (Eds.), *Pain and Itch: Nervous Mechanisms.* London: Churchill, 1959.

Shilder, P. The somatic basis of neurosis. *Journal of Nervous and Mental Dis.* 70:502–519, 1929.

Silva, M.C. Philosophy, science, theory: interrelationships and implications for nursing research. *Image* 9:59–63, Oct. 1977.

Suppe, F. (2nd ed.). *The Structure of Scientific Theories.* Urbana, Ill.: University of Illinois Press, 1974.

Szolcsanyi, J. In D.R. Kenshalo (Ed.), *Sensory Functions of the Skin of Humans.* New York: Plenum, 1978.

Torebjork, H.E. In D.R. Kenshalo (Ed.), *Sensory Functions of the Skin of Humans.* New York: Plenum, 1978.

Welch, A.S., and Welch, B.L. Isolation, reactivity and aggression: Evidence for involvement of brain catecholamines and serotonin. In B.E. Eleftheriou and J.P. Scott, *The Physiology of Aggression and Defeat.* New York: Plenum, 1971.

Chapter 6

Nausea and Vomiting

Catherine M. Norris

Nausea and vomiting are universal and frequent experiences; we can hardly describe the great variety of circumstances under which they occur. At one extreme, these phenomena may reflect simple dietary overindulgence; at the other, their occurrence may signal imminent death. Aside from the common cold, digestive complaints (of which nausea and vomiting are of major importance) are the cause of more employee absenteeism than any other single ailment (Wilbur 1973). It has been suggested that acute, transient attacks of vomiting are so common that they can almost be regarded as the normal way of life (Editorial 1974). Nausea, with or without vomiting, sends one person out of every six to seek medical aid (DiPalma 1965). Almost 80 percent of pregnant women complain of nausea during the first trimester; about half of these women experience vomiting (Fairweather 1968). In England, nausea and vomiting account for 51.7 episodes of illness per 1,000 population each year (Pivesent 1974).

Because of related medical bills and absenteeism, nausea and vomiting exert considerable influence on individual and corporate economics. We would expect to find nursing and medical literature replete with theories, studies, and suggested remedies aimed at reducing these complaints. Of the 11 nausea citations in English listed in 1980, all but 5 are related to drug research; of the 42 vomiting citations, 27 are reports of drug studies. The remainder are reports of vomiting in selected pathologies. Some physiologists (Borison and Wang 1949, 1953) have studied nausea and vomiting. These phenomena have not been spotlighted for intensive study by physicians, nurses, or other clinical workers except by pharmacologists who are studying symptom relief and nausea and vomiting as side effects of potent drugs. Nausea and vomiting are dealt with concomitantly in many medical textbooks, but such treatment lacks the depth appropriate for such prevalent disorders.

There are reports of a few clinical studies of particular phenomena, such as vomiting after gallbladder surgery, but the number of subjects is small and focused on pathology. In the last 5 years, some attention is given to nausea and vomiting as they occur in oncology patients who are receiving chemotherapy or radiation therapy.

Only one report was found to deal with nausea and vomiting as protective (Bell, Emslie-Smith, and Patterson, 1980, p. 64). No reports dealing with nausea and vomiting as health-promoting were found.

Seven published articles related to nursing were found in searching the literature for the last 15 years. Three of these are reports of research related to postoperative vomiting (Dumas 1963a, 1963b, 1964); one is an in-depth literature study clarifying the physiology of vomiting (McCarthy 1964); one is written for nurses, "When Vomiting Signals a Geriatric Emergency" (Daren et al. 1975).

The Dumas study, based on the assumption that postoperative vomiting is undesirable and should be damped, is health-promoting and disease-preventing in orientation. The McCarthy paper was not developed within an explicit nursing framework; the Daren article is an illness-oriented paper. Two nursing-care articles report assessment and intervention options in nursing oncology patients with nausea and vomiting (Lewis et al. 1979; and Welch 1979).

Minow reports a study of nausea and vomiting in which patients with inferior infarction/ischemia had more nausea than patients with anterior infarction (1982).

GENERAL AVERSION TO THE CONCEPTS

The frequency of nausea and vomiting and the misery involved with them, as evidenced by the high percentage of related doctor visits, are incongruent with the amount of descriptive literature and the number of published research reports on these subjects. There is no way to turn off an audience of health workers—nurses included—faster than to pursue a discussion of nausea and vomiting. Vomiting is so repulsive to some people that, upon witnessing a person vomiting, they become nauseated and may vomit themselves. Inability to tolerate vomiting in others has been identified by some as a reason for not opting for a career in nursing. While pursuing this study, this author was reminded by friends and family that she was not welcome at mealtime. One author, seeking a "loathsome" yet descriptive name for one of his works, entitled his book, *Nausea* (Sartre 1964). When this investigator asked many nurses and other people the reason for their aversion, they cited the intolerable sight or odor of vomit. Many also reported that seeing and smelling vomitus made them nauseated. This explanation is not plausible in view of the many foods with similar appearance or more offensive odors that are prized delicacies and are ingested widely and with zest. The explanation has to lie deeper than widespread individual or personal aversion. Powdermaker, in describing the great value of gluttony among the Trobriand Islanders, quotes people as saying in anticipation of a feast, "We shall be glad; we shall eat until we vomit (Powdermaker 1960)."

This kind of statement, made by people whose food supply is scarce, puts a high value on overeating to the point of vomiting and implies that vomiting does not occur on the average day when food is in short supply. Since people in Western cultures notoriously overeat and are notoriously overweight, our aversion to nausea and vomiting may be rooted in guilt for gluttony. The naive statement of the Trobriand natives might generate a speculative hypothesis that people who are overeaters (and those who because they are overweight) have nausea and vomiting more frequently than people of normal weight who eat less. In other words, are nausea and vomiting less problematic to slim-bodied, light eaters?

Before the fall of the Roman Empire, at the height of its decadent affluence, it was common practice to gorge one's self with food, turn from the table, vomit into a receptacle, and turn back to the table to gorge again. It appears from available sources that there was no guilt about body abuse, waste of food, or gluttony (Solomon and Solomon 1977); this practice, therefore, sheds little light on our aversion to nausea and vomiting.

Perhaps having control of organs that connect with body surfaces is one of the last controls or footholds in the loss of physical integrity with loss of bowel integrity representing the final loss. Or perhaps as a civilized people, compared to more primitive peoples, we put a very high value on hiding all excreta from ourselves and others: witness the modern toilet and the paper handkerchief. Vomitus is harder to hide than excrement or mucus. Certainly the emesis kidney basin cannot rival the smooth gestures of flushing a toilet or folding a tissue and putting it in one's pocket. (Some primitive cultures, incidentally, have taboos about putting excreta from one's nose into one's pocket.)

Does vomiting intrude on another's privacy and life space? Or does it remind other people of their own vulnerability? Does it render spectators helpless and guilt-ridden while feeling they should be able to do something about it? Is the aversion a kind of blame or sanction for behaving offensively in public? Could it, as a holdover from pioneer days when food was scarce, represent "a waste of good food"? Or is the aversion to vomiting related to being confronted with the alien work of the body in producing this foreign, odoriferous, uncontrollable mess? Vomiting is so generally repulsive that one suggestion of rape crisis groups is that a woman about to be raped might avoid assault by putting her fingers into her throat and causing herself to vomit (Staraska 1975). This advice originated in the experience of a woman who was dragged into a car by several men who intended to rape her. After she caused herself to vomit, they threw her out of the car. The power of nausea and vomiting in family dynamics in which a member manipulates for power or expresses repulsion using the threat of nausea or the act of vomiting is also well known.

Greenwald (1973) has named a concept, *orgasmic discharge,* to describe dramatic release of accumulated tensions. The mechanisms of "orgasmic discharge" are joy, grief, rage, sexual orgasm, and vomiting. While release is only short-lived, these mechanisms completely dominate the person while they are occurring and are very effective for relieving great emotional stress. Greenwald describes the infant as readily "spitting up" whatever is not agreeable. As the infant grows to childhood, there is increasing reluctance to vomit—whether the stressor is psychic or dietary—because of the risk of losing parental love. The child, when reaching adulthood, does not let the vomiting experience evolve fully, but attempts to damp any evidence of the need to vomit. This theory supports both a fear-of-consequences and a guilt-for-performance explanation of aversion to nausea and vomiting.

Maybe nausea and vomiting are sex oriented. If they are, the orientation is most certainly female. As female it may represent to some a weakness, capriciousness, helplessness, or chronic unwellness. And as weakness, at least, social mores indicate it should be ignored. Or, as female, it may be dismissed with other women's problems as being psychogenic. It appears that some people abreact their own experience with nausea and vomiting and so introject some of the discomfort and wretchedness of others. Exploration of personal, physiological, psychological, and professional aversion to nausea and vomiting is needed if we are to free these areas for unbiased study.

The Appearance of Vomitus

People find vomitus offensive and often respond by becoming nauseated themselves. What about its appearance per se is disgusting? If it looks like sour milk, as does the vomiting done by infants, how does this differ from the proverbial "curds and whey" of Miss Muffet or from some dishes containing sour cream or cottage cheese? Vomitus may appear to be a great mixture of food in various textures and sizes. But in almost all cultures, common dishes, often representing the soul food of the group, contain a conglomeration of grated, sliced, diced, and chopped food particles. Certainly minestrone soup, borscht, or sweet-and-sour cabbage soup require a certain perspective to be seen as attractive. If vomitus is largely bile, how different is its appearance from mustard or curry sauce? If vomitus appears to be slimy, is it any more or less slippery than egg-drop soup, boiled dumplings, or potato-flour gravy? It would seem that, since vomitus resembles foods that are considered attractive and valued, responses to it are learned.

The Odor of Vomitus

Vomitus has a variety of odors that may account for its offensiveness. The most general odor is that of sourness; but is it any more sour-smelling than sour pickles, sauerkraut, or buttermilk? The smell of bile is mild, almost aromatic, and might be perceived as inoffensive. The odor of feces may be no worse than bierkaase (commonly called "dirty sock cheese"), Limburger cheese, or some tripe dishes. Again, response seems to be learned, but whether the response is related to the meaning of vomiting or its appearance and odor is not known. Unlocking the *why* of this response is important for nurses who need to be free in observation, assessment, and intervention in the vomiting phenomenon.

The Language of Nausea and Vomiting

If the way people communicate is the way they live, or if there is a relationship between language and behavior, the language of nausea and vomiting expresses a variety of ideas and feelings. This is a language of hard-sounding consonants spoken in staccato ways that fall on our ears without cadence or lilt. Words such as puke, gag, retch, cat, keck, upchuck, urp, spew, throw up, and vomit can be pronounced to mimic small explosions. In recent years, a few softer-sounding semihumorous terms—"tossing one's cookies," "checking one's groceries," "barf," and "feeding the goldfish"—have come into common usage.

Whether the coining of these phrases signals a greater acceptance of the behaviors or whether they express anxiety or embarrassment is not known. It is interesting to note that the infants' vomiting is called "spitting up" or regurgitation, which provide differences in meaning even though they have hard sounding consonants. Parents will not call "spitting up" vomiting.

If one separates nausea from retching and vomiting, the sounds may be less negatively loaded. Common terms include "the birdies," "the collywobbles," "the weewaws," "qualms in the stomach," "the heaves," and "feeling squeamish."

In addition to the experience of nausea and vomiting in the literal sense, people express several kinds of feelings in the figurative and symbolic sense. Expressions like, "I can't swallow any more of that," "I've got a bellyfull of that person," "I could vomit when I hear you talk like that," "I'm going to puke," or "She makes me gag" are common. People are not saying that they are nauseated, but may be identifying one target organ where they feel or can anticipate feeling stress. And additional use of the language of nausea and vomiting may be to express rage, hate, disgust, revulsion, and general feelings of sickness.

The Words and Their Uses

If nausea and vomiting are the source of misery, the dichotomous aspect of all concepts—the good part of relief from them—should be expressed in terms of good feelings. Actually, people do not usually separate the stomach or abdomen from the rest of the body in expressing feelings of well-being or comfort. People who are nauseated, however, express their goals in alleviating the state in terms that help identify antonyms. People want to "settle" their stomachs; they want to be "easy" on their stomachs; they want food to "go down easy" or food that "will go down easy;" minimally, they want the "food to go down and stay down;" they want their stomachs to "agree" with them and speak of food as "agreeing with me."

People express nausea and vomiting somewhat differently from the ways they express other symptoms or diagnoses: "I am nauseated," or "I am vomiting," "I vomited," or "I feel nauseated." The usual way to express illness is the possessive: "I have a headache," "I have a pain," or "I have diarrhea." Whether nausea and vomiting are so all-absorbing that they encompass the whole individual, the use of "I am" is as understandable as in, "I am dying," which can be used either literally or figuratively. There may be certain conditions under which the affected person feels a sense of control or ownership and says, "I have;" at other times, the victim feels so out of control or so tormented by the stressor that he or she perceives the situation as "I am." Then there are those people who say, "I feel nauseous." Since nauseated is the adverb and nauseous is an adjective, the term *nauseous* usually refers to some noxious agent. Is this person saying, "I am repulsive," or "I feel sick and disgusting to others," or does the person mean "I am nauseated and disgusted by others?" While the use of the word *nauseous* may have some cultural determination, its use as contrasted with the word *nauseated* may communicate a different meaning, that is, how a person feels he or she affects others.

UNIVERSALITY OF NAUSEA AND VOMITING

Contrasted to humans vomiting, dogs who vomit have been observed to have a short period of salivating, licking, retching, and sometimes trembling; then the vomitus is spit up easily and quickly. The dog often ingests it immediately and continues undisturbed. Observation of dogs begs a question about whether response to our own nausea and vomiting is instinctive or whether much of it is learned.

Herbivorous animals and rodents seldom vomit. The horse, in extremely rare circumstances, will vomit through its nostrils. Carnivores and omnivores, except rodents, vomit easily (Smith 1974). Even knowing that the stomachs and digestive enzymes of animals differ in both number and structure, it would be interesting to study whether human vegetarians are less subject to nausea and vomiting than are human omnivores. We could also study whether there are differences between human carnivores, ovolacto vegetarians, and strict vegetarians. When vegetarians who have been omnivorous for a period of time return to a vegetarian diet, they speak of "detoxification" or "going on a detoxification routine." Is reducing the risk of nausea and vomiting one of the aims of detoxification?

Drug research using herbivorous animals needs careful assessment since it does not tell us whether nausea and vomiting are among the side effects of the drugs tested. Research using carnivores in testing for these side effects is much more expensive so it may be limited. Nurses need to be aware of research limitations in observing the side effects of new drugs on patients.

Despite the universality of nausea and vomiting, we do not have substantial data about whether men or women have similar frequencies of them or whether one sex experiences the ailments more often. Children are assumed to vomit more often than adults but why or whether the circumstances vary is not known. It is noteworthy that we lack detailed statistics on hospital patients' vomiting.

What Is Nausea?

One dictionary defines nausea as "sickness of the stomach," and "inclination to vomit." The first definition of sickness in the same dictionary is the word "disease" followed by "nausea" (Stedman 1976). We could thus deduce that nausea is a disease of the stomach but common sense tells us that it is more than a disease of the stomach.

Taber's dictionary (1974) defines nausea as "an inclination to vomit, usually preceding emesis." It is present in seasickness, early pregnancy, diseases of the central nervous system, neurasthenia, and hysteria; it may be triggered by the sight or odor of obnoxious matter or conditions or mental images; it may be present without vomiting.

Nausea is characterized as distress but not as pain although one writer says, "The stimulus which induces nausea . . . is apparently the same as that which causes visceral pain, but of lower intensity (Brobeck 1973)."

Like pain, fatigue, and weakness, nausea is largely subjective, at least in its early manifestations. Communication depends on a small imprecise vocabulary of expressions such as, "I feel distressed," descriptions such as, "I feel as if my stomach were turning over," and similes such as, "I feel as if someone were pushing a lead weight into the middle of my chest."

Nausea is in some senses related to hunger. Some people say that at times they cannot tell whether they are hungry or nauseated; others state that if they get "over-hungry" or let hunger go unsatisfied for too long, they become nauseated. We could postulate that hydrochloric acid levels in the stomach that signal hunger could at some point become an irritant and cause nausea. People who report nausea that is relieved by food may be in a relative bind about the difference between hunger and nausea (which is associated with anorexia).

Nausea is frequently related to anorexia. While anorexia is not nausea, it appears to be a factor in all nausea. Anyone who is nauseated has no desire for food, refusing even prized delicacies. Nausea goes beyond anorexia. In nausea, thoughts of food and eating are repulsive, distressful, and may worsen nausea.

In addition to being disgusted and repulsed by food, there is agreement among people who describe their own nausea that there is concomitant discomfort in both throat and abdomen. They describe the throat as feeling tight or as having a feeling of increased sensitivity in the pharyngeal fauces. Abdominal sensations are described as queasiness, heaviness, uneasiness, or a sinking feeling. At the psychological level, there may be feelings of disgust or revulsion. Some writers describe nausea as a psychic experience only (Borison and Wang 1953; and Isselbacher et al. 1980). When nausea occurs without other physiological events, it often accompanies or follows emotional shock related to unbearable sensory perceptions.

Nausea may be limited to these feelings or it may be accompanied by or progress to include signs of autonomic nervous system response. These signs include vasomotor changes with feelings of being hot or cold, increased perspiration, and pallor. First the pulse increases, then decreases. Increased salivation is nearly always present, accompanied by increased swallowing, licking of the lips, and sometimes, yawning. Nausea may be resolved and not proceed past this point; it may, however, last for hours as in the case of morning sickness in pregnancy (Voda and Randall 1982). Simultaneously with these signs and symptoms, or following them, nausea is characterized by a beginning action phase in which there is forced inspiration, irregular respiration, contraction of the abdominal muscles and diaphragm, and extension of the head and neck. At this point the glottis also closes.

Are gagging and swallowed regurgitation nausea? Since the phenomenon of vomiting requires ejection of material from the mouth, we cannot include either gagging or regurgitation that is swallowed in our definition. Gagging or swallowed regurgitated materials defined within the concept of nausea or defined as a separate concept were not found in the literature; gagging and swallowing regurgitated particles may possibly be phases of nausea. Nausea seems to progress toward vomiting with gagging and swallowed regurgitation being the later stages; nausea might bypass early stages and begin with either gagging or swallowing regurgitated materials. Finally, the vomiting posture is assumed: there is forceful regurgitation into the mouth; respirations cease to protect the respiratory tract during vomiting. Now, vomiting is the only resolution. The posture, cessation of respiration and forceful regurgitation, indicate irreversibility.

This discussion makes clear that presently there are no direct indicators of early nausea and its existence must be predicated upon determination of indirect indicators until the point of gagging is reached.

What Is Vomiting?

Vomiting is defined as "ejecting the contents of the stomach through the mouth." The act is usually reflex, involving coordinated activity of both voluntary and involuntary muscles. In telephone interviews with mothers of young infants (under 20 weeks of age) not one mother could be convinced that spitting up is synonymous with vomiting. The infants' mothers say they would know the difference between spitting up and vomiting and that they would be concerned if their infants vomited, while spitting up is normal.

The simple definition of vomiting does not characterize the nature of the act, nature of the contents of the vomit, or the fact that vomiting is quite often preceded by nausea. Vomiting in its simplest form occurs after overeating, overimbibing alcohol, or after eating food contaminated with large numbers of microorganisms like *Staphylococcus aureus.* In the simplest sense, vomiting represents a disturbance limited to the intestinal tract.

The dictionary definition does not mention "expulsion of gastric contents under pressure." Pressure adds another dimension and other meanings to the act of vomiting. Projectile vomiting, which adds suddenness to force without a change in the contents expelled, often represents a serious condition of the central nervous system.

The dictionary definition of vomiting does not specify the nature of the gastric contents expelled. Blood, feces, or foreign bodies expelled in vomit, indicate complicated vomiting. Other unmentioned variables complicating the vomiting act are odor, duration, frequency, and time related to food ingestion, drug ingestion, a fall, or a blow on the head. Simple vomiting may also be complicated by accompanying signs and symptoms, but these are not part of the dictionary definition.

Certainly, the dictionary definition of vomiting does not indicate that vomiting under certain conditions represents a physiological emergency or, under other conditions, a protective function of the body.

The dictionary does not identify either nausea or vomiting as having interpersonal functions or as being cultural themes. For example, women's worlds are traditionally peaceful and peacemaking worlds. Culturally, women are not empowered to wage war; ruthless business and political competition are still not familiar worlds to women. Could it be that women, powerless in the world at large, wage small wars in their personal domains, using nausea and vomiting as passive weapons? Household activities, family dynamics, social situations, and the family car certainly come to a halt when the convention-bound woman of the house becomes nauseated and vomits.

Last but not least, the simple dictionary definition does not deal with gas as a stomach content or expulsion of this gas. Expulsion of gas from the stomach is called *eructation,* commonly known as belching. In contrast to the act of vomiting, belching is the source of pleasure or at least relief. In some Asiatic cultures, belching after a meal is considered a compliment to the hostess and cook (Waldo 1967).

Antecedents and Concomitants of Nausea and Vomiting

The common vomiting of infants, as has already been noted, is called "spitting up" and occurs shortly after feeding. It is impossible to determine whether infants have symptoms of nausea. The signs of nausea are absent, although vomiting may be preceded by hiccoughs, active shaking, or handling the baby after feeding. It often occurs concomitantly with belching. We question whether the nervous structures required for the experience of nausea and vomiting are fully developed and whether postprandial vomiting in infants is simply spilling-over related to the amount of feeding and environmental conditions surrounding the feeding. Nursery nurses reported that infants' diaphragms contract, that the abdominal muscles do not, and that the overall impression is of a relaxed infant. The nurses discriminated differences in the force of flow with spitting up oc-curring with little force. In other words, spitting up is not an orgasmic experience. The mothers interviewed reported that spitting up stops when their infants are 12 to 15 weeks old. This assertion would seem to support the immature-neural-development theory. On the other hand, some nursery nurses interviewed ob-served that spitting up appears to be an accidental loss of food with the expulsion of swallowed air. We need to systematically study and compare spitting up with vomiting if we are to understand the babies called "spitter-uppers" and those who do not stop spitting up once they reach 12 to 15 weeks. One writer suggests that spitting up is the reversal of the peristaltic flow of the stomach, but no supporting data are given (Smith 1968).

In adults, events, sights, or sounds that disgust, revolt, shock, or otherwise threaten the psyche often cause feelings of nausea and sometimes cause vomiting. Witnessing an automobile accident, watching someone bleed, observing physical violence, hearing a scream of pain, or even seeing someone else vomit are experiences that may trigger nausea and vomiting. Word pictures, bad news, or any intolerable experiences may cause nausea and vomiting. Lack of acceptance of parts of one's own self that one sees dramatized in interaction with others may be expressed as nausea and vomiting.

Psychological nausea and vomiting have cultural dimensions, too. The Navajo, who believes the bear is his brother, is revolted when served bear by an unaware host. The average person in our culture would be revolted by being served a meal of horse meat or skunk; being told what one had eaten after the meal would be even more revolting.

Nausea and vomiting are also responses to the injection of noxious agents like microorganisms, irritating substances, or substances too highly concentrated to be tolerated by the gastric mucosa. "Montezuma's revenge" is well known to many travelers south of the United States' border and elsewhere who, however wary, often succumb to it. Nausea and vomiting may represent a total-body response to overdosage, cumulative effect, toxic response, or side effect of drugs.

Overeating, eating the wrong food, and eating at times that are inappropriate in terms of other behaviors are probably the major causes of nausea and vomiting.

The preferred definition of nausea in some dictionaries, is "sick" or "sickness," and certainly there is no doubt that both nausea and vomiting herald the beginning of many disease conditions as part of the syndrome called "general malaise" and that they are major symptoms in other disease entities. In these situations, nausea and vomiting are adaptive responses to internal toxicity, pressure, injury, obstruction, pain, or other stressors. Specific instances of toxicity might be toxemia, septicemia, uremia, and side effects of drugs. Specific instances of pressure might be overeating, intracranial pressure, severe hypertension, middle-ear disturbances, or inguinal hernia. Obstruction might be characterized by such conditions as intestinal obstruction, congestive failure, or facial sinus congestion. Pain might be either acute or chronic. Whatever the cause of nausea, vomiting, or both, affected persons are quick to admit that they are unable to work or that their job effectiveness is greatly limited. Nausea and vomiting have been called "God's gift to the hypochrondriac." For persons who routinely relate to others through their physical symptoms, nausea as a complaint and vomiting as an act may be used consciously or unconsciously to get attention, to express feelings not communicable verbally, or to establish interaction with others.

Falls, pain, dyspnea, headaches, or disorientation may be antecedents or concomitants of nausea and vomiting. When such added symptoms exist, the nausea and vomiting are probably not limited to psychic processes or gastrointestinal tract disturbances, but involve much more of the total organism. Some clinicians think that nausea is one of the earliest symptoms of depression

Functions of Nausea and Vomiting

The act of vomiting rapidly empties the stomach; it limits the possibility of damage from ingested noxious agents by preventing their access to the major absorptive region of the alimentary tract. Vomiting, according to Borison and Wang (1953), is one of the most primitive of animal functions. Guyton (1976) identifies vomiting as a first line of defense, that is, protective. In general, nausea and vomiting are adjustment and adaptive responses to internal toxicity, pressure, injury, obstruction, pain, or other stressor. And nausea, as the most common phenomenon preceding vomiting, might be called an early-warning system of disease.

The nausea and vomiting in the first trimester of pregnancy have been identified as protective in some as-yet unknown way. In a study of 6,637 live births, female infants of women who had had no nausea and vomiting had a 70 percent higher rate of perinatal mortality than the female infants of women who had experienced nausea and vomiting. Higher perinatal mortality was directly related to the fact that 7.9 percent of the women who did not have nausea and vomiting delivered infants weighing less than 5.5 pounds (the top cutoff for assignment to the low-birth-weight (LBW) category; mothers of LBW infants also had shorter gestations (Brandes 1967). Other investigators associate absence of nausea and vomiting with higher abortion rates (Speert and Guttmacher 1959; Medalie 1957; and Walford 1963).

In addition to protecting, nausea and vomiting warn of impending illness. General recognition of this warning system is found in the common expression, "I must be coming down with something," offered when people feel nauseated. Mothers use their children's nausea and vomiting to assess what communicable diseases are "going around" and who the children have been exposed to. In treatments using drugs, nausea and vomiting warn of cumulative effects and side effects of the drug as well as overdosage, toxicity, and idiosyncrasy.

In severe systemic disease conditions, nausea and vomiting are adaptive responses that do not improve the disease condition even though they may produce momentary comfort. Rather, nausea and vomiting in these diseases are used to measure or identify points along a continuum of increasing seriousness of an illness, progress toward recovery, or lack of progress. In both nausea and vomiting, duration is an important tool, and, in vomiting, the contents of the vomitus is important in assessment.

Since reluctance to vomit is learned, use of vomiting to release long-term and acute psychic tension is probably more limited in Western culture than in some others. Rather than lose the love of significant adults, children will swallow almost anything. The concept of the "bilious" child has fallen into disuse over the last 40 or 50 years, although children with so-called weak stomachs still exist. And, there are still adults who express spontaneous feelings of disgust and chronic tension by vomiting. Vomiting is, to some students of the concept, one of the few ways humans have for "orgasmic discharge," that is, dramatic release of accumulated tensions. This is a direct, normal response to an identified stressor and not related to either anorexia nervosa or bulimia, both of which represent pathology.

Beyond the psychological or physiological functions of vomiting, feelings of relief from acute misery may result. This is not true in cases of systemic disease or morning sickness of pregnancy where nausea persists even after vomiting. In reality, nausea and vomiting may have multiple causes with one cause being more important and stronger than the other causes. A case in point is postoperative nausea and vomiting: while the gastric mucosa may be greatly irritated by the choice of anesthetic, pain, trauma, electrolyte imbalance, systemic effects of anesthesia, fear, or pressure may all work together to produce the symptoms. A coffee-ground-like vomitus is typical and indicative of imminent death.

There are common nausea and vomiting situations for which no function has been found. These include motion sickness, which occurs when we ride a roller coaster and seasickness, which results from the rhythmic rocking of a boat riding the waves. If we go back in time, we learn that nausea related to unstable or unfamiliar situations is hypothesized as a primitive warning system related to stability in space of which remnants still exist and are triggered when we are in certain kinds of motion situations, even though our stability is not threatened (Treisman 1977).

For 5 years the investigator studied almost exclusively within the medical model. Years of functioning in this model were desensitizing and immobilizing. Whenever a new instance or new material was discovered, the immediate response was to label it "symptom" and then wend a way through the medical literature to attach it to a disease condition or otherwise give it respectability. Finally, the investigator became more sensitive in listening about nausea and vomiting and began to hear that nausea is a warning of conditions that people can learn various ways of preventing or warding off. People learn criteria they use to decide whether vomiting would be helpful or whether it should be discouraged. Using the medical model, only two reasons could be found for encouraging vomiting—in the case of oral ingestion of some poisons and for croup. Are there few or many situations when the protective functions of nausea and vomiting need to be supported by nurses? And do new ways need to be sought by nurses to foster these phenomena as protective functions?

Along with the recognition that nausea and vomiting are protective in their basic function it became obvious that everyone is doing a constant assessment of these phenomena on a short-term and long-term basis as one aspect of maintaining body–mind homeostasis. Using past and present experience, values (including cultural values), feelings, and input from others (including media communication), people work out their own and their children's health practices in terms of what produces the best health for each individual.

Nurses, airline passengers, and patients questioned while clarifying the concept provided the following evidence of minute-by-minute, day-by-day, self-care assessment activities:

> I get nauseated when I get overtired; I must not get overtired.
> When I think of the crookedness of my boss, I could vomit. I must just do my work and keep out of office politics.
> I get airsick when I fly; I have to take dimenhydrinate (e.g., Dramamine).
> I get carsick if a window isn't open in the car. I warn everyone who rides with me that this is the way it is. Or, I don't ride with people I don't know well.
> If I were to eat horsemeat, I would vomit it. I make sure I know what I'm eating.

When I have three martinis, I get sick and vomit; I always limit myself to two.

When I have three martinis, I get sick and vomit; but last Friday night I needed that third martini, so I had it and hoped I wouldn't have to pay the price.

The sight of blood makes me nauseated. I could never work in a hospital; I even have to force myself to visit sick friends.

I'm just like my mother. I get nauseated when I have to change a soiled diaper; I just have to steel myself and get over it if I'm going to have children.

My four-year-old son was very uncomfortable and wanted to vomit but could not. He cried and groaned all the while saying he wanted to but couldn't vomit. I told him to relax and just let it come. He did and hasn't had any difficulty since.

I hate to vomit; it takes a lot out of me, so I'm careful about what I eat and drink and try not to get too stressed.

I have to eat when I have an alcoholic drink or I get sick.

I vomit easily and feel better afterwards. I don't hesitate to tickle my uvula to make myself vomit.

I vomited once in public; I was so embarrassed I wanted to die. I'm making sure that doesn't happen again.

If someone tries to rape me, I hope I can make myself vomit.

If I drink even water after working in the extreme heat for a couple of hours, I get nauseated and sometimes vomit.

My three-year-old is a bilious child; I wonder why.

Often, I feel nauseated and think I would feel better if I could vomit.

The odor of Limburger cheese makes me sick to my stomach; my husband likes it, so I am trying to overcome my reactions enough to taste it.

People, and most animals, smell both food and drink before ingesting.

The first sign that my three-year-old is ill is if she vomits.

Study of the range of assessments made in the examples cited above includes decision making. People make decisions that ward off nausea and vomiting, avoid nausea and vomiting, initiate vomiting, or influence or manipulate others' behavior. Some people make a conscious decision to risk nausea and vomiting; others make a conscious effort to become habituated to seeing vomiting and vomitus, as nurses or medical aides might do, while certain individuals try to become habituated to their own nausea and vomiting, as in early pregnancy or oncology therapy. Some people grow through accepting their sickness; others become much more sensitive to their health needs; some become wise in the management of their health needs and are able to be nonchalant rather than hypochondriacal. Personal growth results in higher levels of integration in managing the processes of living. An appropriate area of study for nurses is the constant assessment–decision making process that promotes health.

Relationship of Nausea to Vomiting

When both nausea and vomiting occur, they occur in sequence. Nausea precedes vomiting and may accompany it. No reference was found in the literature nor did anyone report cases of vomiting preceding nausea. Nausea often occurs, as much as half the time, without vomiting. Vomiting may also occur without nausea, but this is less frequent. Estimates indicate that one-half of the women who experience nausea in pregnancy vomit (Fairweather 1968; and Zeigel and Van Blarcom 1976), but it is not known what percentage of the general population or any illness population have nausea without vomiting. When forceful vomiting occurs alone and spontaneously, without nausea or other warning, it is often a sign of central nervous system pathology.

Mechanism of Nausea and Vomiting

Despite their clinical importance and universal appearance, the precise mechanisms initiating nausea and vomiting are not well understood (Borison et al. 1953). For a long time, clinicians postulated that "reverse peristalsis" accounted for nausea and vomiting, but research has not borne this out (Inglefinger et al. 1942; and Isselbacher et al. 1980).

We now know that nausea and vomiting are based on complex reflex action controlled and coordinated by the vomiting center in dorsolateral reticular formation in the medulla (Borison et al. 1959). Efferent pathways relay impulses through the phrenic nerves to the diaphragm and to the abdominal muscles and viscera by way of spinal nerves.

Afferent pathways from the duodenum, labyrinth, and many other possible sensory receptors in the gastric mucosa, abdominal viscera, olfactory epithelium, and testes reach the vomiting control center. Since emetic responses also occur in response to emotions, some afferent fibers relay impulses to the vomiting center through the limbic system. Circulating chemical agents (drugs and toxins) create impulses mediated through the chemoreceptor trigger zone for vomiting in the medulla. Vomiting, then, is integrated and controlled by two different medullary centers—both of them *vasovagal*—but coordinated by one, known formally as the vomiting center.

In nausea, the phase of general discomfort and uneasiness in the stomach area is associated with diminished functional activity and altered motility of the duodenum and small intestine. This vasovagal syndrome is accompanied by gastric discomfort. At this early stage, intestinal muscles relax while the pyloric antrum contracts and forces its contents into the body of the stomach. In some instances, intestinal contents also may be forced into the stomach. The fundus of the stomach, the cardia, and the esophagus become flaccid at this point.

As nausea becomes more pronounced, the diaphragm descends on the stomach and the lower border of the stomach descends 1 or 2 inches because of a sudden relaxation of the abdominal muscles. This action tends to stretch the esophagus and gastric walls, thus exerting tension on the nerve endings (Brobeck 1973). The duodenum then undergoes a generalized contraction; the onset of severe nausea occurs simultaneously with this contraction. The intensity and duration of severe nausea approximates the degree and duration of the duodenal contraction (Inglefinger et al. 1942). Antral and duodenal contractions are closely synchronized (Johnson 1973).

If nausea continues, *retching* occurs. Retching denotes the labored, rhythmic respiratory activity that frequently precedes vomiting (Isselbacher et al. 1980). Abdominal muscles start to contract; internally, the nasopharynx is isolated by the soft palate; the glottis is closed by contraction of the appropriate muscles; the fundus and cardia of the stomach and the esophagus remain flaccid, while the pyloric region of the stomach remains contracted and gastric contents remain in the body of the stomach. In retching, the mouth is closed and the vomiting posture is not present even though there is contraction of the abdominal muscle.

As the course progresses, movements suggestive of vomiting are observed. The head and neck become extended; knees are flexed; the mouth is opened widely with no expulsion of vomitus (Borison et al. 1953). This is the typical posture for vomiting, the exception being those turning to one side in bed.

Vomiting begins as contractions of the abdominal muscle increase, exerting pressure on the stomach, thus becoming a major force. Finally, a strong, simultaneous contraction of the diaphragm and abdominal muscles accompanied by a very deep inspiration of air occurs. Respirations cease in mid inspiration, and the stomach empties.

The respiratory system also plays an important role in retching and vomiting. While no rhythmic hyperactivity of the respiratory musculature is observed (Borison et al. 1953), the diaphragm contracting in unison with abdominal muscles has already been noted. The large inspiration that occurs just before ejection helps to prevent aspiration by allowing time for vomiting to occur before hunger for air forces another breath. Inspiration during the act of vomiting would uncover the glottis and allow gastric contents to enter respiratory passages. Pneumographic studies, in which central stimuli were applied, demonstrated that inspiratory response fell continuously during vomiting. Subjects' vocal accompaniment during central stimulation indicated that thoracic viscera were under positive pressure during vomiting (Borison et al. 1953).

Concomitantly with the contraction of abdominal wall and diaphragmatic muscles, there are annular contractions of the pylorus. So, a small part of the musculature of the stomach plays a role in the expulsion of gastric contents. Gastric contents may play an active role in vomiting, but it is generally agreed that the stomach itself plays a passive role in the vomiting process with the major ejection force coming from the abdominal musculature, which, in full contraction, creates a rapid increase in intraabdominal pressure. Curare injected into the striated muscles of the abdominal walls of study animals makes them unable to vomit (Selkirk 1971).

In summary, many nausea and vomiting receptor messages are received from the vomiting chemoreceptor trigger zone, limbic system, and afferent sympathetic pathways to be coordinated by a complex reflex center in the dorsolateral reticular formation that initiates and essentially controls nausea, retching, suggested vomiting, vomiting, and recovery. While the stomach plays a minor role, the striated muscles of the abdomen and smooth muscle of the diaphragm are major causal agents for feelings of nausea and the act of vomiting. While there is no consensus on the exact roles of specific entities and the sequence and activities involved in vomiting, researchers agree on the importance of the respiratory apparatus in the act of vomiting (Borison et al. 1953).

EFFORTS AT CONTROLLING NAUSEA AND VOMITING

Some Damping Practices

Sometimes diversion resolves the complaint of nausea. Whether it ceases or is merely superceded perceptually is not clear. Among clinicians, it is commonly recognized that there are times when the urge to vomit is reversed. It may be so distressing that regurgitated gastric contents are swallowed, or the person may lie or sit quietly, determined not to vomit. One nurse, Mary Jo Hoftiezer (1977), observed that application of ice to the stomach region of the abdomen often lessens the subjective experience of nausea; best results are obtained when the nauseated person rests on the ice pack in a semilateral, supported position. Hoftiezer (1977) has also noted that cold, moist cloths to the forehead are often helpful in reducing nausea. Whether these interventions are diversionary or whether there is some reflex action affecting receptors in the stomach, other receptors, or reticular formation itself is not yet known.

Ingestion of some foods, especially high in protein, is said to reduce or prevent morning nausea of early pregnancy (Voda and Randall 1982). Other damping practices for morning nausea range from dry soda crackers to dill pickles and are very individualized. Alcohol has been found useful by some people receiving chemotherapy for cancer (Voda 1979).

Some Fostering Practices

Commonly, we may wish to vomit to get relief from an upset stomach, a sour stomach, or one that is full beyond toleration. Sometimes a person's volition is strong enough to initiate the act of vomiting. If this fails, touching the soft palate (uvula) or the pharyngeal fauces to stimulate the gag reflex is effective. The effectiveness of volitional vomiting is related to a particular individual's attitude about vomiting.

According to the medical model, nausea and vomiting must almost always be damped, even when there might be some danger to the patient. For example, the side effects of prochlorperazine (Compazine), which has often been used for treating these phenomena, include the danger of heart block. Taking such drug-related risks is understandable when vomiting presents danger to patients, as in the case of threatened evisceration. But for much of the nausea and vomiting experienced by patients, the use of inhibiting or preventive means may say more about the needs of health care workers to produce comfort or meet the patients' expectations for a discomfort-free existence. Personnel's perceptions of nausea and vomiting as disgusting cannot be discounted since we have no data about decision making. There are several effective and safe pharmacotherapeutic agents for the control and treatment of nausea and vomiting (Bergerson 1979).

It is interesting to note the practice of 19th-century Mexicans, who gave vomitaries (emetics) to "clean out the stomach" when it was afflicted by discomfort or illness (Kay 1979).

Synthesis

Data on nausea and vomiting were synthesized in several ways. First, operational definitions of nausea and vomiting were created. Then the concepts were moved to a higher level of abstraction. The theory of adjustment–adaptation was used to relate the concepts to a larger world of knowledge. A short developmental operational definition of emotionally determined nausea and vomiting followed (Figure 6-1). Next, a beginning typology of nausea (Table 6-1) was worked out, using a time-sequence-of-events approach. A beginning typology of vomiting (Table 6-2) was created, using a degree-of-seriousness approach. An early attempt to summarize all of the data in a model using an adjustment–adaptation conceptual framework is presented in Figures 6-2, 6-3 and 6-4. Conjectures and questions are discussed as one way of projecting possibilities for future studies.

OPERATIONALIZING NAUSEA

Because there were no direct indicators of early nausea and the experience is largely subjective, two operational definitions seem called for—one for the early,

Figure 6-1 Developmental Definition of Nausea and Vomiting with
Emotional Origin

1. In infancy "spitting up" is the natural, expected, and accepted way to rid the stomach of food, gas, or other overload.

2. As neural development occurs, vomiting may perform the same function as "spitting up."

3. The child may learn to use vomiting to control feelings of helplessness.

4. With the development of speech, disapproval for vomiting and gagging, especially after the fact, is common. The child is scolded, sent to bed, or spanked about the need to vomit.

5. The child learns to control the need to vomit.

6. The child learns other ways to handle revulsion, disagreement, and helplessness by learning, for example, to accept whatever parents say, conform to parents' demands, obey the rules, or accept punishment.

7. The child gets approval for not vomiting and for being a good child.

8. Censure against vomiting becomes stronger as the child gets older and gives it up almost entirely.

9. Nausea and vomiting may return in adulthood as childhood situations are duplicated.

10. The adult may then use nausea and vomiting to control, manipulate, and get attention.

---

more subjective phase and one for the late phase, when rhythmic respiratory contractions, gagging, retching, and assumption of the vomiting position can be observed. On the other hand, the signs and symptoms of parasympathetic stimulation, which can be to some extent objectively assessed, combined with subjective complaints would provide some verifiable indicators of nausea. So three operational definitions were created. Only one of these—late-stage nausea—is verifiable.

Operational Definitions of Nausea

Definition 1.

1. Verbal statement by subject of queasiness, uneasiness over area of stomach, esophagus, and pharynx associated with the subject naming it "nausea."
2. Verbal statement by subject of heaviness, pressure, or sinking feeling over area of stomach or sternum associated with the subject naming it "nausea."
3. Verbal statement by subject of inclination to vomit.

Table 6-1 Nausea: Beginning Typology

	Definition	Symptoms
Phase I	Simple, psychological	Queasy feelings in gastric area Feeling of repugnance Feelings of disgust Feelings of revulsion Feeling helpless, unable to tolerate, unable to cope Feeling overwhelmed Feeling unwilling or unable to move Feeling of not wanting to be touched Sinking feeling, heaviness, uneasiness over abdomen Tightness in throat
Phase II	Autonomic phase	Vasomotor disturbances: feeling hot, feeling cold, perspiring, pallor Increased pulse rate followed by decrease Dizziness Increased salivation Yawning Licking lips Increased rate of swallowing
Phase III	Beginning action phase	Forced inspiration Irregular respiratory movements Extension of head and neck Diaphragm and abdominal muscles contracting Glottis closed Nasal passages closed by uvula
Phase IV	Action phase	Retching with mouth closed Gagging with mouth closed Regurgitation with swallowing regurgitated material Deep respirations
Phase V	Suggestive vomiting	Head and neck extended Vomiting posture—mouth opens but nothing ejected Forceful regurgitation into mouth Cessation of respirations until pause in vomiting or until cessation Contraction of abdominal muscles
Phase VI	Nausea (Any of Phases I, II, III, IV) with complications	Nausea with pain Nausea with hypertension Nausea with hypotension Nausea with dehydration Nausea with electrolyte imbalance

Table 6-1 Continued

Definition	Symptoms
	Nausea with elevated temperature
	Nausea after history of blow on head
	Nausea accompanied by altered levels of consciousness
	Nausea after drug or poison ingestion
	Prolonged nausea
	Nausea accompanied by hiccoughs

Note: The patient may progress from phase to phase, may experience only one or two phases, may progress rapidly from phase to phase in 1 or 2 minutes, or may progress slowly for 1 1/2 hours. Some nausea, including morning nausea, may last most of the day. Nausea may first appear in Phase VI.

Definition 2.

1. All of the above plus
    a) Vasomotor changes, that is, diaphoresis, feelings of being hot or cold.
    b) Increased salivation.

Definition 3.

1. Forced inspiration.
2. Retching, that is, labored, rhythmic respiratory activity.
3. Rhythmic contraction of abdominal muscles.
4. Vomiting posture, that is, head and neck extended, mouth open.

Operational Definitions of Vomiting

The dictionary definition of vomiting is deficient in two respects as a guide to observers who wish to call vomiting by name when they see it. Ejecting the contents of the stomach through the mouth, a common dictionary definition, has three elements: (1) ejecting, (2) contents of the stomach, and (3) through the mouth. The contents of the stomach may be gas and ejecting this gas would not be called vomiting. So the first correction needs to specify that either what is ejected is nongaseous or that it is liquid or semisolid in nature. The manner of ejecting stated in the dictionary does not permit the observer to differentiate between spitting up and vomiting. In order to make this differentiation, we understand that the abdominal and diaphragmatic muscles must be contracted during vomiting. These muscles usually contract in preparation for vomiting, but do not generally do so in spitting up.

Table 6-2 Vomiting: Beginning Typology

	Definition	Symptoms
Class I	Primitive mode or reflex immaturity	"Spitting up" or "wet burp" of infants.
Class II	Simple	Expulsion of gastric contents into a receptacle Feeling repulsed as after overeating or at the beginning of pregnancy Vomitus characterized by sour odor or odor of alcohol, contains undigested food particles Preceded by feelings of nausea Motion and sea (kinesthetic) sickness
Class III	Vomiting with pressure	Sudden, almost unexpected expulsion of gastric contents before time to reach or call for a receptacle Vomitus characterized by sour odor or odor of alcohol, contains undigested food particles
Class IV	Projectile vomiting	Forceful expulsion of gastric contents landing three to six feet from point of expulsion Vomitus characterized by sour odor, undigested food particles, gastric juices, or gastric juices and bile Without nausea and with very little warning
Class V	Complicated vomiting	Abnormal contents such as blood, frank or coffee grounds, feces, foreign bodies Abnormal odor such as fecal, fetid, fruity, acidotic Abnormal duration and frequency such as frequent vomiting related to ingestion of food or drugs, picnic foods or leftovers, cream foods, food with questionable odor or taste 48 to 72 hours after initial dose of drugs such as digitalis, xalidixic acid (negative gram), opiates, chloroquine, HCl, lidocaine HCl, salicylates, ammonium chloride, potassium tablets Accompanied by migraine headache, hypertension, pain in abdomen or angina, ear infection (or pain), diabetic acidosis, depression, bladder distention, difficult breathing, epileptic seizure,

Table 6-2 Continued

	Definition	Symptoms
		pancreatitis, dehydration, or electrolyte imbalance
		Following blow on head, radiation therapy
Class VI	Emergency vomiting	Vomiting blood or feces
		Vomiting and abdominal pain or angina
		Vomiting and distention
		Vomiting and respiratory difficulty or aspiration
		Vomiting and diabetic acidosis
		Vomiting and hypertension
		Repeated vomiting and electrolyte imbalance or dehydration
		Projectile vomiting
		Vomiting following a blow on the head

Operational definition of vomiting.
1. Liquid and/or semisolid matter that represents the stomach contents is ejected through the mouth.
2. Simultaneously with this ejection, the diaphragm and abdominal muscles contract in unison.

DISCUSSION

Many questions are raised in the text, which, in turn, open speculations about research possibilities. While this does not itself generate testable hypotheses, more descriptive work has the potential for yielding some hypotheses that would be useful in studying nursing.

Both men and women questioned in this study thought women vomited more than men; this is an unknown. Another unknown is whether men and women vomit under different circumstances. There was a feeling expressed, often by innuendo, that women more often vomit related to emotional stress than do men, but no studies were found except for those on pathological conditions—for example, anorexia nervosa and bulimia—to support this conjecture. Women subjects interviewed agreed that children vomit more than adults but there was no consensus about whether girls vomit more frequently than boys. We might speculate about sex differences in culturally accepted behaviors related to vomiting, but such research has not yet been done.

Figure 6-2 Adaptation to Nausea and Vomiting

1. Every living organism is susceptible to injury.

2. Agents capable of causing injury to all living organisms are those that interfere with the cellular metabolic processes of the organism.

3. Agents may be external to the organism or emerge from within it. The nature of the external agents may be physical, chemical, or biological; the nature of the internal agents may be chemical or physical.

4. The injurious agents incur physiological change or may destroy either the structure or the function of the organism if the agents are not neutralized.

5. Every living organism has ways to defend itself against injury.

6. Every living organism has ways to heal or otherwise cope with injury.

7. Major defenses against injurious agents also involve physical, biological, or biochemical processes. Physical processes include moving away from the agent. Biological and biochemical processes include ejecting or removing the agent, neutralizing or destroying the agent, adjusting to injury, and increasing strength to cope with the agent.

8. Vomiting is one primitive protective function with which all omnivorous animals are endowed.

9. In the human organism, vomiting functions as a first-line defense against injury and as a first-line reflex for coping with situations interpreted as injury.

10. Injurious agents entering the gastrointestinal tract through the mouth may be ejected by vomiting before they are absorbed through intestinal mucosa into the body proper.

11. Nausea may precede vomiting to warn the organism of attack or impending attack by injurious agents.

12. When injurious agents enter the body through intestinal absorption or emerge from the internal surfaces or workings of the body, the organism may still attempt to eject the agents through vomiting.

13. It is possible to use nausea and vomiting to anticipate systemic injury, determine degree of injury, and select methods of treating the injury. Nausea and vomiting may, for example, be prodromal to onset of disease, creating electrolytic imbalance or dehydration, indicating severity of diabetes or pancreatitis, signaling increased cerebrospinal pressure or impending death.

14. Nausea and vomiting may signal rapid physiological change and may be perceived as a threat of injury to the body, but may in reality be a normal physiological adjustment mechanism as, for example, the nausea and vomiting of pregnancy.

15. When no function can be found for a physiological phenomenon, as with nausea and vomiting in motion sickness, meaning can often be found in the evolutionary development of the species.

A carefully designed study, replicating as far as possible Dumas' work (1963*a*, 1963*b*, 1964), might be useful in studying postoperative vomiting as an indicator of unresolved emotional stress. This would be useful especially to test specific techniques for preoperative anxiety resolution and stress reduction. Vomiting is such a common event in postsurgery care and such a source of discomfort that studying nursing measures of relief is paramount. Pharmacotherapeutic measures while often effective, all have side effects and are not applied until after vomitive behavior has occurred.

Nausea and vomiting have a range of meanings for nurses. The full extent of this range and the most frequent meanings are not yet completely understood. Assuming that the meaning these phenomena have for nurses influences nursing behavior, choice of intervention, and even attitude toward patients, baseline data like range and mean of meaning would be required before predictive studies could be carried out.

Nausea and vomiting also have a range of meanings in Western culture and among other cultures; meanings may have changed over the last century. Meanings and changes in meaning influence nausea and vomiting behavior and peoples' experiences of their behavior. We need studies that identify these meanings and the extent to which meaning may have been altered over time.

Vomiting occurs at the peak of a long inspiration. We wonder if nurses should not study whether encouraging deep breathing during nausea would make vomiting safer for ill patients. If the blood is well oxygenated, the drive to breathe during the vomiting act would be lessened; this, in turn, would reduce the risk of aspiration. But until relevant studies are completed, this remains conjecture.

If it is important for nurses to predict whether a patient will vomit—and it might be necessary to procure equipment, protect clothing, support stitches, or prevent esophageal damage—it may be that the person who is nauseated is a more reliable predictor than nursing observations or symptoms elicited from patients. This is also conjecture, but is an area that lends itself to study.

If there is lack of precision about differentiating anorexia, nausea, and taste alteration, intervention decision making will be imprecise. Studies of what patients report when they name these behaviors and studies of the ways nurses clarify what people mean by these names might modify intervention. This may be especially true with oncology patients on chemotherapy who may report a "tinny" or "oily" taste as nausea or anorexia (lack of appetite). Nursing interventions might be developed to deal specifically with taste alteration and anorexia as opposed to subsuming these phenomena under nausea.

The questions of whether an empty stomach reduces feelings of nausea and vomiting behavior is another potential area of study for nurses. Nurses reporting on their observations of morning nausea indicate that some nauseated pregnant women, at least, feel better after ingesting simple, high-protein foods. If it is more comfortable when nauseated to empty the stomach, is drinking water until

Figure 6-3 General Adaptation and Adjustment Model

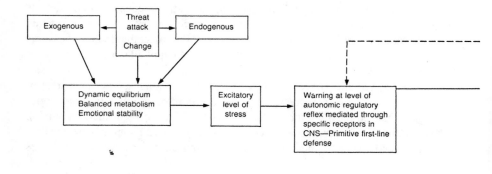

Figure 6-4 Adaptation and Adjustment Model for Nausea and Vomiting

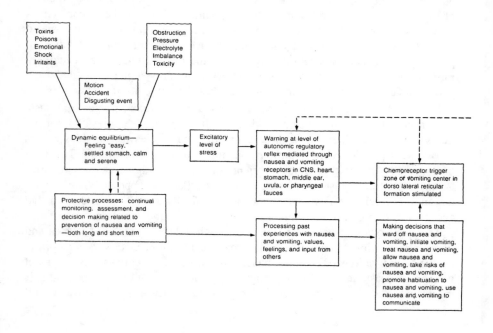

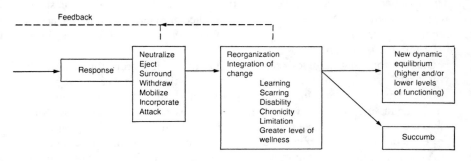

Note: WHO's use of terms is applied here: adjustment is the resetting of control systems without the presence of disease; adaptation represents changes made in response to disease or illness.

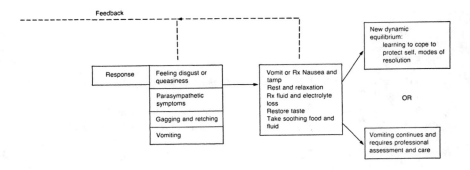

Note: WHO's use of terms is applied here: adjustment is the resetting of control systems without the presence of disease, adaptation represents changes made in response to disease or illness.

vomiting desirable thoroughly to "clean it out"? And if this is useful under some circumstances and not others, what are the respective circumstances? In earlier days of the profession, nurses believed postanesthesia patients who were nauseated should really empty their stomachs in order to convalesce more rapidly. This practice coincided with the use of tight abdominal binders when anesthesia was in its infancy. Nurses have not yet studied postsurgery vomiting and its relation to rate of recovery or quality of convalescence; therefore, we do not have reliable information.

Observations that herbivorous animals do not vomit (except for horses, who vomit rarely through their noses) stimulate speculation about whether vegetarian humans vomit less than their omnivorous counterparts. If so, are there ways nurses could use this diet with human carnivores to prevent vomiting? Since there are large groups of people who are strict vegetarians and other groups who are ovolactovegetarians, obtaining normative study data should be feasible.

As stated earlier, the basic function of nausea and vomiting is protective. We might ask whether there are ways nurses can utilize this concept in practice. Obviously this will not be possible until studies are done that discriminate between when the phenomena are performing their protective function and when they have failed and become merged with an illness process. We could speculate that if vomiting is protective, there would be occasions in which known specifications about the phenomena would be part of nurses' decision to support or initiate vomiting behavior, but this is many research studies away.

There is evidence of a continuing assessment of behavior based on an ongoing input of ideas, values, and facts that influence safety or protective behavior, risk-taking behavior, or self-abuse behavior in relation to nausea and vomiting. As yet, there are not adequate amounts of normative data to describe this self-monitoring and decision-making behavior. If nurses intend to develop a health-promoting body of nursing knowledge, studies in this area should also be undertaken.

REFERENCES

Bell, G.H., Emslie-Smith, and Patterson, C.R. *Textbook of Physiology*. New York: Churchill, Livingstone, 1980.

Bergersen, B.S. *Pharmacology in Nursing* (14th ed.). St. Louis: Mosby, 1979.

Borison, H.L., and Wang, S.C. Physiology and pharmacology of vomiting. *Pharmacol. Rev.* 5:193–230, 1953.

Borison, H.L., and Wang, S.C. Functional localization of central coordinating mechanism for emesis in cats. *J. Neurophysiol.* 12:305–312, 1949.

Brandes, J.M. First-trimester nausea and vomiting as related to outcome of pregnancy. *Obstet. Gynecol.* 30:429, 1967.

Brobeck, J.M. (Ed.). *Best and Taylor's Physiological Basis of Medical Practice* (9th ed.). Baltimore: Williams & Wilkins, 1977.

Daren, J.C., Grossman, H., and Klotz, A.P. When vomiting signals a geriatric emergency. *Nurs. Update* 6:12–13, June 1975.

DiPalma, J.R. (Ed.). *Drill's Pharmacology in Medicine* (3rd ed.). New York: McGraw-Hill, 1965.

Dumas, R.G. Psychological preparation for surgery. *Am. J. Nurs.* 63:52, August 1963.

Dumas, R.G., and Leonard, R.C. The effect of nursing on the incidence of postoperative vomiting. *Nurs. Res.* 12:12–15, Winter 1963.

Dumas, R.G., and Anderson, B.J. Psychological preparation beneficial—If based on individual's need. *Hosp. Top.* 42:79, May 1964.

Editorial. More about d and v. *Br. Med. J.* 4:1, Oct. 5, 1974.

Fairweather, D. Nausea and vomiting in pregnancy. *Am. J. Obstet. Gynecol.* 102:133–175, Sept. 1968.

Greenwald, J. *Be the Person You Were Meant To Be*. New York: Dell, 1973.

Guyton, A.C. *Textbook of Medical Physiology*. Philadelphia: Saunders, 1976.

Harrison, R.J. *Textbook of Medicine* (7th ed.). New York: Wiley, 1977.

Hoftiezer, M.J. Personal communication, 1977.

Inglefinger, F.J., and Moss, R.E. The activity of the descending duodenum during nausea. *Am. J. Physiol.* 136:561–566, 1942.

Isselbacher, K.J., Adams, R.D., Braunwald, E., Petersdorf, F.G., and Wilson, J.D. *Harrison's Principles of Internal Medicine* (9th ed.). New York: McGraw-Hill, 1980.

Johnson, A.G. Gastroduodenal motility and synchronization. *Postgrad. Med. J.* (Suppl. 4) 49:29–33, 1973.

Kay, M. Personal communication, 1979.

Lewis, F., Cannell, S., and Parsell, S. Clinical tool development for adult chemotherapy patients: Process and content. *Cancer Nurs.* 2:99–108, Apr. 1979.

McCarthy, R.T. Vomiting. *Nurs. Forum* 3:48–59, 1964.

Medalie, J.H. Relationship between nausea and vomiting in early pregnancy and abortion. *Lancet* 273:117–119, July 20, 1957.

Minow, S. Nausea in Myocardial Infarction. In C.M. Norris (Ed.), *Concept Clarification in Nursing*. Rockville, Md.: Aspen Systems Corp., 1982.

Pivesent, R.I.F.H. More about d and v (editorial). *Br. Med. J.* 4:410, Nov. 16, 1974.

Powdermaker, H. An anthropological approach to the problem of obesity. *Bull. NY Acad. Med.* 36:286–295, 1960.

Sartre, J.P. *Nausea*. New York: New Directions, 1964.

Selkirk, E.E. In G.H. Bell, J.N. Davidson, and H. Scarborough (Eds.), *Textbook of Physiology* (3rd ed.). Boston: Little, Brown, 1971.

Smith, A. *The Body*. London: Ruskin House, 1968.

Smith, D.M., Kirk, G.R., and Shepp, E. Maturation of the emetic apparatus in the dog. *Am. J. Vet. Res.* 35:1281–1283, 1974.

Solomon, J., and Solomon, J. *Ancient Roman Feasts and Recipes Adapted for Modern Cookery*. Miami, Fla.: Seeman, 1977. P. 21.

Speert, H., and Guttmacher, A.F. Frequency and significance of bleeding in early pregnancy. *J.A.M.A.* 155:712–715, 1959.

Staraska, F. *How To Say No To a Rapist and Survive*. New York: Random House, 1975.

Stedman's Medical Dictionary (23rd ed.). Baltimore: Williams & Wilkins, 1976.

Taber, C.W. *Encyclopedic Medical Dictionary* (24th ed.). Philadelphia: Davis, 1974.

Treisman, M. Motion sickness: An evolutionary hypothesis. *Science* 197:498–505, July 29, 1974.

Voda, A., and Randall, M.P. Nausea and Vomiting of Pregnancy: Morning nausea. In C.M. Norris (Ed.), *Concept Clarification in Nursing*. Rockville, Md.: Aspen Systems Corp., 1982.

Voda, A. Personal communication, 1979.

Waldo, M. *International Encyclopedia of Cooking*. New York: Macmillan, 1967. Vol. 2, p. 45.

Walford, P.A. Antibiotics and congenital malformations. *Lancet* 2:298, 1963.

Welch, D. Nursing the patient with advanced liver metastasis. *Cancer Nurs.* 2:297–303, Aug. 1979.

Wilbur, D.L. New dimensions in digestive disease (editorial). *Postgrad. Med.* 54:33, Sept. 1973.

Zeigel, E., and Van Blarcom, C.C. *Obstetric Nursing* (6th ed.). New York: Macmillan, 1972.

Chapter 7

Nausea and the Patient with Myocardial Infarction

Susan G. Minow

Nurses deal with nauseated patients every day. Because nausea is a nursing phenomenon, its description is basic to nursing theory and practice. While the concept of nausea needs to be studied intensively in various settings, I am interested mainly in nausea that occurs in patients with myocardial infarction (MI). The term *nausea* almost always appears in descriptions of symptoms for MI, but the literature provides little information concerning a physiological link between the two.

Acute MI accounted for 357,844 deaths in the United States in 1976; this breaks down to 224,718 deaths in males and 133,126 deaths in females (Vital Statistics 1976). A variety of parameters have been used to predict the risk of death in patients with acute MI (Kleiger et al. 1975), but as yet it is still difficult to predict the outcome of patients suffering from MI.

Observations of clinical coronary-care nurses seems to indicate that they are more concerned about patients who have nausea and pain than those who have pain alone. Why? Could nausea be an alarm system, warning nurses of a possible ominous outcome in MI patients? Literature on nausea related to myocardial infarctions is almost nonexistent. My ever-present apprehension for patients with MI-presenting nausea, in addition to other symptoms, prompted me to formulate some basic knowledge.

PERSPECTIVE ON MYOCARDIAL INFARCTION

Coronary heart disease involves the pathologic process of deposition of lipid material in the intima layer of the coronary arteries. These lesions, which later include calcifications, are called *atherosclerotic plaques*. The pathologic process is progressive, leading to varying degrees of interference of free blood flow to the myocardium. More severe obstructions of blood can lead to chest pain (angina pectoris) or ischemia; total occlusion of a major artery can result in MI (Singer 1976).

Three major areas as follows are considered in diagnosing a MI:

1. The characteristic clinical picture includes substernal chest pain, heaviness, burning, aching or pressure, shortness of breath, diaphoresis, weakness, nausea, vomiting, and severe anxiety.
2. Enzyme changes. The enzymes are serum glutamic oxacetic transaminase (SGOT), serum lactic dehydrogenase (LDH), serum creatinine phosphokinase (CPK), and serum creatinine phosphokinase–cardiac fraction (CPK-MB) (Wallach 1970).
3. Classic electrocardiographic (EKG) readings (Andreoli 1971).

MIs are also subdivided according to their electrical location. The first location is entitled *anterior*, which shows wave changes in leads V_1, V_2, and V_3. The next location is called *inferior* and involves wave changes in leads II, III, and AVf. Another location is *lateral* and shows changes in leads I, AV1, V_5, and V_6. The last location is pure *posterior*, with wave changes seen in leads V_1 and V_2 (Andreoli 1971).

COMPLICATIONS OF ACUTE MYOCARDIAL INFARCTION

In patients who fail to survive an acute myocardial infarction, a number of pathologic states are evident postmortem. Some deaths may be related to known mechanisms, while in others the exact mechanism is not known. In many instances, death does not occur because of the presence of necrotic tissue but as a complication of the surviving muscle. A common cause of death is acute coronary insufficiency due to ventricular fibrillation or cardiac arrest (Hurst 1977).

Congestive heart failure is a common complication of MI. This usually begins as acute left ventricular failure with symptoms of dyspnea, tachycardia, tachypnea, orthopnea, pulmonary rales, or rhonchi (Romhilt and Fowler 1973). The patient may also experience restlessness, insomnia, or weakness. Cardiac failure can lead to the sudden onset of pulmonary edema, in which the patient literally drowns in his or her own secretions (Hurst 1977). Patients with heart failure may also exhibit gastrointestinal symptoms, including anorexia, nausea, vomiting, abdominal distension, fullness after meals, or abdominal pain (Hurst 1977).

Cardiogenic shock is another complication of MI. Its diagnosis is made according to a systolic blood pressure below 80 mm Hg or evidence of decreased perfusion of the skin, brain, or kidney. Patients may have cold, clammy skin, decreased urinary output, impairment of cerebral function, or abdominal pain

(Romhilt and Fowler 1974). Hypotension can cause nausea and vomiting (Mellenkamp and Wang 1977).

Another major complication of acute MI is cardiac rupture, which is a major cause of death. The prevalent type of rupture is the rupture of the free left wall of the ventricle; the patient may experience new or prolonged pain before death ensues (Romhilt and Fowler 1974). Less common types of rupture include ventricular septal ruptures and papillary muscle ruptures. Ventricular septal ruptures usually occur within the first week following the infarction and often lead to shock or congestive heart failure (left or right), the degree of which depends upon the size of the defect (Romhilt and Fowler 1973). Papillary muscle ruptures can result from many disease states, but they are most commonly due to coronary insufficiency or MI (Burch, DePasquale, and Phillips 1968). The papillary muscles receive their blood supply from the large branches of the coronary arteries; thus they are susceptible to injury if blood flow is impaired (Romhilt and Fowler 1973).

Pericarditis is a complication that is usually restricted to infarcts of the transmural variety. Usually, pericarditis is of no major functional significance; it can be important, when, for example, hemorrhagic effusion occurs into the pericardium, resulting in cardiac tamponade (Hurst 1977). Pericarditis may occur without pain, although pain is the most prominent symptom. Pain may be precordial or it may be confined to the trapezius area, neck, shoulders, or upper arm, especially on the left side. The pain is usually aggravated by deep inspiration. Cough may also be a complaint and low-grade fever is frequently present (Hurst 1977). Pain can cause the symptoms of nausea and vomiting (Mellenkamp and Wang 1977).

Additional sequelae of acute MI include thromboembolic complications, which result from thrombus formation over the infarcted endocardium or within the pelvic or leg veins. Recognition of pulmonary emboli without pulmonary infarction is difficult. Recurrent episodes of weakness, dyspnea, tachypnea, sweating, tachycardia, and arrhythmias in the absence of extension of the MI are, however, suggestive. Systemic arterial embolism can cause infarction of any organ and may not produce pain, coldness, numbness, and discoloration to an extremity (Hurst 1977).

Ventricular and atrial arrhythmias are common after an MI. There is a high incidence of premature ventricular contractions occurring in about one-third of the patients, causing symptoms in about 10 percent (Romhilt and Fowler 1974). Premature ventricular contractions can lead to ventricular tachycardia, and persistent ventricular tachycardia may, in turn, produce serious impairment of cardiac function. With rapid ventricular rates, cerebral blood flow can be reduced by 40 percent. Ventricular tachycardia can deteriorate into ventricular fibrillation resulting in zero cardiac output (Hurst 1977). Atrial flutter and fibrillation occur less frequently following the infarction than do the ventricular arrhythmias (Romhilt and Fowler 1974). But any atrial or ventricular arrhythmia that leads to hemodynamic impairment can cause hypotension or shock. And as previously mentioned, this may result in the symptoms of nausea or vomiting.

Second- and third-degree heart block complicates an MI in about 8 to 10 percent of affected patients. Heartblocks are also found more frequently in inferior-wall infarcts than in anterior-wall infarcts since the atrioventricular node arises from the right coronary artery in approximately 85 percent of the patients (Romhilt and Fowler 1974). Second-degree heart block may or may not cause symptoms. At high grades and low rates, dizziness and syncope may result (Hurst 1977). Third-degree heart block can result in various degrees of symptoms, from asymptomatic to serious. Symptoms include lightheadedness, palpitations, tiredness, severe and fatal Adams-Stokes attacks, and heart failure (Hurst 1977).

PHYSIOLOGICAL LINK BETWEEN NAUSEA AND MYOCARDIAL INFARCTION

Located behind the atrioventricular node are a number of autonomic ganglions (Hurst 1977) that are presumed to be vagal ganglions. These and the adjacent structures are thought to act as receptors (James 1968). The most common pathologic change to this area occurs because of ischemia or infarction. In Thoren's study (1972) with cats, it was found that the receptors increased their activity during short-term general asphyxia and during transient occlusion of one of the coronary arteries. The coronary artery supplying the atrioventricular node in 90 percent of the people is the right coronary artery. The occlusion of this artery results in a posterior MI (Hurst 1977). Changes of ischemia or infarction are picked up by the receptors, travel to the reticular formation (where the vomiting center is located), and eventually result in syncope or a more prolonged loss of consciousness; additional manifestations include diaphoresis, increased salivation, a defecation reflex, and a high incidence of nausea and/or vomiting. All these symptoms can be caused by excess vagal stimulation (Hurst 1977).

The origin of this vagotonia has been questioned. But work done by Juhasz-Nagy and Szentivanyi (1961) and James (1968) suggested that the neural strictures at the posterior border of the atrioventricular node may be the site. If this is true, the vagal actions of a posterior MI are the human counterparts of the Bezold-Jarisch reflex seen in experimental animals (Hurst 1977).

The Bezold-Jarisch reflex is an experimental reflex that originates from unknown chemoreceptors in the heart and has afferent and efferent pathways in the vagus nerve (Krayer 1961). A wide variety of chemicals like veratrine, nicotine, and 5-hydroxytryptamine may initiate this reflex in certain animals (Dawes and Comroe 1954). The results of stimulating this reflex are sinus bradycardia, hypotension, and peripheral vasodilatation (Hurst 1977).

Hurst (1977) stated that a reflex corresponding to the Bezold-Jarisch reflex may be present in some patients, especially those with a posterior or inferior MI. Ischemia would cause an activation of the autonomic ganglion receptors resulting in a vagal reflex, which causes a high incidence of sinus bradycardia, heart block, hypotension, nausea, bronchospasm, and tracheal burning as seen in these types of infarctions.

In addition to the Bezold-Jarisch reflex, there is supporting evidence for the opinion that there are sensory stretch receptors in the ventricles. These are receptors that are excited by a rise in intraventricular pressure, left ventricular distension, or ischemia, and whose afferent fibers run in the vagi. When excited, these fibers cause a reflex fall in blood pressure and heart rate and cause peripheral vasodilatation (Dawes 1963).

It has also been shown that activation of nonmyelinated vagal afferents emanating from the left ventricle of the heart can, besides causing reflex bradycardia and hypotension, elicit a marked reflex relaxation of the stomach. This gastric relaxation can be produced by electrical excitation of the vagal cardiac afferents (Abrahamsson and Thoren 1973).

PERSPECTIVE ON NAUSEA

Nausea is found in association with patients with an MI. As has been described, nausea can result directly from the ischemia or infarction or indirectly from a variety of complications resulting from the infarction, or both.

What is nausea? Definitions include "a stomach disturbance characterized by a feeling of the need to vomit, strong aversion, repugnance, disgust" (Morris 1969) and "a sickness of the stomach, producing dizziness and an impulse to vomit, a feeling of loathing in general" (*Funk and Wagnall's* 1973).

Within an etymological dictionary (Klein 1967), it was found that nausea or "nausia" was first used by the Greeks meaning "ship sickness." It was derived from the word *nautical*—"pertaining to ships or navigation." Possibly the Greeks originated the word to describe how they felt when they became sick at sea— seasickness–motion sickness.

Treisman (1977) put forth some interesting theories on how motion sickness, with its related nausea and vomiting, came about. He stated that motion sickness is widespread among humans and is also found in a number of other animals. The author contends that the unbeneficial, unpleasant phenomena of nausea and vomiting could not have occurred so widely by accident; rather, he suggests that it was a part of some evolutionary process that originated as a mechanism for survival.

Treisman's (1977) reasoning began with the concept that all animals from birth must organize their movements and this organization produces the animals' "spatial framework." The animal ventures into the environment according to this framework, using proprioceptive input, vestibular input, and visual input; all of these factors are coordinated. If for some reason the system is interrupted, the framework must realign itself. Motion sickness would occur if the system were bombarded by repeated challenges, exceeding its adaptation capacity, or if the coordination or correlation between the input systems was broken, interrupting their flow.

But why should this phenomenon cause vomiting in an individual? Treisman believes vomiting began as an evolutionary defense against ingested toxins. When an indiscriminate eater consumed toxins, these toxins affected the nervous system, which in turn affected sensory input and motor output. An emetic response to this would be advantageous. So the same interruption to the spatial framework caused by ingesting toxins is caused by motion; riding in cars, planes, and ships evokes the same response. "Motion sickness is an adaptive response evoked by an inappropriate stimulus (Treisman 1977, p. 495)."

Why does nausea occur? Treisman (1977) stated that when encountering a toxin, an animal should not only eliminate it but avoid it in the future. He named this tactic "aversion conditioning." Thus, the sight, sound, or occurrence of something like pain or injury may trigger the same toxin-early-warning system.

An accepted explanation (Brobeck 1973; and Mellenkamp and Wang 1977) for the multiplicity of causes for nausea and vomiting is the presence of a "vomiting center." In 1949 H.L. Borison and S.C. Wang established, through experiments with cats, the presence of a vomiting center located in the dorso-lateral border of the lateral reticular formation (Borison and Wang 1949; and Borison and Wang 1950). This can be seen in Figure 7-1.

In 1977, a number of articles on nausea appeared in *Drug Therapy*. Mellenkamp and Wang (1977) reiterated the presence of the vomiting center; they stated that the vomiting center is the final common pathway that receives stimuli from a number of afferent pathways (Figure 7-2). Many of these pathways have been identified with the use of various agents or processes known to cause nausea and vomiting including orally ingested compounds that act on the intestinal tract, tactile pharyngeal stimulation, distension or traction of the viscera, increased intracranial pressure, pregnancy, stimulation of the inner ear, pain, hypotension, electrolyte disturbances, and psychic factors. This variety of agents implied that there are many different afferent pathways to the vomiting center, all of which have not yet been identified.

A chemoreceptor trigger zone (Borison and Wang 1953, 1972; and Mellenkamp and Wang 1977), which is sensitive to blood-borne compounds yet distinctly separate from the vomiting center was also found. Stimulation of the chemoreceptor trigger zone activates the vomiting center, which is insensitive to blood-borne stimuli. Therefore, the vomiting center receives information from three sources: the chemoreceptor trigger zone; the heart, stomach, and intestines; and the higher centers of the cortex (McCarthy 1964).

Figure 7-1 Location of Vomiting Center and Chemoreceptor Trigger Zone

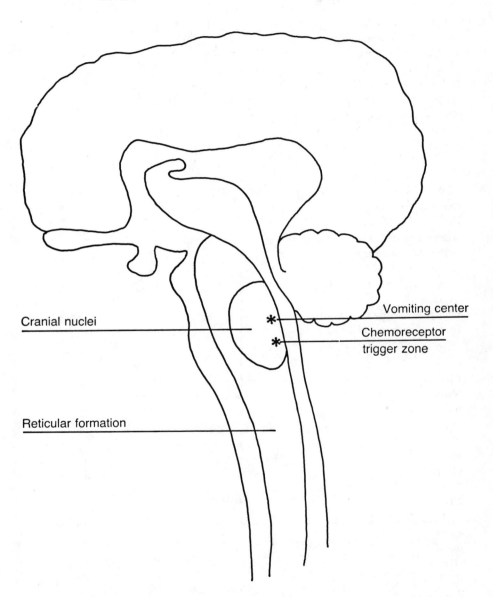

Note: Permission to publish modification of location of Vomiting Center obtained from Dr. Richard Wang.

Figure 7-2 Afferent Pathways to the Vomiting Center (Mellenkamp and Wang 1977)

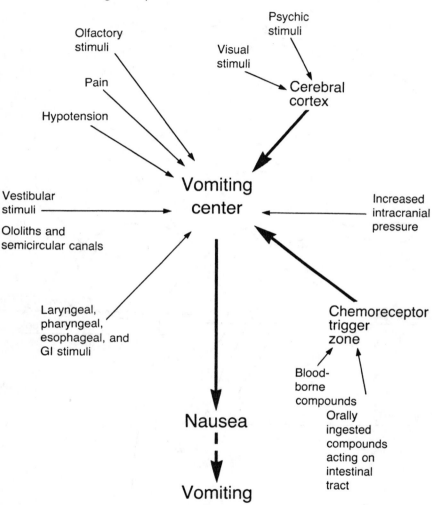

The vomiting center is also located close to autonomic nuclei such as the respiratory and vasomotor centers, excitatory and inhibitory ascending tracts of the reticular formation, and the salivary and vestibular nuclei (Mellenkamp and Wang 1977). Therefore, strong neural discharges on the vomiting center will affect the surrounding area producing related symptoms such as, for example, increased salivation, diaphoresis, defecation reflex, and/or dizziness.

When toxic compounds are ingested or pain occurs or certain sights, sounds, or smells are present, impulses travel by different pathways to the vomiting center. This elicits the emetic response by stimulating the efferent pathways that influence (1) the sensation of nausea and (2) the motor act of vomiting. The influence extends to the phrenic nerves of the diaphragm, the spinal nerves to the abdominal and intercostal muscles, the visceral fibers of the vagus and sympathetics, and the voluntary muscles of the pharynx and the larynx (McCarthy 1964).

In summary, ischemia or infarction of the myocardium could stimulate (1) direct receptors, (2) chemoreceptors, (3) stretch receptors, and/or (4) nonmyelinated afferents originating from the heart to send impulses to the vomiting center. This center in return could produce the sensation of nausea and, if the impulses are strong enough, produce the motor act of vomiting. Also, if the impulses are strong enough, adjacent autonomic ganglia may be affected, causing increased salivation, a defecation reflex, diaphoresis, and/or dizziness (Figure 7-3). In addition, complications arising due to ischemia or infarction of cardiac muscle can elicit the symptom of nausea. Both directly and indirectly, nausea in the patient with MI could be the result of an evolutionary process.

Figure 7-3 Model of Nausea and Ischemia or Myocardial Infarction

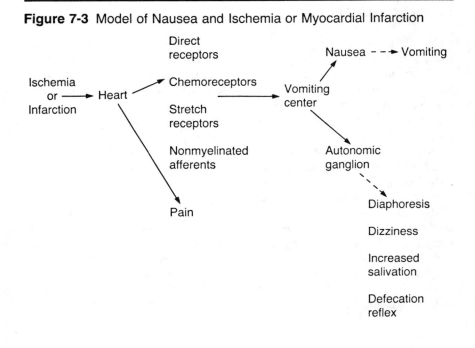

INCIDENCE OF NAUSEA IN MYOCARDIAL INFARCTION

Two studies have been done on the incidence of nausea in MI. Reports of these studies appear in Italian publications accompanied by abstracts in the English language. The following information is derived from those abstracts.

The first study was done in 1968 by Verdun di Cantogno, Vizzeri, and Orione. They found that epigastralgias (gastric complaints) occurred in 7.1 percent of 450 cases of MI. Epigastralgias were observed generally during rest and were less marked than the symptom of angina; epigastralgias were associated with dyspnea. The second study was completed in 1971 by the same researchers. Nausea and vomiting were present in 75 cases (14.6%) of 500 cases of MI (Verdun di Cantogno, Vizzeri, and Orione 1968; and Verdun di Cantogno, Vizzeri, and Orione 1971). From the available data, it was not possible to specifically document the incidence of nausea alone.

One Exploration of Nausea in Patients with Myocardial Infarct

An attempt was made to ascertain the following:

1. Subjective complaints and objective signs of patients with MI or ischemia who experience nausea and/or vomiting.
2. Criterion attributes of nausea or vomiting.
3. Complications that arise in patients experiencing nausea prior, during, and/ or following MI or ischemia.

All 10 English-speaking patients admitted to the CCU in one hospital over an 8-day period with diagnoses of MI or myocardial ischemia agreed to be studied.

All patients' charts were reviewed for information related to demographic factors and current illness variables. Those patients who became nauseated or vomited were also closely observed.

A two-part study was derived from factors deemed significant in MI. Part one asked for demographic and current illness-related information including date, admitting diagnosis, location of MI or ischemia, age, sex, serum enzymes, and whether the patient was nauseated on admission. Part two was used to study related complaints of nausea and vomiting attributed to the current illness; the goal was to explore the temporal aspects of nausea and vomiting, that is, time of day, number of hours following admission, and relationship to chest pain. It also included descriptive aspects, such as how patients appeared during the nausea/vomiting event, in an attempt to identify criterion attributes. This tool included a checklist of complications that might be associated with nausea and vomiting: hypotension, pain, pain-medication reactions, atrial arrhythmias, junctional arrhythmias, ventricular arrhythymias, congestive heart failure, pulmonary edema, left ventricular failure, and cardiac arrest. This part of the study also included identification of subjective complaints associated with nausea, since nausea is a subjective as well as a physiologic phenomenon. The severity of nausea was rated on a six-point scale ranging from the simple complaint of nausea to the motor act of vomiting.

Chart review. Since no one could predict which patient would become nauseated, charts were reviewed for all 10 patients who agreed to be studied.

Observations. Observations were done by four registered nurses plus myself. Investigators were briefed on the conceptual framework and the data-collection tools before starting their observations. I was also present with each of the other nurses when they made their first observations to increase the consistency and reliability of the study. One observer was present on a 24-hour basis to observe patient actions during the total period of data collection. So a patient who became nauseated or vomited was observed.

Information and descriptions obtained were influenced by some conditions in the situation and some limitations in what was observed. All patients admitted to the CCU were routinely given pain medication, which in itself might cause nausea and/or vomiting. Emotional reactions, such as anxiety, which might cause nausea or vomiting, were not included in the observations. The number of observers reduced the reliability of the data. Also, the data collectors had no control over the medical or nursing care the subjects received.

Demographic and Illness Data

Ten patients, three females and seven males, ranging in age from 48 to 79 years with a mean age of 62.9 years, were admitted to the CCU during the 8-day period of the study with the diagnosis of "rule out MI" (Table 7-1). The listed diagnoses were made at the time of discharge from the CCU.

Five patients (A, B, D, F, I) were subsequently diagnosed as having a MI; their mean age was 62.6 years. Diagnoses were made using presenting signs, symptoms, EKG analysis, and a cardiac enzyme profile. The remaining five (C, E, G, H, J) with a mean age of 63.2 years, were diagnosed as having myocardial ischemia, using the same diagnostic categories.

Criteria for Diagnosis

Definitive diagnosis of the MI was not made until serum enzymes were elevated. With the exception of one subject (H), three sets of serum enzymes were measured, one on admission and the others on the next two consecutive mornings. Patients A, B, D, F, and I showed definitive enzyme changes that differentiated MI from myocardial ischemia (Table 7-2).

Table 7-1   Age, Sex, and Diagnosis by Patient (10)

Patient	Age	Sex	Diagnosis
A	68	F	Inferior MI
B	66	M	Anterioseptal and lateral MI
C	60	M	Inferior ischemia
D	62	M	Anteriolateral MI
E	62	M	Substernal chest pain
F	69	M	Anterioseptal MI
G	62	F	Substernal chest pain
H	53	M	Unstable angina
I	48	M	Inferior MI
J	79	F	Inferior ischemia

Diagnosis and Time

Seven of the ten patients reported nausea prior to admission (at the time the initial infarction or ischemia took place). Three subjects (A, C, J) also experienced nausea on admission and four subjects (A, F, I, J) experienced nausea after admission (Table 7-3).

Temporal Aspects

Nausea occurred before, with, and after the chest pain and alone. Table 7-4 shows the frequency of nausea; half of the patients reported chest pain occurring with the nausea. In five instances, nausea occurred before the chest pain.

Nausea—Criterion Attributes

Criterion attributes associated with nausea range from diaphoresis to the motor act of vomiting. The frequency distribution of criterion attributes are shown in Table 7-5. Diaphoresis occurred in all instances and in all patients. No patients reported being hot and though the defecation reflex occurred in three instances, only one patient experienced it.

Additional observed criterion attributes follow for patients C, F, I, and J.

Patient C on admission   Pale.
                                          Forehead diaphoretic.
                                          Bent over slightly.
                                          Holding stomach with one hand.

Table 7-2 Serum Enzyme Profiles at Three Points in Time on Patient (10)

Patient	Diagnosis	Time Taken	SGOT (4–20)	LDH (20–70)	CPK (20–90)	CPK-MB (0)
A	Inferior MI	1*	264	210	1354	133
		2†	107	220	831	119
		3‡	126	241	351	58
B	Anterioseptal and lateral MI	1	118	94	882	176
		2	177	217	1174	127
		3	70	262	1044	45
C	Inferior ischemia	1	31	62	62	0
		2	13	51	52	0
		3	14	48	46	0
D	Anteriolateral MI	1	9	48	94	0
		2	56	93	720	5
		3	40	139	237	130
E	Substernal chest pain	1	15	39	30	0
		2	14	38	20	0
		3	4	30	17	0
F	Anterioseptal MI	1	20	55	89	0
		2	89	148	255	141
		3	13	52	45	27
G	Substernal chest pain	1	54	43	12	0
		2	23	30	10	0
		3	12	27	10	0
H	Unstable angina	1	7	42	25	0
		2	6	39	25	0
I	Inferior MI	1	14	36	90	0
		2	41	46	548	137
		3	15	100	967	—
J	Inferior ischemia	1	13	66	26	0
		2	22	67	19	0
		3	24	65	19	0

*Admission.
†First morning.
‡Second morning.

Patient F after admission

Holding emesis basin with other.
Taking deep breaths intermittently.
Concentrating look.
Trying to burp.
Said, "I feel sick to my stomach."
Coarse tremor to hands.

Table 7-3 Diagnosis and Time of Nausea in 10 Patients

Patient	Diagnosis	Nausea before Admission	Nausea on Admission	Nausea after Admission
A	Inferior MI	X	X	X
B	Anterioseptal and lateral MI			
C	Inferior ischemia	X	X	
D	Anteriolateral MI	X		
E	Substernal chest pain			
F	Anterioseptal MI	X		X
G	Substernal chest pain	X		
H	Unstable angina			
I	Inferior MI			X
J	Inferior ischemia	X	X	X

Table 7-4 Association of Chest Pain with Nausea

Occurrence of Nausea	Nausea Self-report	Observed	Number of Patients
Before chest pain	2	3	2 (C, J)
With chest pain	5		3 (A, F, G)
After chest pain	1		1 (D)
Without chest pain		2	2 (F, I)
Chest pain without nausea			4 (B, E, H, I)

Table 7-5 Patients' Criterion Attributes Associated with Nausea

Criterion Attribute	Nausea Self-report	Observed	Number of Patients
Vomiting	2	1	3 (A, C, J)
Diaphoresis	8	5	7 (A, C, D, F, G, I, J)
Increased salivation	4	3	3 (A, F, J)
Increased swallowing	5	4	4 (A, C, F, J)
Heat	0	0	0
Cold	5	2	3 (A, G, J)
Dizziness	6	4	5 (A, C, D, F, J)
Defecation reflex	3	0	1 (A)

	Thick tongue.
	Respiratory rate 20 and dyspneic.
	Diaphoretic.
	Pale.
	Wanting bed at higher angle but not straight up.
	Eyes staring.
	Swallowing frequently.
	Complaining of being lightheaded.
Patient I after admission	Complaining of gassy, burning feeling in stomach.
	Trying to burp.
	Belching.
Patient J on and after admission	Complaining of nausea.

Patient I after admission

Thick tongue.
Respiratory rate 20 and dyspneic.
Diaphoretic.
Pale.
Wanting bed at higher angle but not straight up.
Eyes staring.
Swallowing frequently.
Complaining of being lightheaded.
Complaining of gassy, burning feeling in stomach.
Trying to burp.
Belching.

Patient J on and after admission

Complaining of nausea.
Forehead and palms diaphoretic.
Swallows frequently.
Spits out excess saliva.
Takes deep breath then swallows.
Lying flat on back.
Bed at 60-degree angle.
Moves head and body together.
Hand trembles holding emesis basin.
Holds tissue in other hand.
Wipes lips frequently.
Pale.
Complains of room spinning.
Sits up abruptly, says, "I'm going to be sick," vomits.
Diaphoretic, gown damp and clingy.

Nausea—Subjective Complaints

Additional criterion attributes were identified verbally as complaints at the time the nausea occurred. These complaints are mostly related to the gastrointestinal tract. Other subjective material related to a variety of other organ systems. These are shown below for patients A, C, F, G, and I.

Patient	Complaints
A	Shaky.
	Weak.
	I don't feel like moving.
	I don't want to lie flat.

Patient	Complaints
C	Weak.
	My stomach hurts.
	No real chest pain.
F	Indigestion.
	Gassy feeling in stomach and under my [left] ribs.
	It feels like the gas keeps shifting.
	I want to burp, but gas never comes up.
G	Headache.
	I feel sick to my stomach, it comes in waves.
	. . . it's not so bad I need to vomit.
I	For the past 4 days I've had stomach pain, a burning pain from my stomach to throat.
	Indigestion.
	Upset stomach.

Nausea—Severity

Nausea/vomiting episodes were rated on a six-point scale (Table 7-6). A rating of "one" reflected the subjective complaint of nausea; a rating of "six" indicated the performance of the motor act of vomiting. Note the tendency for nausea to be rated as more severe in inferior infarction/ischemia than in anterior infarction.

Nausea—Associated Complications

Seven MI and ischemia patients who had nausea and vomiting experienced complications ranging from epigastric burning to ventricular tachycardia (see Table 7-7). No grave complication was found in any of the seven patients. Pain occurred in three patients, sinus bradycardia in two patients, and premature ventricular contractions in two patients.

Discussion

Seven of the ten patients studied experienced nausea at some time. Whether the nausea was caused directly from the MI/ischemia or indirectly from the pain associated with the MI/ischemia could not be identified. The important fact is that nausea did occur in seven out of ten myocardial disease patients.

The observations made of these patients permitted identification of criterion attributes associated with the event. The remainder of the discussion examines how these attributes relate to the conceptual framework, how they make the description of nausea more precise, and how they foster the generation of hypotheses for future testing.

Table 7-6 Severity and Frequency of Nausea by Patient and Diagnosis

Severity	Frequency	Patient	Diagnosis
6	3	A, C, J	Inferior MI, inferior ischemia, inferior ischemia
5	2	A, A	Inferior MI, inferior MI
4	3	F, J, J	Anterioseptal MI, inferior ischemia, inferior ischemia
3	1	C	Inferior ischemia
2	2	F, G	Anterioseptal MI, chest pain
1	2	D, I	Anteriolateral MI, inferior MI

Table 7-7 Complications Associated with Complaints of Nausea

Patient	Location	Complications
A	Inferior MI	Pain, sinus bradycardia, right bundle branch block
C	Inferior ischemia	Epigastric burning
D	Anteriolateral MI	Pain, premature ventricular contractions, 1 run of ventricular tachycardia
F	Anterioseptal MI	Pressure in chest, medication reaction
G	Substernal chest pain	Pain
I	Inferior MI	Burning, gassy feeling in stomach
J	Inferior ischemia	Sinus bradycardia, premature ventricular contractions, dull aching in sternum, neck and shoulders

Summary Statements

1. *Nature of Diagnosis.* The patient with an inferior infarction/ischemia was more likely to have nausea than the patient with an anterior infarction. If the postulated location of the cardiac receptors for nausea is correct, then a patient with an inferior infarction/ischemia would be expected to have more nausea than someone with an anterior infarction. In at least 90 percent of the people the atrioventricular node (cardiac receptors are located here) arises from the right coronary artery. Occlusion of the right coronary artery results in inferior ischemia or infarction. Therefore, the receptors are triggered and impulses are transmitted to the nausea–vomiting center. The intensity of the impulses elicits nausea or nausea and its criterion attributes.

2. *Severity of Nausea Related to Location of Infarct.* The nausea was rated as more severe in the patient with an inferior infarction/ischemia than a patient with an anterior infarction. An inferior infarction/ischemia would be more likely to trigger both the cardiac nausea receptors and the pain receptors, resulting in a more forceful impulse to the nausea–vomiting center, while an anterior infarction may only trigger pain receptors. It is possible that if an anterior infarction does trigger the cardiac nausea receptors, it does so to a lesser degree than an inferior infarction does.

3. *Temporal Aspects of Nausea.* Seven patients experienced nausea. All experienced it prior to admission. Only four patients experienced nausea after admission. In five instances occurring in 2 patients nausea appeared before chest pain; four patients experienced nausea with or after the chest pain; four patients experienced chest pain with no nausea. The symptom of nausea in patients with MI/ischemia has often been linked to the symptom of pain. Postulated myocardial receptors sensitive to infarction/ischemia transmit this information to the nausea–vomiting center. It is possible that nausea is a primary entity as well as a secondary phenomenon related to pain. Another point needs to be made. Though pain medication has the ability to block the pain sensation, it does not halt the ischemic process; the ischemia or infarction may continue. Nausea after admission may be due to the cardiac nausea receptors being activated.

4. *Diaphoresis.* Diaphoresis occurred in all instances of nausea. Impulses emanating from either the cardiac nausea receptors or pain, if strong enough, can affect the autonomic ganglion adjacent to the vomiting center. The autonomic ganglion can then produce diaphoresis. All nauseated patients experienced diaphoresis yet all did not experience vomiting. This suggests that there may be a whole spectrum of responses dependent upon the number and/or strength of impulses reaching the vomiting center.

5. *Complications.* The complications associated with the nausea were primarily pain and vagal sequelae (i.e., bradycardia). Again, pain and cardiac nausea receptors may be working synergistically or separately to produce the sensation of nausea. The cardiac receptor link to the vomiting center is through the vagi. The impulses traveling from the myocardium to the vomiting center may affect the efferent pathways resulting in blocks and bradycardias.

Conceptual Model

The conceptual model was derived from selected review of literature with its proposed theories and the findings of the clinical exploration (Figure 7-4). Three categories of criterion attributes associated with nausea are presented in the model. Criterion Attributes I consist of age, sex, and serum enzymes. It is

Figure 7-4 Conceptual Model of Nausea and Ischemia or Myocardial Infarction

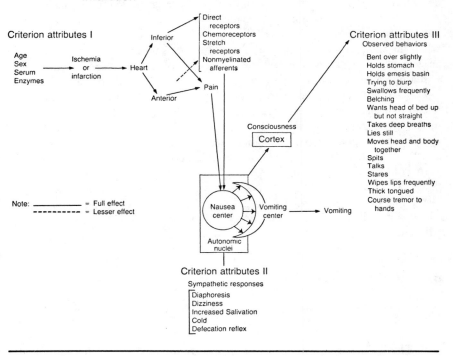

possible that these variables affect the diagnosis and severity of the MI or ischemia.

Ischemia or infarction of the myocardium takes place due to partial or complete occlusion of one or more of the coronary arteries. Depending upon the location of the damage, the ischemia/infarction is labeled. In this study, inferior and anterior ischemia/infarction were the two primary locations.

In 90 percent of the people, an inferior infarction would affect the atrioventricular node and the surrounding area, thought to be where the cardiac nausea receptors are located. An anterior infarction usually does not affect this area but it does affect the left ventricle. It is further postulated that ischemic damage or stretch to the left ventricle may also cause transmission of impulses to the nausea–vomiting center. The model depicts both inferior and anterior infarction/ischemia as having the ability to stimulate cardiac receptors. The inferior location, however is shown as having more influence based on the location of the direct receptors.

Whenever the myocardium is deprived of oxygen, pain occurs. Both locations, inferior and anterior, appear on the model as sources of pain. Both cardiac nausea receptors and pain receptors have afferent pathways to the nausea–vomiting center. Synergistically or separately, impulses are transmitted to the center. The model depicts the nausea center separate from the vomiting center; it is in the nausea center that the sensation of nausea is produced. Nausea would be caused when the number and/or strength of impulses transmitted and subsequently received were low. If the number and/or strength of the impulses increases, the vomiting center would then be activated and vomiting would occur.

Located adjacent to the nausea–vomiting center are a number of autonomic nuclei that also become activated when the number and/or strength of impulses increases. Criterion Attributes II are based on this fact as represented by the sympathetic response to pain/ischemia/infarction. These include diaphoresis, dizziness, increased salivation, cold, and a defecation reflex.

In addition, the model suggests that when nausea reaches the conscious level, people react instinctively or behave in learned ways that have been helpful in alleviating past nausea and avoiding vomiting. Whether such behaviors are instinctual or learned is open to question. Behaviors labeled in Criterion Attributes III are directly from observations made of nauseated patients in this study.

Hypotheses for Testing

The following hypotheses are generated by this exploratory study:

1. The incidence of nausea prior to admission in patients with an inferior MI is more frequent than in patients with an anterior infarction.
2. Serum enzyme levels are significantly increased in patients who experience nausea compared to those who do not experience nausea.
3. Serum enzyme levels are significantly increased in patients who have nausea and an inferior infarction compared to patients who have nausea and an anterior infarction.
4. Severity of an inferior infarction, and therefore severity of the nausea, decreases with age.
5. The severity of nausea in an inferior infarction is greater in older females than in older males.
6. The frequency of nausea increases in a linear fashion to the severity of an inferior infarction.
7. The incidence of nausea occurring before chest pain is greater than the incidence of nausea occurring with or after chest pain.

These hypotheses indicate one direction for further study related to nausea of patients with myocardial infarction.

REFERENCES

Abrahamsson, H., and Thoren, P. Vomiting and reflex vagal relaxation of the stomach elicited from heart receptors in the cat. *Acta Physiol. Scand.* 88:433–439, Aug. 1973.

Andreoli, K.G. *Comprehensive Cardiac Care* (2nd ed.). St. Louis: Mosby, 1971.

Borison, H.L., and Wang, S.C. Functional localization of the central coordinating mechanism for emesis in the cat. *J. Neurophysiol.* 12:305–313, 1949.

Borison, H.L., and Wang, S.C. The vomiting center. *Arch. Neurol. Psychiatr.* 63:928–941, 1950.

Borison, H.L., and Wang, S.C. Physiology and pharmacology of vomiting. *Pharmacol. Rev.* 5:193, 1953.

Borison, H.L., and Wang, S.C. A new concept of organization of the central emetic mechanism. *Gastroenterology* 22:1–12, Sept. 1972.

Brobeck, J.R. (Ed.). *Physiological Basis of Medical Practice* (9th ed.). Baltimore: Williams & Wilkins, 1973.

Burch, G.E., DePasquale, N.P., and Phillips, J.H. The syndrome of papillary muscle dysfunction. *Am. Heart J.* 75:399–415, 1968.

Carnevali, D. Conceptualizing, A Nursing Skill. In Pamela Holsclaw Mitchell (Ed.), *Concepts Basic to Nursing*. New York: McGraw-Hill, 1977.

Dawes, G.S. Cardiovascular Reflexes and Myocardial Infarction. In Thomas James and John Keyes (Eds.), *The Etiology of Myocardial Infarction*. Boston: Little, Brown, 1963.

Dawes, G.S., and Comroe, J.H. Jr. Chemoreflexes from the heart and lung. *Physiol. Rev.* 34:167–201, Apr. 1954.

Donaldson, S.K., and Crowley, D. The discipline of nursing. *Nurs. Outlook* 26:113–120, Feb. 1978.

Funk and Wagnall's Standard Comprehensive International Dictionary. Chicago: J.G. Ferguson, 1973.

Hurst, W.J. (Ed.). *The Heart* (4th ed.). New York: McGraw-Hill, 1977.

Jacox, A. Theory construction in nursing: An overview. *Nurs. Res.* 23:4–12, Jan.–Feb. 1974.

James, T.N. The coronary circulation and conduction system in acute myocardial infarction. *Prog. Cardiovasc. Dis.* 10:410–445, Mar. 1968.

Juhasz-Nagy, A., and Szentivanyi, H. Localization of the receptors of the coronary chemoreflex in the dog. *Arch. Intern. Pharmacodyn.* 131:39–42, 1961.

Kleiger, R.E., Martin, T.F., Miller, J.P., and Oliver, G.C. Mortality of myocardial infarction treated in the coronary care unit. *Heart Lung* 4:215–226, Mar.–Apr. 1975.

Klein, E. (Ed.). *A Comprehensive Etymological Dictionary of the English Language.* New York: Elsvier, 1967.

Krayer, O. The history of the Bezold-Jarisch effect. *Arch. Exp. Pathol. Pharmakol.* 240:361–368, 1961.

Kritek, P.B. The generation and classification of nursing diagnosis: Toward a theory of nursing. *Image* 10:33–40, June 1978.

McCarthy, R.T. Vomiting. *Nurs. Forum* 3:49–59, 1964.

Mellenkamp, E., and Wang, R. The patient with nausea: Causes. *Drug Ther.* 7:28–32, Apr. 1977.

Morris, W. (Ed.). *The American Heritage Dictionary of the English Language.* New York: Houghton Mifflin, 1969.

Norris, C. (Ed.). *Concept Clarification in Nursing*. Rockville, Md.: Aspen Systems Corp., 1982.

Romhilt, D.W., and Fowler, N.O. Physical signs in acute myocardial infarction. *Heart Lung* 2:74–80, Jan.–Feb. 1973.

Romhilt, D.W., and Fowler, N.O. Initial signs and early complications in acute myocardial infarction. *Hosp. Med.* 10:8–20, Nov. 1974.

Singer, R.B. *Medical Risks: Patterns of Mortality and Survival*. Lexington, Mass.: Lexington Books, 1976.

Thoren, P. Left ventricular receptors activated by severe asphyxia and by coronary artery occlusion. *Acta Physiol. Scand.* 85:455–463, 1972.

Treisman, M. Motion sickness: An evolutionary hypothesis. *Science* 197:493–495, Jul. 29, 1977.

Verdun di Cantogno, L., Vizzeri, E., and Orione, G. Frequency and characteristics of cardiovascular symptoms preceding the acute episode in 450 cases of myocardial infarction. *Minerva Med.* 59:3607–3614, Sept. 5, 1968.

Verdun di Cantogno, L., Vizzeri, E., and Orione, G. Modes of onset and clinical symptoms in 500 myocardial infarct crises. *Minerva Med.* 62:1618–1624, Apr. 18, 1971.

Wallach, J. *Interpretation of Diagnostic Tests*. Boston: Little, Brown, 1970.

Chapter 8

Nausea and Vomiting of Pregnancy: "Morning Sickness"

Ann M. Voda and Mary Pat Randall

INTRODUCTION

The topic selection, nausea and vomiting of pregnancy, for this chapter came about because of the significance of the concepts to us. Voda's research interest is female reproductive physiology, specifically, postovulatory menstrual cycle events during the so-called premenstrual syndrome, events surrounding the closure of menstrual life, menopause, and events associated with the phenomenon of first-trimester nausea of pregnancy. According to Voda, women and phenomena associated with their reproductive functions have been conceptualized out of an *illness* rather than *wellness* model. To menstruate or gestate is generally *not* to be sick, nor is menopause, a normal growth and developmental process, a disease. Out of a wellness framework, Voda has conceptualized nausea of first-trimester pregnancy. The conceptual model developed by her and Randall shows clearly the interrelationship between the normally functioning menstrual and pregnancy cycles. Hypotheses generated out of the model suggest that first-trimester nausea is not only explainable, but predictable because of normal physiological adjustment mechanisms that occur within the maternal organism. Only when normal adjustment mechanisms do not occur does nausea culminate in the motor act of continuous, severe vomiting; at such times therapeutic intervention is necessary.

Randall's interest in the phenomenon has a dual origin: (1) She was pregnant while writing her part of the chapter and experienced both nausea and vomiting. (2) She is a maternal–child community health nurse, who disagrees with the labeling of nausea and vomiting of pregnancy as a "sick-illness" or psychological problem; she also considers the phenomenon to be long under-researched.

Both authors agree that the incidence, prevalence, degree of misery, discomfort, pain, loss of work, and economic impact of morning sickness are unknown. Most important, since this is a phenomenon unique to women, persistent ques-

133

tions for both authors are whether first-trimester nausea might be a universal experience and, if so, whether it might be a useful predictor of fetal outcome.

The extent of misery women experience with morning sickness and how they cope with it in ways other than using drugs is of considerable concern to both of us. Generally successful nonpharmacologic coping strategies are virtually unknown. Thus, nausea of first-trimester pregnancy continues to be viewed largely out of a sickness-disease framework; that is, women are treated with a drug—Bendectin—to suppress nausea even though that drug is highly suspect for causing birth defects.*

DESCRIPTIONS OF THE PHENOMENON OF MORNING SICKNESS

The following interviews were conducted with primipara in their early twenties, all of whom said they had wanted to become pregnant.

Interview with D.R.

How many months' pregnant are you?

My last period was the 15th of June. My nausea started on August 2nd. I had a urine pregnancy test before that, but it was negative. I didn't get a positive report until the Friday after August 2nd. This is September 5th; my period was due about July 12th. I'm very regular. That means I probably got pregnant around July 1, the time I would have been ovulating. So I guess I'm about 2 months pregnant.

---

*Bendectin is one of the more commonly used drugs of pregnancy. It has been on the market for 23 years. The drug manufacturer (Richardson-Merrill Inc.) estimates that 25 percent of pregnant women in the U.S. take the drug; it is also popular in other countries. Doubts about its safety arose only recently; specifically, the Harvard School of Public Health found a weak association between Bendectin and congenital heart defects. On September 15 and 16, 1980, an FDA panel met to review data about the drug. While no definitive stand was taken against Bendectin, the FDA panel did note that the drug is probably overprescribed; its intended use is only for intractable vomiting. Under this criterion, fewer than 10 percent of pregnant women in this country should require Bendectin (Kolata 1980). Bendectin is considered a "safe drug" for use in pregnancy. Studies in rats and rabbits, which were given $90\times$ the minimum human dose showed no drug-induced fetal abnormalities. Bendectin contains 10 mg of doxylamine succinate (an antihistamine) and 10 mg of pyridoxine hydrochloride (Vitamin B_6) (*Physician's Desk Reference*. Oradell, N.J.: Medical Economics Company, 1977. P. 1109.). The mode of action of the antihistamine is believed to be suppression of the vomiting center, which has been proven to be a successful treatment for both nausea and vomiting. The place of pyridoxine hydrochloride as an antiemetic is less secure. (Biggs, J.S.G. Vomiting in pregnancy: Causes and management. *Drugs* 9:299–306, 1975. P. 305.)

When did you have the test for pregnancy?

It was the last week of school, the first week in August.

How did you know you were pregnant?

Oh, my breasts started swelling.

Do they normally swell during your menstrual period?

No, not very much.

Were you trying to get pregnant?

Yes.

Did you become nauseated after you discovered you were pregnant?

No.

Before?

Yes, after the first test, which was negative, but before the second test, which was positive on August 2nd.

Would you describe your nausea?

It is like a queasy feeling in your stomach, in the pit of your stomach and a feeling up here . . . and a tightness right above the sternum. It's a feeling that just sits there in the back of your throat; it's not the same feeling as when you have the flu and you want to vomit. You know you're going to vomit then. With this, you just have this overwhelming feeling that you're going to vomit. It's an uneasy feeling. You know you don't feel exactly right. And, when I do vomit, I have this uneasy feeling, but I don't get the urge to vomit. Smells make me gag . . . if I even think of food it makes me gag. That's when I vomit . . . it's a very strong gag reflex.

Have you vomited?

Yes.

When you vomit, do you vomit a lot?

No. Hardly anything, maybe just a little phlegm. I have eaten crackers before I've gotten up, and then after getting up. I still have felt uneasy. If I then went to fix my breakfast, the smell of an egg cooking made me gag and I had to go vomit; but I'd only vomit a very tiny amount of the crackers I had eaten. It's not like I empty my stomach. It's just like a gag that you keep gagging and gagging but only a little bit comes up. Then, as soon as you have that up, the feeling is gone for a little while. But, the thing that triggers it is thinking of food. I can't stand the thought of cooking. I haven't cooked hardly at all because I just can't. When I get up in the morning I think, "I should take something out to eat for tonight." But I can't make myself do that because the thought of any kind of food makes me sick.

How are you handling your meals now? Do you go out to eat?

Yes, we eat out a little. But my husband comes home and takes something out and then he cooks, because I won't do it. It just makes me sick; the thought of cooking makes me sick and the smell of it makes me sick.

Is it just when you wake up in the morning?

No. It's all day long.

All day long?

I have it when I first wake up. I've tried eating crackers . . . it doesn't help; it's still there. I can eat cold cereal; that doesn't gag me. But if I have to cook toast, just the smell of toast cooking, or an egg cooking . . . that makes me gag and that's when I gag and vomit. But it's not really vomit. You do vomit a little bit, but it's just a gag.

So you don't get rid of a lot of food that you take in?

Oh, no.

The "queasy feeling" doesn't stop you from eating?

I don't feel like eating, but I do eat. Before I was pregnant I used to be hungry all the time. I just don't feel hungry now but I can get food down. I know I have to eat, so I eat something.

Tell me how you feel right now, at 10 A.M.?

Right now my stomach feels empty, and I had cold cereal and milk this morning. I just feel empty, but I don't feel nauseated, but then . . . I took two of the Bendectin* before I went to bed. I was just taking one and that did not help at all. So then I quit taking it at all; I thought, "This is ridiculous to even take this pill because it's not helping." But then I tried two for the last two days, and when I wake up I don't feel nauseated. Bendectin is an antinausea drug. . . . It's the only drug that has been proven safe in pregnancy, I've been told, and I've taken a lot of it.

Do you ever get nauseated when you're lying down? Do you have the gagging feeling then?

It's just kind of there with you all the time. It's like it predominates your mind—that's all you can think of—it's just that you have this uneasy feeling here in your throat and in your stomach. You just know it's there and when it starts getting worse, you automatically start breathing through your mouth. It's just like an automatic reaction; you want to breathe through your mouth. It gets worse when I go outside when it's really hot. When I have to run around in the car I come in to where it's really cool. I just *need* this cool air, but then I get an overwhelming nausea. When I've been in the heat and come in to sit down and rest . . . then the feeling becomes nausea, when you know you're going to vomit anytime soon. Those are the times when I actually vomit a little more. But usually, it seems like my stomach is empty. Do you know what I mean? When I actually vomit—even if I have eaten not too far before—it seems like there's nothing in my stomach to vomit!

We went to the mountains this weekend where it was cooler, but I still had the nausea. But I didn't ever have that overwhelming desire to vomit like I get when it's hot. Also, the nausea seems to get worse if I don't eat. If I don't eat something every so many hours, then I go through . . . "yuk" . . . it's strange. . . . I have pains in my stomach like I'm hungry, but the thought of food doesn't appeal to me; then I don't want to eat. It's funny, I can tell my stomach is empty and that I need to eat something, but just the thought of eating anything is repulsive. Nothing sounds like it's good to eat. Nothing!

Tell me about the change in your breathing that you referred to earlier.

You know how it is when you have the flu: You're going to vomit, you want to vomit, and you vomit. With this, I don't want to vomit. I get this uneasy feeling and, as it gets stronger, I just automatically want to breathe through my mouth. I just keep breathing through my mouth, but it's not like I'm panting.

You're taking deep breaths?

Yeah, through my mouth. It just seems to help this feeling somehow. Overall, it seems like the Bendectin is working better now. But I don't know if it's working better or I'm getting towards the end of the nausea, when I won't be feeling like I do now. I am more than two months pregnant now.

Interview with L.W.

When do you think you became pregnant?

The first week in September.

This is October 26.

I'm about 10 weeks on the pregnancy wheel, more like eight weeks, but it's counted as 10 weeks.

Have you been nauseated?

When I've been nauseated, I've really been nauseated. It's not a constant, continual thing. When I am, it's a very bad nausea. It's like no type I've ever had with flu, food poisoning, or anything like that.

When did you first have the queasy nauseated feeling?

About a month ago.

That would have been . . . the end of September. You think you got pregnant about September 1. That would place it about five weeks after your last period that the nausea started.

But it just happened for one day. Then I didn't have it for three or four days. Then I had it again. Then it came a little bit more frequently.

Is this a planned pregnancy?

Yes.

You and husband wanted a baby?

Yes. I went off the pill . . . I didn't get pregnant when I went off the pill. I've been off the pill for almost two years. I got pregnant this summer and had a miscarriage and I had to have a D and C. It wasn't a full D and C . . . the end of July or August first, somewhere around there. Then I got pregnant again. The pregnancy works out better this way because now I can finish my degree. The baby should come two weeks after I'm done and two weeks before my husband gets his Ph.D. at Berkeley.

This pregnancy comes at a perfect time. I didn't want to be pregnant here in the summer. I just couldn't stand being pregnant here in the summer. I just think it would be terrible. If I'd let it go too long, I doubt if I could have gotten to Berkeley. Eight and a half months' pregnant.

Can you tell me what your nausea is like? Can you describe it or draw a word picture?

It reminds me of being seasick, a very queasy feeling, where, no food tastes good. No food seems to really calm it down.

Does your nausea feel like a knot in your stomach, is it . . . ?

It is not a knot. It's an empty feeling. It's kind of like being seasick, being really rocky. Anything that you would take in would make it worse.

Can you stand on your feet? Are you dizzy?

No. Not dizzy.

When you're seasick, you're dizzy. You're not dizzy with this?

No. I can stand up, and I can function pretty well, but I'm just. . . . It reminds me of, like, when after you've done a lot of somersaults. You kind of get up and . . . the room kind of moves around. It's that kind of feeling. It's a very . . . I want to say queasy, but that doesn't describe it for you.

Do you have a tightness in your chest or your throat?

Always in my stomach.

Does your stomach jump around, like it has butterflies in it? Is that what you're trying to say?

Yes, very much so.

What about smells? Smell of bacon cooking, smell of something baking . . .

I haven't done any cooking. If I don't feel like eating, I don't cook it.

What about your husband, does he cook?

Well, he doesn't eat breakfast, so I'm not around food in the morning. If I think a food is going to make me nauseated, then I don't prepare it for him. He eats what I eat.

Are you nauseated when you're lying down in bed?

Yes, in the morning.

On the days you get up and are nauseated, can you recollect what time you went to bed the night before?

Probably between 9:00 and 9:30 P.M.; that's the time I go to bed every night.

Since you've been pregnant?

Yes. The nausea doesn't bother me as much as the fatigue does. I figure the nausea will go away. The fatigue does not; it stays with you all day. Sometimes it will be bad in the morning. Then it will clear up—the nausea. I'll just be a little tired all day. Then it will be worse at night after dinner.

After you've eaten?

Yes.

Have you ever had to throw up?

Yes. I've thrown up about three times.

Have you thrown up food?

Yes.

Really vomited up the dinner that you had?

Yes.

Most of the time, what is it like? Do you really vomit?

From the toes up.

Food, each time?

No, not food each time. But when I do vomit, it seems like everything that's ever been in my stomach comes up.

But vomiting is the uncommon situation for you?

Yes. Mostly it's just the nauseated feeling. When it does finally trigger the vomiting, everything comes up, then nothing will stay down, not even ice water—once the vomiting trigger gets off.

Eating small, frequent meals wouldn't stop it?

No.

Do you do anything at night before you go to bed to prevent nausea?

I'll sometimes have a glass of milk—only because I'm hungry, and milk seems to taste good. Coffee and tea seem to be the stimuli for the nausea; they make it much worse, so I've given them up. I never have been one to drink colas or 7-Up. My main thing has been trying to find something that will taste good.

You've never smoked?

No.

The smell of food cooking, the thought of food, or just seeing food on television seems to trigger nausea for some women. You say this doesn't bother you?

No, but I kind of have a hard stomach. It's hard to get me to upchuck. It takes a really powerful stimulus. Food doesn't do it, that I know of.

But foods you've eaten for a long time taste different to you? Would you explain what foods? Milk tastes good?

Yes, milk tastes very good. Coffee and tea have a different taste. Cooked vegetables, like fresh broccoli and fresh spinach, don't taste very good, for some reason. I think another thing is prenatal vitamins. They're high in Vitamin B, and iron, folic acid. They give you terrible breath. I think they change the taste in your mouth. I always have like a coating on my tongue. I can't get rid of it, no matter how I brush it. I've noticed it just since I started taking the prenatal vitamins.

The taste alteration?

I think it's partly from the vitamins.

You think you can bring on the vomiting? It never really progresses to vomiting unless you have coffee or tea, for sure?

Sometimes it would go on to vomiting . . . I put on fishsticks for dinner one time. Fish, baked fish was a stimulus one time.

Just eating the food, not smelling it made you vomit?

I ate it. It could have been a combination.

Have you ever had dry heaves?

I've had a couple of dry heaves, but nothing has ever come up. No mucus ever came up. But it felt like dry heaves. It didn't last very long, just a couple of times.

When you first had this nauseated feeling, did you think you were pregnant right away?

I suspected it. Number one, being late was one of the things because I never have been late. Even after the pill, like clockwork. Very regular. So by the time I was a week late, I was beginning to suspect it. By the time I was three weeks late, I was very fatigued, and hungry. I've never really been hungry in my whole life. Never had a real craving for food. I would eat breakfast, an egg, an English muffin, glass of milk, and coffee. At ten o'clock, I was starving.

Was this before you became nauseated?

Yes . . . at ten o'clock I would be starving. I would just have fruit and a piece of cheese for lunch in Illinois. Now I was having sandwiches, and fruit, and everything; then I was hungry again at two o'clock and hungry again at four. A lot hungrier. But by the time I got to the fifth or sixth week, that tapered off and the nausea started. Then I went and got a home pregnancy-testing kit. It was positive and I had it confirmed by the doctor.

Does activity seem to trigger the nausea? I know you're fatigued, so you can't do what you used to do. Let's just say routine housework, chores.

Well, I used to jog every morning. That never bothered me until a couple of weeks ago—didn't bother me with the nausea. If I were nauseated when I went out to jog, the jogging didn't make it any worse. If I felt fine when I went out and jogged, when I came back I felt fine, too. So the jogging didn't make any difference. I can barely make a mile anymore, I'm just exhausted. I have to go home and go back to bed.

You don't go to bed nauseated or sick every night after you eat?

Not every night, but probably four nights a week I go to bed feeling queasy and shaky. If I can go right to sleep, it seems to settle down. I have a dry cracker every morning.

Does that help?

It seems to.

But you don't eat breakfast?

I try to eat a little bit. I don't eat anything that I think is going to make me sick. I will, like, have a piece of toast, and that's all. Then at 9:30 or 10:00 o'clock I'll have a piece of fruit or a glass of milk, or something like that. I eat a little bit gradually in the morning; if I don't eat something, I think I feel worse.

Do you think keeping something in your stomach helps keep the feeling suppressed?

Yes. Otherwise I get too hungry, and I feel like I'm getting kind of hypoglycemic-feeling, really jittery and shaky. That makes the nausea much worse. I always try to eat a little bit of something and then just eat gradually until 11:00 A.M. Then I get a full breakfast. Because it's not what you eat; if you're going to eat 100 grams of protein a day and throw it all up, you're back to square one. It's better to eat a little bit as you go, and keep it down. Because what you keep down is what counts.

So you eat because you think you need to eat because you're pregnant, or because if you don't eat you're going to be sick and you'll pay the price?

Both. I've been very careful not to take even an aspirin.

You're not on any antinausea medication?

No, the doctor asked me if I wanted that and I refused it, because I think it's risky. I figure this is something I'll just have to live with and it will get better. . . . I think it's going to get a lot worse before it gets better. Not necessarily the nausea—what I mean is the other things that go with pregnancy, the physical discomforts. These are going to get worse before they get better. This is something I'm going to have to learn to live with, without resorting to medication. I'm hoping I'm going to be over the nausea in a couple of weeks, maybe three more weeks. I'm hoping it won't last too much longer. If I had a full forty-hour-a-week job I wouldn't be able to do it—not from nausea, but from fatigue.

Interview with P.K.

How many weeks' pregnant are you?

I went to the doctor today and he says 12 weeks, 3 months.

Have you been nauseated?

Yes.

When did your nausea start?

The first time was just after we moved here, which was August 2nd. It was about two weeks after I skipped my first period. I was looking nausea up in my nursing books because I wondered how long it would last. The book said that's when it usually starts, two weeks after you get pregnant, so I knew it was right on time.

Were your periods usually regular?

Yes, very regular. I was sure when I skipped that I was pregnant. It's just a feeling that started in the morning with a lot of fatigue. Getting up in the morning and having a feeling of nausea.

What is the nausea like?

It's hard to describe. . . . just a feeling in my stomach that I was going to vomit or that I couldn't eat. It was hard to know what I wanted to eat. Just looking at food or smelling it, even thinking about it or seeing it on television would make me have this feeling in my stomach. It's not really like a pain; it's just an uncomfortable feeling.

Did you salivate with it?

No, I've been really kind of thirsty. I've been able to drink a lot of milk. I started to feel better for three or four days and I thought, "Oh good, it's going away." Then it came back and I had the same feeling. I called my doctor and he gave me a prescription for Bendectin. He said to take two at night and one midmorning for awhile. I was doing okay. After I'd eat breakfast, I'd start to feel nauseated again, so I would take a pill midmorning and that would help the rest of the day. Then I was nauseated in the morning too, so I had to start taking them at night and they really helped. When I get up, I don't feel nauseated. I feel a little tired, but I'm able to go and eat breakfast and get going in the morning.

Prior to the time you took the Bendectin when you got nauseated, did it ever culminate in vomiting?

Yes. The second week I started working at the hospital I woke up one morning and I had this terrible headache and was really nauseated; and I did vomit. I wasn't sure if I had the flu or something else because I hadn't been this sick to my stomach in the few weeks I'd been nauseated. That day I felt pretty bad all day. It lasted for a day and I did vomit twice.

Did you vomit food?

I tried to eat breakfast, thinking that I'd feel better. When I get up and feel nauseated I eat breakfast . . . just force myself. It was better if my husband fixed it, so I wouldn't have to look at it. I just have a scrambled egg or a poached egg on dry toast and some milk—just get something in my stomach. Then usually if I just sit quietly for an hour I feel better. I can get going and go to work and I feel fine most of the rest of the day, except when I get hungry; then the nausea comes back. If I don't eat at least every couple of hours, I start to feel hungry and the nausea starts to come with it. Then I have to drink some milk or eat a sandwich . . . something to make that feeling go away.

Can you describe it any more specifically? Is it like when you had nausea and vomiting with the flu or a gastrointestinal upset?

The only way I could compare it to the flu would be like that one morning when I did vomit and then I thought I had the flu. I don't know for sure. A couple of other mornings I thought I really had to get to the bathroom to vomit . . . but I didn't. I don't know how to describe it. You feel that it's coming. You're right on the verge. Your stomach muscles tighten and you feel you're going to vomit. It's right there. I've had that feeling a couple of times but then I'm not able to vomit. That's as close as you can get to vomiting and that feeling is like the flu. It's not like the flu in that with the flu you feel the symptoms for several hours. You know it's coming on. You know you've got the flu. You have to lie down. You just can't eat anything. With this nausea, I feel good, and I think I'd just feel fine if I just had a little more energy. I guess I would just call the way I feel as a low feeling in the bottom of my stomach, like a knot or something.

I know it's hard to describe. If you kept your stomach full do you think the feeling would stop?

Yes. I've felt that when I started to feel better it was because I had eaten. Like, before I went to bed I'd had a cheese sandwich and some milk. That was something I could eat that wouldn't bother me. I think it helped me through the night. If I went to bed at 11:00 P.M. or midnight and ate before I went to bed, I wasn't as hungry when I woke up in the morning and I wasn't as nauseated. For awhile when I started orienting at the hospital, I was tired. I worked the day shift. I was going to bed at 8:00 P.M. and going without eating until 5:00 in the morning. I felt really sick when I got up. I told my husband that maybe if I got up and ate something, I'd feel better. But of course, I didn't want to get up in the middle of the night.

Do you think now the symptoms are subsiding because you're on the Bendectin?

Yes, I'm sure it's the Bendectin. I wonder if I should go off it for a couple of days and see what happens. Maybe I'll wait a little while longer.

What does this whole thing mean to you? This nausea of pregnancy? Did you anticipate it?

No. I know they say it can be in your head. You can have psychosomatic illnesses. I didn't really think about it. I wanted to get pregnant, and it happened. I got pregnant right away, the first month we tried. I have been using the ovulation method. I was able to watch my mucus—just count my days, because my cycles were extremely regular. I've never had any problems. It was easy to count the days and watch the mucus and go from there. I didn't think I'd get pregnant so easily. We wanted to have children, so we figured if it doesn't work right away, fine, but we wanted to try it. The first month we went off the method I was pregnant and that was fine. I was excited about it. I never really thought of being sick until it happened.

And when did it happen, specifically?

Two weeks after I skipped my period. If I had looked in my books and started reading about it, maybe I would have thought, "I'm going to get sick in a couple of weeks." It wasn't like that. I never thought of it. After we moved here and I got my books unpacked I thought, I'm going to start looking things up and see how long this is going to last. Then I saw I was going by the book. The nausea started right on time.

Did your husband want the baby, too?

Yes.

How do you feel today?

I feel great today, although I'm kind of tired. I took two Bendectin before I went to bed about midnight, and I got up this morning and ate breakfast. I got ready to go to the doctor, and I was able to walk to the doctor's and felt just fine. Before I took those pills, it would take me all morning to get going. I'd feel the nausea and I'd have to lie down and rest. If I ate, I'd have to sit for half an hour, and then I'd feel real tired. Now I feel great.

Do you think that the nausea is a positional kind of thing? In other words, when you're lying flat in bed, and then sit up—is that when you experience the nausea?

Usually when I wake up I feel nauseated. My husband always asks me the first thing, "Well, how do you feel today?" He hopes I'm feeling better. I usually say, "I don't really know yet." I feel tired lying there. The more I think, the more I think the feeling will come on when I get up. It was really worse when I tried to cook . . . just the smell of food and sight of food . . . going grocery shopping . . . it was all I could do just to look at food. Anything I looked at made me feel like I was going to be sick. It's awful because usually when you go shopping you look forward to buying things . . . trying out new recipes. . . . It's really hard!

You don't remember when you were at the worst of your nausea whether or not you'd sweat?

I was really sweating that day I thought I had the flu. Maybe it was just a bad day.

You say that the nausea you experience is a lump in your stomach?

Yes. When it gets worse, I run to the bathroom and it doesn't come. It just settles. I wondered if when I started working and the tension of moving, getting a new job, getting settled in a new apartment, things like that . . . I wondered if some of the anxiety from all that was causing it, too. Usually when you start a new job, you're kind of nervous, maybe have butterflies, but I don't know I . . . felt good about my work, everyone was so friendly there. I felt like I just got right into it. I didn't really think that it would be making it worse . . . I didn't feel tense about going to work or anything. Also, because I kept thinking, "We want the baby." It's not something I would be really against. And that would make me feel sick or something.
    When I've had the flu, I've felt just kind of general malaise. I feel awful all over. With the flu, you just feel like you can't be up and around. But with this nausea, if I don't feel like I'm going to vomit, I get that feeling when I get hungry. But I feel like I could still work. I could walk around, take care of patients, and do things even though that feeling was there—as when you have the flu you just don't want to get up or do anything. You just feel terrible all over. With this nausea, I knew if I got it at work, I just needed

to eat. When hunger came the nausea came with it. If I just even grabbed a glass of milk, that would curb it.

I'm going to call my mother tonight. I don't remember her ever saying she had morning sickness. I'm curious now to ask her about it. I feel like I've had a bad case. I was wondering if it were hereditary. It is discouraging enough to make you feel that you don't want to get pregnant again for quite awhile because you don't want to have to go through this again. But then I feel that in the end, I'll have my baby. That compensates. You do feel awful, though, when you can't get things done at home.

You haven't missed any work?

Just that one day when I did vomit. I thought maybe I had the flu and stayed home. That day I stayed in bed all day. Otherwise, when I had to get up in the mornings and I felt bad . . . once I forced myself to eat and rest a little while I'd be able to get going to work. Going to work got my mind off it, too. Once I got up and got going I had a little more energy. On my days off, I would sit home and it would take me forever to get going. I wouldn't get anything done. I'm glad I'm able to work. I need that.

ETIOLOGY

Specific etiology of morning sickness in pregnancy is unknown even though nausea and vomiting have been associated with early pregnancy throughout the history of the civilized world. The phenomenon was known in early Egypt, according to a description recorded on a papyrus dated 2000 B.C. (Fairweather 1968). In ancient Greece, Hippocrates knew of the problem. In Rome, considerable literature on the subject was written before the end of the second century A.D. Soranus, a practicing physician in Rome, wrote *Soranus's Gynecology*, epitomizing the best gynecological and obstetrical practices of the ancient world (Temkin 1968); Soranus's views and practices remained highly influential until the 16th century. In the 17th century, concurrent with the renaissance of science, many French, German, and English physicians studied and reported on the phenomenon of early-pregnancy morning sickness. During both the 17th and 18th centuries, there was considerable preoccupation with etiology. Only at the end of the 18th century was vomiting addressed in its mild and pernicious forms by an Englishman named Vaughn. During the next 100 years, the study of hyperemesis gravidarum—its incidence, causes, and treatment—had priority. Research in the 20th century focused on the psychological, psychosomatic, and sociocultural aspects of both "morning nausea" and hyperemesis gravidarum. Past and present-day clinicians and scholars have postulated that hormones (progesterone, estrogen, testosterone, chorionic gonadotropin, anterior pituitary), disturbed carbohydrate metabolism, vitamin deficiency (B-complex), and allergies may cause morning sickness. To date, research supports no theory or specific etiology (Fairweather 1968).

Many theories about the etiology of morning sickness have been proposed. While Soranus does not offer a theory of etiology, he states that if the fetus is male the tendency to vomit will be much greater (Temkin 1968). In the 17th and 18th centuries, various stomach humoral theories were proposed; "longings" recognized by some were seen as early recognition of possible emotional causes. One physician during this period believed vomiting was related to menses and that distended blood vessels pressed on nerves of the diaphragm. Other theoreticians believed the vomiting to be protective, ridding the patient of superfluous food, thus preventing increased turgor of visceral blood vessels; still others thought that it rid the body of decomposed and undigested foods. Stretching of the uterus was commonly viewed as the cause of nausea and vomiting up until the 19th century. Late in the 19th century, there was an attempt to classify the theories of etiology. At first, the following seven categories were identified:

1. "sympathy" with the uterus
2. congestive inflammation and great tenderness of the os and cervix uteri in the later months
3. some irritable condition of the cervix
4. ulceration of the cervix uteri
5. morbid irritation of the uterus and inflammation of the deciduous membrane
6. distention and evolution of the uterine fiber or pelvic irritation
7. displacement and flexions of the uterus.

Eventually, there was agreement on three categories—reflex, neurotic, and toxemic (Fairweather 1968).

In 1932, a symposium of the current literature was published by the Bi So Dol Company and believed to represent the gist of current medical opinion on morning sickness and toxemia of pregnancy (hyperemesis gravidarum) in which hyperemesis gravidarum was described as "the disease of theories" (Bi So Dol 1932). In terms of etiology of morning sickness, both physical and psychological causes were advanced: neuroses, displaced uteri, cervical erosions, adhesions, and constipation. From the psychological point of view, the thesis was advanced that some women felt that nausea and vomiting were a real part of pregnancy: ". . . When one of these women misses a period, she eagerly looks for the onset of morning vomiting to clinch the proof that she is pregnant." From the purely physical point of view, during the 1920s and 1930s pregnant women generally were looked upon as being in an extremely unstable condition in regard to metabolism and subject to sudden deviations in normal bodily functions.

The focus of recent research has been on hyperemesis gravidarum. There is, however, a small group of researchers interested in morning sickness. One group identified an inverse relationship between gastric acidity and chorionic gonadotropin secretion; gastric hypoacidity was associated with maximal chorionic gonadotropin secretion. This is said to diminish gastric motility and produce nausea and vomiting (Way 1945).

In terms of fetal outcome, some studies suggest that the *absence* of nausea and vomiting of pregnancy is associated with a high abortion rate (Speert and Guttmacher 1959; Medalie 1957; and Walford 1963). Another study also speaks of fetal outcome: Female infants ($N = 6,637$) of women who had no nausea and vomiting had a 70 percent higher rate of perinatal mortality than female infants of women who had nausea and vomiting. This higher perinatal mortality was entirely due to the fact that the 7.9 percent of women who did not have nausea and vomiting delivered infants weighing less than 5.5 pounds (the top cutoff point for assignment to the low-birth-weight category). These same women had shorter gestations and delivered a higher male sex ratio (117.4:100) at termination of the pregnancy (Brandes 1967); this concurs with Soranus's observations that if the fetus is male, the mother's tendency to vomit will be much greater than if the fetus is female (Temkin 1968).

Psychosomatic researchers acknowledge that the percentage of all pregnant women who suffer from nausea, with or without vomiting, appears to be too high to be caused solely by personality disorders. Even so, theoreticians continue to believe that nausea in pregnancy has strong roots in the psyche. Two studies indicate that there are no significant psychological differences among pregnant women who vomit, except in women who have hyperemesis gravidarum (Semmens 1971; and Netter-Munkett, Mau, and Konig 1972).

Chertok (1972) conducted a study with pregnant women in France in which he tested, among others, the hypothesis that vomiting is positively correlated with ambivalent attitudes of the mother toward the fetus. One hundred women were first interviewed during the *third* month of pregnancy from which Chertok ascertained the "original attitude of the women" and concluded that, "vomiting may therefore represent the *expression* of a conflict between wanting and rejecting the child." This apparently cause-and-effect relationship was not proved. But for those women who *were* ambivalent, it is not hard to imagine how having had nausea and vomiting for two months might cause them to have second thoughts about their pregnancies. Chertok did not suggest that the higher incidence of ambivalence in pregnant women who vomit may be due to this discomfort and not the pregnancy itself. Nausea was not taken into account at all in Chertok's study.

Ziegel and Van Blaricom (1972), also proponents of emotional etiology for nausea, stated, "Nausea may very likely be due to a state of tension." They believe that nausea disappears after the first trimester because the emotional as well as the physical adjustments have been made by that time. According to the stress-and-ambivalent-tension theory, prevention of morning sickness might be rest and relaxation since these measures reduce tension; but, in practice, these measures do not prevent the problem. Emotional factors are but one area of many factors affecting the severity of morning sickness.

INCIDENCE OF NAUSEA

Morning sickness is not a rare phenomenon. Mild nausea and vomiting, the so-called morning sickness, are said to constitute the most common disorder of the first trimester of pregnancy (Reader et al. 1976). Prevalence estimates range from approximately 20 to 50 percent of all pregnancies (Kolata 1980; and Ziegel and Van Blaricom 1976). Incidence of the phenomenon seems to have cultural variability with low or no incidence reported in Eskimo, native African, or American Indian populations (Benson 1966; and Louw 1966). Further, the incidence is said to be greatly reduced in wartime.

The incidence of hyperemesis gravidarum (severe, pathological nausea and vomiting) may be as high as five percent, although studies do not bear this out. There seems also to be a wide variation of incidence among countries and even among cities in the same country. For example, incidence of hyperemesis gravidarum is also low among Eskimo and African as compared to European and American populations. The incidence in urban centers may differ from that in smaller communities, and time period influences the incidence. During both World War I and II it occurred rarely according to studies done in Germany. Hyperemesis gravidarum also occurs rarely in times when food is scarce. During stable periods, the incidence of hyperemesis gravidarum in the United States, England, Germany, and France is reported to be between 1.5 and 3.5 cases per 1,000 total births. Accurate determination of incidence is confounded by sampling problems and case-definition problems (Fairweather 1968).

The onset of morning sickness and hyperemesis gravidarum is said to occur nearly simultaneously, but authors differ about when the onset of nausea and/or vomiting occurs. Some researchers state that it starts one or two days after the first menses is missed, while others state it in terms of conception, beginning up to 40 days after conception. Sterk et al. (1971) found that one-half of the pregnant women ($N = 9,202$) started vomiting in the first month of pregnancy.

Morning sickness, once initiated, may last five months, but the more common pattern is nausea beginning after the first month and subsiding by the beginning of the fourth month. Actually, morning sickness may be a misnomer. Even though morning sickness is associated with a particular time of day, that is, some women have their symptoms upon awakening and at breakfast only, others have symptoms that persist through the noon meal, and an occasional woman is said to have nausea and might possibly vomit in relation to the evening meal. Women who experience nausea and vomiting in the evening may have some disturbance of appetite also. Food cravings and antipathies may cause nausea and revulsion.

SYMPTOMS AND COURSE

Morning sickness has not been studied for associated symptomatology, but through the centuries a variety of associations have been made. First and foremost, the pregnant woman is said to have some first-trimester nausea and vomiting. It is estimated that one-half of the women defined as having morning sickness have nausea without vomiting, but that all hyperemesis gravidarum patients vomit (Fairweather 1968).

In morning sickness there is no appreciable weight loss, no ketosis, and no disturbed nutrition. This is in marked contrast to the woman with hyperemesis gravidarum, who has constant vomiting and may dribble saliva from her mouth. Women with hyperemesis gravidarum may have a five percent or greater weight loss; their urine becomes scanty and concentrated and the pulse rate is somewhat accelerated. Other symptoms associated with morning sickness are headache, loss of appetite, sleepiness, inertia, fatigue, irritability, dizziness, constipation, change in libido, gastric bloating, painful breasts, and swollen breasts. The incidence of these symptoms and their relationship to morning sickness is unknown.

Morning sickness is usually resolved during the first trimester of pregnancy with only minor adjustments in living and dietary habits. Without competent intervention, however, hyperemesis gravidarum may cause delirium, coma, and life-threatening convulsions, which before this century often caused death.

In addition to the descriptions of nausea and vomiting provided by the three women we interviewed, we spoke with 14 other women in our attempt to clarify the symptoms and define the course of the phenomenon. Eleven of the fourteen women reported that they had experienced "morning" nausea at different times during the day, and four women complained of having "morning sickness" all the time, while still another woman's "morning" nausea began in the afternoon. The woman whose nausea appeared in the afternoon believed that her experience was probably attributable to the fact that she worked the night shift and had a different biorhythm than other women.

The experiences of women interviewed do not appear to differ from most descriptions of women with morning nausea found in the literature, except for the four women who experienced nausea and vomiting throughout the entire day. Only one report noted "an increasing number of patients who complain of severe nausea in the evening and even vague nausea during all waking hours" (David and Doyle 1976).

As far as what triggers the nausea is concerned, several women mentioned that what they ate before going to bed might affect their nausea in the morning. Milk seemed to increase nausea as did high-carbohydrate, very sweet foods. One interviewee said that food in her stomach at night relieved her morning nausea. None of the women could associate any emotional stress or problem with the onset of nausea and vomiting. One woman was having some marital difficulties but did not feel that this was the cause of her nausea. Another remarked that she felt as though her emotions were on a seesaw; one minute she was quite happy, the next she was depressed and crying. This same woman said her nausea began before she noticed the emotional swings and before she missed her first period. One woman recalled vomiting in a shopping center while another vomited at work. Exercise seemed to precipitate nausea, especially in the morning. One rule of thumb employed by the women was to postpone making the bed and other activities until noon.

Several women reported that cigarette smoke (their own or someone else's) stimulated or increased nausea. Drinking alcohol, even wine, caused nausea and vomiting in two cases. Fatty foods, especially oily salad dressings, caused problems for all but one woman.

TREATMENT

Advice given to women early in this century to combat nausea was intended to treat a hyperacidic situation. Specifically, "Simple cases (of nausea and vomiting) can usually be helped by eating frequently in small amounts; by not rising in the morning on an empty stomach; by the use of laxatives and by such simple remedies as bicarbonate of soda, milk of magnesia, cerium oxalate, or a simple mixture of cerium oxalate, bismuth and ginger. They find ginger ale in small amounts most helpful (Bi So Dol 1932)." Hard, dry biscuits were particularly recommended on awakening before raising one's head off the pillow; this form of treatment is also recommended in current literature (Temkin 1968; Ziegel and Van Blaricom 1972; David and Doyle 1976; Hellman et al. 1971; Boston Women's Health Book Collective 1976; and Shervington 1974). Other unorthodox solutions cited in recent literature are hibernotherapy, intravenously administered honey, husband's blood, and husband's sex hormone (testosterone) (Hellman et al. 1971).

Does the Advice Work?

Eating dry crackers in bed before arising was tried by every woman who we interviewed who experienced morning sickness. It was not helpful for any woman.

Five women resorted to medication (Bendectin) for relief of the nausea and vomiting but did not obtain total relief, and four of the five felt guilty for taking a drug. Four women obtained relief after having a protein snack at bedtime. All women reported symptoms of malaise, constipation, and exhaustion and said that "fatigue, an empty stomach, or disagreeable odors" all increased nausea.

The two women who did not have nausea and vomiting expressed their own ideas about why they did not: One said, "I am in perfect physical shape" and the other, "I have an iron stomach; nothing bothers my gut." The second woman, who smoked, stopped when she was two months pregnant. Smoke, however, never nauseated her; none of the women interviewed smoked during their pregnancies.

Treatment of the nausea and vomiting for each woman was, as Hellman, Pritchard, and Wynn (1971) describe, "seldom . . . so successful that the mother is afforded complete relief." In addition to eating crackers and avoiding fatty foods, several women tried eating dry meals or eating small, frequent meals as the women we interviewed indicated and which seemed to be the most helpful solution. In general, all women stated that it was very difficult to eat anything at all when they felt nauseated, but that keeping food in the stomach often warded off nausea. Only three women claimed to have found a solution for morning sickness that worked: Rather than eating high-carbohydrate food as recommended in books on pregnancy, these women ate food high in protein and low in carbohydrate and fat. All three stated that this gave them immediate relief in most instances. One woman ate a high-protein snack before going to bed at night and found this decreased her morning nausea immensely.

Exactly what physiological processes are altered in morning nausea remains speculative. One text consulted discussed protein as a treatment for nausea and vomiting; increased protein intake was said to increase blood sugar by gluconeogenesis (Hartman 1975). Reinken and Gant (1974) found a relationship between altered protein metabolism in 24 women with hyperemesis gravidarum and an increased need for Vitamin B_6. Weidenbach (1967) speaks of a change in carbohydrate metabolism. Ziegel and Van Blaricom (1972) report an increase in metabolism in general. Krause and Hunseher (1972) also suggest a need for increased dietary protein due to an overall increase in metabolism.

Finally, some women admitted feelings of ambivalence toward the baby during the first trimester. Only one woman felt guilty about these feelings. She and her husband had planned the pregnancy and she could not understand why, at times, she did not want the baby. McBride (1973) explains ambivalent feelings of expectant mothers as "real love and real hate at one and the same time, not some watered-down neutral feelings." Ambivalence is normal, she states, and further, "living with your own ambivalence is a good preparation for dealing with the mixed feelings that your child is bound to have toward you in the future."

A PROPOSED PHYSIOLOGICAL ETIOLOGY OF MORNING NAUSEA

The physiological changes that occur in the maternal organism are widespread and complex and, as the literature indicated, they are established often fully during the early weeks and months of pregnancy. Some workers suggest that because there are so many changes occurring in maternal metabolism, the pregnant female is almost another species (Hytten and Leitch 1964).

No longer tenable, however, is the hypothesis of maternal changes being due to the "stress" of the fetus or to a depletion of maternal reserves. Many changes appear to occur so very early that they cannot be responses to an immediate need; rather, they represent early, preprogrammed, fundamental maternal adjustments (hormonally induced) that are necessary to safeguard the fetus in later stages of gestation. This explanation implies that the maternal changes are initiated at the time of conception, or, to be more accurate, after ovulation.

Homeostasis

One of the most important aspects of homeostasis is concerned with water and its role as the internal environment in which all metabolic reactions occur. The principle of physiological homeostasis requires that blood-electrolyte levels, sodium particularly, be maintained and regulated within very narrow limits in this internal water environment. The regulation of water and electrolytes is a complex process, the end goal being to maintain a constancy of concentration of body fluids in which metabolic reactions can occur. This control in the nonpregnant state is achieved mainly by the synergistic action of two hormones—posterior pituitary antidiuretic hormone (ADH) and aldosterone, the adrenal mineralocorticoid. Serum osmolality, which is a function of the number of particles in a solution, is maintained at about 290 mOsm/kilogram (mOsm/kg) in the nonpregnant state and is done so largely as a result of the regulatory activity of ADH and aldosterone.

Normally, a prolonged increase or decrease in the body fluids results in pathology to the organism. An increase or decrease in concentration of blood plasma ($>$ or $<$ 290 mOsm/kg) is termed *hemoconcentration* or *hemodilution*; either condition has its clinical or sick correlates. Hemodilution is probably better known to nurses since it is a common clinical entity encountered in postoperative patients due to a stress-induced, inappropriate secretion of both antidiuretic and aldosterone hormones (Bland 1963; and Moran et al. 1964). Hemodilution clinically is referred to as a *dilutional hyponatremia*. Common symptoms of this condition are confusion, headache, anxiety, restlessness, nausea, vomiting, apathy, and fatigue (Hayes 1968).

All pregnant women increase total body water to expand the plasma volume. The overall physiological effect of plasma volume expansion is to decrease the serum osmolality; that is, a relative hemodilution occurs and it is known that serum osmolality in pregnant women decreases to about 280 mOsm/kg (from 290 mOsm/kg in the nonpregnant state) (MacDonald and Good 1971, 1972; and Robertson and Cheyne 1972) early in pregnancy with no further significant change throughout the remainder of pregnancy. Robertson and Cheyne (1972) suggest that osmolality change occurs during the first eight weeks. MacDonald and Good (1971) disagree; they hypothesize that the change occurs more abruptly—about two to four weeks after ovulation. No work has been done to test their hypotheses. Once the osmoreceptors are finally reset to those lower levels, they are maintained at a fairly constant level for the remainder of pregnancy. Thus, we can hypothesize that it is at this time that the nausea and vomiting of pregnancy should subside.

Recently updated knowledge of the normal events associated with the menstrual cycle, particularly the natriuretic (salt-losing) action for the gonadal hormone, progesterone, has changed long-held assumptions that progesterone was a salt-retaining hormone. We now know that the postovulatory luteal-phase progesterone increase in women is associated with increased circulating levels of aldosterone, the adrenal mineralocorticoid (Katz and Romfh 1972; Sundsfjord and Aakvaag 1972; Schwartz and Abraham 1975; and Voda 1980). The mechanism of action by which progesterone affects peripheral aldosterone levels to promote salt loss is postulated to be that of competitive inhibition of aldosterone by progesterone. Specifically, progesterone may prevent the stimulation of sodium transport by effectively competing for receptor-binding sites in the renal tubule (Landau and Lugibihl 1958). This inhibits the peripheral action of the mineralocorticoid in the renal nephron. The inhibition of aldosterone is explained on the basis of the structural similarity of steroids; that is, they possess three six-membered rings and one five-membered ring. Knowledge of structural similarity and the fact that steroids can bind to target-cell receptors to inhibit the action of other steroids is the basis for the effective use of synthetic-steroid analog antagonists. Spironolactone (Aldactone) is an example of an aldosterone antagonist. Aldactone is thought to bind with the aldosterone receptor to prevent salt reabsorption and promote salt loss. Both aldosterone and progesterone levels are known to increase and stay at high levels during pregnancy (Hytten and Leitch 1964). Along with ADH increase, aldosterone functions to increase and maintain an absolute increase in circulating plasma volume during pregnancy. It has already been mentioned that the exact time of onset of these hormone-initiated maternal adjustments is unknown. MacDonald and Good (1971, 1972) place the onset at or shortly after conception. This would place the onset of volume increase squarely in the luteal phase of the menstrual cycle. The effects of volume increase are experienced by many women during the premenstruum as edema, bloating, or some degree of premenstrual tension. If a woman should conceive during a particular ovulatory cycle, the symptoms of edema-initiated premenstrual tension are prolonged. Until such time that adjustments are made, the woman is in a state of biochemical disequilibrium that manifests itself as nausea as well as other symptoms associated with the premenstrual syndrome.

A proposed physiological model to explain these changes and associated behaviors is shown in Figure 8-1.

Figure 8-1 Physiological Model Postulating 1) Adjustment Mechanisms That Occur To Produce First Trimester Nausea and Vomiting and 2) Relationship of the Physiology of the Menstrual Cycle to the Pregnancy Cycle in Terms of Adjustment Mechanisms. See Text for Detailed Explanation.

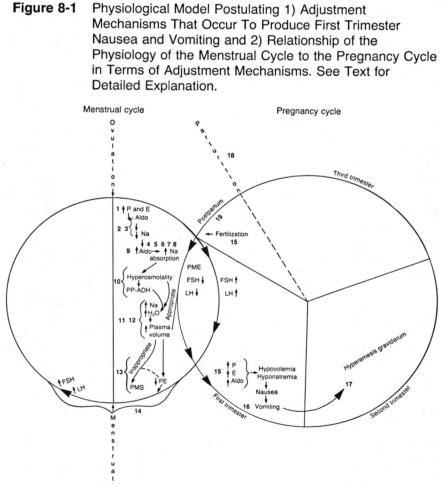

Model Explanation

1. After ovulation, if the corpus luteum is functional and steroidogenic (progesterone [P] plus estrogen [E] synthesis), steroid hormone levels increase in the circulation.
2. As blood progesterone concentration increases, more of this hormone is delivered through the blood to the renal nephron with increased diffusion of progesterone into the distal renal tubule cells.
3. Progesterone binds to the cytosol aldosterone receptor. This inhibits the action of aldosterone to reabsorb sodium (Na^+) (through synthesis of postulated sodium-binding protein), resulting in a progesterone-induced sodium diuresis. The mechanism is probably due to competitive inhibition of aldosterone receptor by progesterone. Maximal diuresis may occur at the midluteal phase of the menstrual cycle.
4. Sodium diuresis may be of two kinds: *Isosmotic,* resulting in a hypovolemic state, or *hyperosmotic,* which results in a hyponatremic state.
5. *Hyponatremia* is a potent stimulus for aldosterone secretion through low sodium levels bathing the adrenal gland and kidney glomrulus, particularly the juxtaglomerular (JGA) apparatus.
6. *Hypovolemia* itself is a potent stimulus to the JGA through a drop in mean blood pressure.

   Both hyponatremia and hypovolemia are potent stimuli for renal renin release (a proteolytic enzyme). Renin catalytically converts liver-synthesized angiotensinogen to angiotensin I.
7. Angiotensin I (a decapeptide) is converted in the lungs to an octapeptide, angiotensin II, which is further converted to the heptapeptide, angiotensin III.
8. Angiotensin II is trophic to the adrenal gland (glomerulosa region) to direct aldosterone synthesis and secretion. Low sodium in the blood bathing the gland also stimulates aldosterone synthesis and secretion. Both mechanisms function to increase blood aldosterone concentration so as to increase sodium reabsorption, which ultimately restores serum osmolality to normal range as well as restores blood volume.
9. As blood aldosterone increases, hypothetically, the competitive inhibition by progesterone is overcome. As sodium concentrations increase, the blood becomes hyperosmolal. This physiological compensation is aided by some women's craving for and ingestion of salty foods.
10. Hyperosmolality of blood plasma bathing hypothalamic supraoptic nuclei cells is postulated to be a potent stimulus for release of ADH; cells shrink due to dehydration, causing them to fire. The message for ADH release is transmitted by the pituitary neural tract to the posterior pituitary (PP); ADH is released as a neurosecretion by secretory granules into the blood.

11. ADH is trophic to the cells of the distal renal tubules and collecting ducts. Through an unknown mechanism (mediated by cyclic adenosine monophosphate [cAMP]), these renal cells become more permeable to water. The net result of simultaneous ADH and aldosterone activity is to increase plasma volume, which may culminate in a combined hypervolemic hyponatremic state (if aldosterone continues to be inhibited by progesterone; increased blood aldosterone concentration is known to follow progesterone in a time-lag fashion [Voda 1980]).

12. An appropriate compensatory response of aldosterone/ADH secretion is to restore an isosmotic eunatremic state, which may result in a condition called "premenstrual edema" wherein a woman experiences weight gain, and/or a subjective feeling of "bloat." Premenstrual water retention is seen as an *appropriate* or normal physiological adjustment mechanism in all women who have ovulatory cycles.

13. An *inappropriate* or overshoot type of compensation may result in the condition called "premenstrual syndrome" (PMS) in which a woman experiences fatigue, negative affect, inability to concentrate, irritability, painful breasts, and so forth.

14. If conception does not occur, gonadal hormone levels fall, due to an atretic nonfunctional corpus luteum. The compensatory aldosterone/ADH activity subsides, since progesterone no longer inhibits aldosterone; menstruation commences and gonadotropic hormone concentration increases to begin a new menstrual cycle.

15. If, however, a woman conceives, the synergistic activity of ADH/aldosterone persists and the woman begins the pregnancy cycle. Plasma volume continues to increase as well as total body sodium until the osmoreceptors are reset to lower levels ($\sim$280 mOsm/kg), supposedly around the end of the first trimester. During this time, a woman may continue to experience some symptoms associated with the premenstruum. Nausea may appear due to ADH-induced hypervolemia and a relative hyponatremia. The nausea may be abetted by eating.

16. Responses to the physiological compensatory-adjustment mechanisms of pregnancy occur so rapidly that exaggerated nausea may proceed to the motor act of vomiting. At this point, medication may be necessary if vomiting becomes uncontrollable.

17. Inappropriate adjustment mechanisms may prolong the vomiting, which, if it continues into the second trimester may result in hyperemesis gravidarum.

18. Subsidence of first-trimester nausea and vomiting culminates in a normal pregnancy and passage through the pregnancy cycle, terminating in an uncomplicated parturition.

19. Postpartum gonadal hormones return to prepartum levels. The woman now reenters the menstrual cycle and will complete this cycle unless fertilization recurs.

CONCLUSION

The focus of contemporary investigations regarding etiology of nausea and vomiting of pregnancy seems to be leaning more toward the psychosomatic aspects. This may, in part, represent an abdication by medical–physiological researchers of a problem that causes considerable human misery without threatening health.

Subscribers to the psychological–etiological theory believe that women know, guess, or feel they are pregnant before experiencing morning sickness. These researchers essentially subscribe to the psychological–etiological position. Even though gastroacidity changes, chorionic gonadotropic changes, and/or plasma biochemistry changes may coincide with the onset of morning sickness, much more work is needed to answer the question, "Is knowing one is or feeling pregnant a prerequisite for morning sickness?"

The literature is very vague on the question of onset of morning sickness; from the clinicians' point of view, the range given seems wide. Such baseline data would be invaluable to biochemical studies if we could answer the question, "How long after conception does morning sickness occur?" Clinicians' estimates range from two to forty days postconception.

The physiological model presented is based on the assumption that some premenstrual fluid retention is a normal consequence of physiological adjustment mechanisms in all women during ovulatory menstrual cycles. Also implicit in the model is the assumption that volume-adjustment mechanisms of pregnancy are initiated during the postovulatory phase of the menstrual cycle. The feeling of abdominal bloat accompanied by premenstrual weight gain and fatigue are seen as indications that necessary prepregnant adjustment mechanisms have been initiated. These premenstrual volume adjustments may endow mammalian species with survival capabilities: The only prerequisite necessary for these changes to occur is that the female ovulate and have a steroid-hormone-synthesizing corpus luteum.

Opponents of the proposed physiological explanation of nausea of first-trimester pregnancy based on menstrual cycle changes may challenge on the grounds that not all women complain of premenstrual bloat or experience weight gain. The fact that women do not have symptoms may be explainable in part from knowledge that not all menstrual cycles are ovulatory cycles. In the past, inclusion of young women in menstrual-cycle studies with small samples who were anovulatory* probably accounts for the variability in reports by women of the prevalence of premenstrual symptoms, particularly water retention and weight gain.

In order to validate a biochemical hyponatremic–hypovolemic hypothesis for the etiology of the first-trimester pregnancy, we need to pinpoint the exact time of onset of nausea. From the model, the following questions can be generated and need to be answered:

1. Did nausea occur during the woman's menstrual cycle?
2. When does morning nausea start? That is, how far removed in time from the estimated date of ovulation and/or conception does nausea occur?
3. Can the nausea be correlated with indirect indicators of hormone activity such as weight gain and lowered sodium levels?
4. Are there associated changes in eating habits during the menstrual cycle? Is more or less food or fluid consumed? Are preferences and avoidances more pronounced? Are foods high in sodium, protein, and/or low in carbohydrate and fat selected?
5. Are similar changes in eating habits found early in pregnancy?
6. Is the woman who has first-trimester pregnancy nausea the woman who complained of premenstrual bloat, weight gain, and/or fatigue?
7. Is the woman who experiences premenstrual syndrome the woman whose morning nausea culminates in the motor act of vomiting?
8. What is the premenstrual experience of the woman who has no nausea during first-trimester pregnancy?
9. Does the woman with nausea have altered taste and/or olfactory perception during pregnancy and her menstrual cycle?
10. Is nausea or absence of nausea in pregnant women related to fetal/maternal outcome?

Finally, if women do experience morning sickness, and indeed, if reliable statistics were available on the prevalence and incidence of the phenomenon, we might find that some variation of nausea is experienced by *all* pregnant women. In this context, the first-trimester nausea might be indicative that normal physiological adjustment mechanisms associated with pregnancy are occurring in the maternal organism. This kind of conceptualization of "nausea" of first-trimester pregnancy places the phenomenon within a *wellness* rather than an *illness* framework. But the foregoing may not be the case at all. Some women may *not* have nausea, have a normal pregnancy, and deliver a healthy baby.

---

*Most psychological and sociological research on the menstrual cycle has equated menstruation with ovulation. In young women 18–22 it is known that about 20% of the cycles may be anovulatory and this age group (college women) is the captive group on which most of the work has been done.

Variability in the type of nausea in human females as well as prevalence during pregnancy and its value relative to pregnancy outcome may be explainable in terms of evolution. We can speculate that long ago, when our mammalian predecessors were evolving into organisms selecting for intrauterine gestation, it was those organisms that had the most "suitable" intrauterine environment to receive fertilized ova that survived and delivered viable, strong offspring. That is, intrauterine adaptation was most likely accompanied by the biological evolving of mechanisms to increase the capacity (volume) of the vascular system to facilitate the delivery of nutrients to and eliminate metabolic waste from the developing embryo/fetus. Thus, periovulatory onset of plasma-volume increase may be an evolutionary characteristic of mammalian organisms. This has not been substantiated in the literature, however. While nausea in the pregnant human female does not seem consistent with the Darwinian postulate of adaptive changes occurring to increase the chance of "survival of the fittest" of the species, it may be explained if one considers the concept of *pleiotropy*. In pleiotropy, changes in a gene may have many different effects in the phenotype that may be manifest in a multiplicity of ways—both physiologically and developmentally (Lewontin 1978). The explanation of first-trimester nausea in terms of pleiotropy is that natural selection operates to increase the frequency of a particular gene because of a desired effect that has survival value (i.e., to increase maternal plasma volume prior to implantation) with pleiotropic or unrelated effects (nausea or altered taste and/or olfactory perception) simply being carried along.

That some women do not have nausea and have successful pregnancies may be explainable, in part, by another evolutionary concept. More than one gene may influence the expression of a desired survival characteristic (plasma volume increase) so that there may be several alternative ways genetically to achieve a desired effect. This may explain the reported low or nonexistence of nausea in African and Eskimo women versus the high incidence in Caucasian women.

Answers to questions regarding the universality of the phenomenon—that is, "Do all women experience nausea in pregnancy?" or more important, "Must all women experience nausea?"—will come from work designed to test the questions generated in this paper as well as hypotheses derived from other conceptual models. We think that occurrence of the nausea phenomenon in Caucasian pregnant women has biological significance.

Finally, it is noteworthy that of all women interviewed who experienced nausea, all delivered healthy babies; of the two women who did not have nausea, one had a male fetus that died in utero during the fifth month of pregnancy.

REFERENCES

Benson, R.C. *Handbook of Obstetrics and Gynecology*. Los Altos, Calif.: Lange Medical Publications, 1966.

Bland, J. *Clinical Metabolism of Body Water and Electrolytes*. Philadelphia: Saunders, 1963.

Boston Women's Health Book Collective. *Our Bodies, Ourselves*. New York: Simon & Schuster, 1976.

Brandes, J.M. First-trimester nausea and vomiting as related to outcome of pregnancy. *Obstet. Gynecol.* 30:429, 1967.

Chertok, L. The Psychopathology of Vomiting of Pregnancy. In J.G. Hoveles (Ed.), *Modern Perspectives in Psycho-Obstetrics*. New York: Brunner/Mazel Publishers, 1972.

David, M.L., and Doyle, E.W. First-trimester pregnancy. *Am. J. Nurs.* 76:1945–1948, 1976.

Fairweather, D. Nausea and vomiting in pregnancy. *Am. J. Obstet. Gynecol.* 102:135–175, 1968.

Hartman, R.E. *Exercise for True Natural Childbirth*. New York: Harper & Row, 1975.

Hayes, M.A. Water and electrolyte therapy after operation. *N. Eng. J. Med.* 278:1054–1055, 1968.

Hellman, L.M., Pritchard, J.A., and Wynn, R.M. *Williams Obstetrics* (14th ed.). New York: Appleton-Century-Crofts, 1971.

Hytten, F., and Leitch, I. *The Physiology of Human Pregnancy*. Philadelphia: Davis, 1964.

Katz, F., and Romfh, P. Plasma aldosterone and renin activity during the menstrual cycle. *J. Clin. Endocrinol. Metab.* 34:819–821, 1972.

Kolata, G.B. How safe is Bendectin? *Science* 210:518–519, 1980.

Krause, M.V., and Hunseher, M.A. *Food, Nutrition, and Diet Therapy* (5th ed.). Philadelphia: Saunders, 1972.

Landau, R., and Lugibihl, K. Inhibition of the sodium-retaining influence of aldosterone by progesterone. *J. Clin. Endocrinol. Metab.* 18:1237–1245, 1958.

Lewontin, R.C. Adaptation. *Sci. Am.* 239(9):213–230, 1978.

Louw, J.X. Aspects of vomiting in the African. *S. Afr. Med. J.* 40:957, 1966.

MacDonald, H.N., and Good, W. Changes in plasma sodium, potassium and chloride concentrations in pregnancy and the puerperium with plasma and serum osmolality. *J. Obstet. Gynaecol. Br. Common.* 78:798–803, 1971.

MacDonald H.N., and Good, W. The effect of parity on plasma sodium, potassium, chloride and osmolality levels during pregnancy. *J. Obstet. Gynaecol. Br. Common.* 79:441–449, 1972.

McBride, A.B. *The Growth and Development of Mothers*. New York: Harper & Row, 1973.

Medalie, J.H. Relationship between nausea and vomiting in early pregnancy and abortion. *Lancet,* 23:117–119, July 20, 1957.

Moran, W.H., Jr., Miltenberger, F.W., Shuayb, W.A., and Zimmerman, B. The relationship of antidiuretic hormone secretion to surgical stress. *Surgery* 56(1):99–107, 1964.

Netter-Munkett, P., Mau, G., and Konig, B. The dimension of neuroticism as a modifying factor in the association between biological conditions and nausea in pregnancy. *J. Psychosom. Res.* 16:395–404, 1972.

Reader, S.R., Luigi, M., Martin, L.L., and Fitzpatrick. E. *Maternity Nursing* (13th ed.). Philadelphia: Lippincott, 1976.

Reinken, L., and Gant, H. Vitamin B_6 nutrition in women with hyperemesis gravidarum during the first trimester of pregnancy. *Clin. Chim. Acta,* pp. 101–102, Aug. 1974.

Robertson, E.G., and Cheyne, G.A. Plasma biochemistry in relation to oedema of pregnancy. *J. Obstet. Gynaecol. Br. Common.* 79:769–776, 1972.

Schwartz, U.D., and Abraham, G.E. Corticosterone and aldosterone levels during the menstrual cycle. *Obstet. Gynecol.* 45:339–342, 1975.

Semmens, J. Female sexuality and life situations: an etiologic psycho-socio-sexual profile of weight gain and nausea and vomiting in pregnancy. *Obstet. Gynecol.* 38:555–563, 1971.

Shervington, P.C. Common Pregnancy Disorders and Infections. In D.F. Hawkins (Ed.), *Obstetric Therapeutics: Clinical Pharmacology and Therapeutics in Obstetric Practice*. Baltimore: Williams & Wilkins, 1974.

Soranus. In O. Temkin (trans.), *Soranus Gynecology*. Baltimore: Johns Hopkins University Press, 1956. Excerpted in *Am. J. Obstet. Gynecol.* 102:135–175, 1969.

Speert, H., and Guttmacher, A.F. Frequency and significance of bleeding in early pregnancy. *J. A. M. A.* 155:712–715, 1959.

Sundsfjord, J., and Aakvaag, A. Plasma renin activity, plasma renin substrate and urinary aldosterone excretion in the menstrual cycle in relation to the concentration of progesterone and oestrogen in the plasma. *Acta Endocrinol.* 71:519–529, 1972.

Voda, A. Patterns of Progesterone and Aldosterone in Ovulatory Women during the Menstrual Cycle. In A. Dan, E. Graham, and C. Beecher (Eds.), *The Menstrual Cycle—A Synthesis of Interdisciplinary Research*. New York: Springer, 1980.

Vomiting of Pregnancy. New Haven, Conn.: Bi So Dol, 1932.

Walford, P.A. Antibiotic and congenital malformations. *Lancet* 2:298, 1963.

Way, S. Relation between gastric acidity and the anterior pituitary-like content and urine in pregnant women. *Br. Med. J.* 2:182, 1945.

Wiedenbach, E. *Family-Centered Maternity Nursing*. New York: Putnam's, 1967.

Zeigel, E., and Van Blarcom, C.C. *Obstetric Nursing* (6th ed.). New York: MacMillan, 1972.

Chapter 9

Thirst Phenomenon and Fluid Restriction

Guadalupe S. Olivas

INTRODUCTION

Thirst in the fluid-restricted patient is a clinical phenomenon that challenges nurses. The challenge is particularly great in the thirst as well as the drinking behavior of fluid-restricted patients with chronic renal failure and those having cirrhosis of the liver with associated ascites. The clinical significance of thirst in these two disease states arises from the interdependent dynamics of (1) the physiology of thirst itself, (2) the pathophysiology of these conditions in terms of water balance, and (3) the therapeutic regimen of fluid restriction. An underlying assumption is that thirst, as a symptom, will be more useful to clinicians if they are cognizant of the interplay among these three factors. This awareness can direct their efforts to more effectively assist the fluid-restricted patient population in adhering to the regimen in addition to satisfying the basic thirst drive.

The purpose of this work is to present a descriptive correlation of the thirst phenomenon in both renal failure patients and liver failure patients within the theoretical framework of thirst. A combined inductive and deductive investigative approach was used to clarify the concept of thirst. Pertinent relationships in the clinical phenomena of thirst, including hypotheses that might be tested about thirst, are identified.

THE PROBLEM

As already noted, when fluid restriction is part of a treatment regimen, as in liver or renal failure, thirst becomes a major clinical problem. More specifically, noncompliance with the prescribed regimen because of the occurrence of thirst is the problem. The problem is evident in clinical observations in the identified patient population. Anecdotes about hospitalized patients with liver or renal failure, when summarized, illustrate some characteristic behaviors as follows:

1. A marked preoccupation with the desire to drink, and associated with this the following:
   a) cheating on restrictions, that is, sneaking drinks
   b) bargaining to get fluids, that is, refusing to eat or take medication unless a drink is given
   c) lying to get increased fluids
   d) complaining of dry mouth
   e) abusive behavior, both verbal and physical
   f) frequently requesting and pleading for a variety of fluids
2. Anxiety, restlessness, and anger when continually denied control of fluid intake. Preoccupation with drinking increases.
3. Preoccupation with drinking subsides with increasing disorientation as levels of blood urea nitrogen (BUN) and creatinine rise.

Clinical observations of chronic renal failure patients on hemodialysis demonstrated the following characteristic patterns of behaviors:

1. Greater weight gain between dialysis treatments than recommended. The range of weight gain was 3.5 to 8.5 pounds. Average weight gain was 5.5 pounds (2.5 kg). Acceptable weight gain is 0.5 kg per 24 hours between treatments (Gutch and Stones 1975). In the two- to three-day intervals between dialysis treatments, the recommended weight gain is 1.0 to 1.5 kg. This is a difference of 1.5 kg between actual weight gain and recommended weight gain. This weight gain is interpreted as excess fluid intake (Brundage 1976). Patients having greater weight gain complained of more thirst and were labeled fluid "abusers"; patients with increased weight gain usually have edema also.
2. Another behavior pattern noted was habitual ice consumption, either predialysis or during dialysis. In attempting to validate this finding, most patients reported that they were not experiencing thirst. One subject admitted to the sensation of continual thirst. Another patient said he ate ice probably out of boredom. Still another chose to drink fluids during the first two hours of dialysis because of the fluid restriction on nondialysis days.
3. Thirst was experienced during nondialysis days. Those who followed their therapeutic regimen closely quenched their thirst by drinking frequent small amounts, evenly spaced throughout the day. Several hemodialysis nurses reported that some patients did not consider ice to be a fluid, so it is used in quenching thirst. One nurse observed that some patients "cheat" on their restrictions the night before dialysis treatment because they know the ill effects will be eliminated during dialysis the next day, that is, alcohol might be consumed the night before dialysis and not on any other day.

4. Serum sodium ranged from 134 mEq to 144 mEq, with the average of 139 mEq. (Normal range is 136 to 145 mEq.)
5. Predialysis blood pressures revealed a range of:
   a. systolic 130 mm Hg to 180 mm Hg.
   b. diastolic 70 mm Hg to 110 mm Hg.
6. Postdialysis there was a decrease of 10 mm Hg to 60 mm Hg systolic and 0 mm Hg to 40 mm Hg diastolic blood pressure.
7. Urinary output ranged from small amounts (less than 500 ml per 24 hours) to moderate amounts (only one patient had a moderate amount).
8. Hematocrit values were characteristically low, with a range of 22 to 42 percent, and an average of 30 percent. Brundage (1975) reports that patients have the ability to tolerate relative hematocrit levels of less than 14 percent.
9. BUN, creatinine, and potassium were high.

QUESTIONS FOR NURSING

The patient behaviors provide evidence that clarification of the clinical phenomenon of thirst is warranted. Questions related to the two specific groups studied that directed this inquiry include

1. Why is the complaint of thirst so prevalent in fluid-restricted patients? What determines the activation of the thirst experience and subsequent drinking behavior in these patients? Are all the factors primarily physiological or do they include psychosocial aspects?
2. Assuming that drinking is goal-directed behavior, what are the control mechanisms? Since the nurse is most often the health-team member who is left to enforce the fluid-restriction regimen, the following questions were also posed:
   a) What are the subjective and objective criteria that allow nurses to infer that a patient is experiencing thirst? Is it the observation of drinking behaviors and/or the patient's communication of the sensation that leads the nurse to infer that thirst is present?
   b) Do all nurses use the same criteria for making inferences about thirst? Are the inferences based on the same specific characteristics?

These questions must be answered if nursing interventions directed to these patients are to be based on a sound theoretical foundation. The discussion will, therefore, focus on these questions.

DEFINITIONS AND PROPERTIES OF THIRST

Thirst has been defined as a motivational state in which there is a sensation of a need or desire for water (Guyton 1976; Metheny and Snively 1974; and

Fitzsimons, Peters, Peters-Haefeli 1975). Thirst as a sensation of "need," resulting from certain changes in body fluids, is considered to be "regulatory" in nature. Thirst sensation based on "desire," on the other hand, is "nonregulatory," in that there are not necessarily any changes in body fluids (Fitzsimons et al. 1975; and Wong 1976). Thirst as a result of need is considered *true thirst,* whereas the thirst as a result of desire is termed *false thirst* (Wolfe 1958).

Thirst sensation (whether based on need or desire), in turn, leads to the motivated behavior of drinking (Fitzsimons et al. 1975). Drinking, in essence, is the operational mechanism of thirst. Drinking, as a motivational activity, "reflects the ability of the organism to adapt to changes in its physical and social environment. For this reason, motivated behavior may be characterized as being goal-directed and purposive" (Wong 1976). Thus, motivated behaviors are products of the interaction between the organism and its environment.

An analysis of both internal and external variables (and interaction between them) that elicit the activity of drinking is warranted. *Motivated behavior* is defined by Denny and Ratner (1970) as acts that regularly consummate or terminate a recurring sequence of behaviors.

The activity of drinking is considered to be consummatory and is generally preceded by relatively stereotyped sequences of orienting activities (Wong 1976). That is, drinking as a consummatory activity, involves a further sequence of responses directed toward the goal object. Specifically, before drinking occurs, the following series of activities is needed: obtaining the fluid desired or requesting the fluid and pouring it into the mouth. The person toward whom drinking is directed is relieving the sensation of either need or desire.

In the clinical setting, drinking behavior is most often both the patient's and the clinician's point of reference. Both desire and need for fluid may direct patients' drinking behavior. Accordingly, clinicians need to develop an understanding of drinking-motivated behavior in light of interaction of biological with environmental factors in regulating this motivated behavior.

Such an analysis of behavior requires consideration of interactions among neural, endocrine, and experiential factors. The underlying premise is that motivational acts are considered products of complex interaction, involving the

1. Internal state of the organism
2. Effects of environmental objects, called *stimuli*
3. Evaluation of such interactions of previous encounters with similar conditions or with other organisms
4. General contextual setting (Wong 1976).

Clinicians need to be able to depict the complex interrelation of the factors influencing motivated behavior of thirst and drinking as a basis for evaluating thirst, drinking, and fluid restriction as well as for designing appropriate interventions.

CONTROL MECHANISMS FOR THE DEVELOPMENT OF TRUE THIRST

The mechanisms underlying control of water intake and excretion of water and electrolytes, which are the determining factors in the development of *true thirst* are discussed in this section. These mechanisms include the brain, kidneys, and behavioral adjustments.

Inducing Stimuli

Two physiological changes in body water signal the need for water and thus the sensation of thirst. Both are changes in the water balance controlling thirst and both are consequences of water loss; each change is characteristic of the body compartment involved, intracellular or extracellular. Depletion or volume loss from both intracellular and extracellular compartments that provoke thirst independently was expressed in the "double-depletion hypothesis" of thirst (Epstein 1976; and Epstein, Kissileff, and Stellar 1973). This hypothesis has been supported by research in which reductions of fluid have been produced in animals in only one of the two water components; thirst occurred in both induced cellular dehydration and in hypovolemia (Fitzsimons 1961; and Stricker 1966).

Specific evidence supporting the double-depletion hypothesis is in Fitzsimon's (1961) and Stricker's (1966) investigations on rats. These researchers used bleeding procedures in which only extracellular fluid compartments were reduced. The procedure rendered an absolute dehydration state in which intracellular and extracellular fluid volumes were reduced without obvious changes in the proportion between the two (in osmotic pressure between the extracellular fluid compartment and intracellular fluid compartment). This induced absolute reduction of extracellular fluid, caused by increased drinking in the rats. Anderson (1971) labels this type of regulation of water intake *volumetric*, in light of the loss of fluid volume. The major mechanism inducing thirst in absolute dehydration is the reninangiotensin system triggered by reduced kidney perfusion. This mechanism will be discussed in detail later in this chapter.

The double-depletion hypothesis is also supported by a finding indicating that osmolality is a second important parameter in water regulation. Thirst, and therefore drinking, may be induced because of changes in osmotic pressure of extracellular fluid. As early as 1947, Verney postulated that the brain contains osmoreceptors that detect changes in solute concentration of extracellular fluids. His viewpoint was that some large cells in the hypothalamic area respond to increased extracellular osmolarity by swelling. Verney further postulated that this swelling would stretch the dendrites of neighboring neurons and signal osmolality (Epstein et al. 1973). Blass and Epstein (1971), as well as Peck and Blass (1971) found that local dehydration of the lateral preoptic area (LPO), a portion of the forebrain in the anterior part of the hypothalamus just above the optic chiasm, aroused thirst. Damage to the subfornical organ (SFO) on the hypothalamus resulted in activation of the hormone that is a major component of thirst in hypovolemia. (The SFO is in a very different region of the brain than the LPO [Blass and Epstein 1971; and Peck and Novin 1971]).

Increased extracellular solute concentration (especially sodium) causes a shift of water from the cell to the extracellular fluid. This causes a "relative dehydration," or cellular dehydration. Thirst is said to be induced by this osmoreceptor mechanism (Anderson 1971; Epstein 1976; and Epstein et al. 1973).

The Mechanism

The two types of true thirst, *cellular* or *relative dehydration* and *absolute dehydration* (hypovolemia) differ markedly in the nature of the physiological mechanisms in operation (Epstein 1976; and Epstein et al. 1973). Cellular thirst is thought to be simple in respect to the receptors that provoke it. Stimulation of these osmoreceptors regulates the release of ADH as a result of cellular dehydration of the osmoreceptors themselves. ADH (vasopressin), though produced by neurosecretory cells in the hypothalamus, is stored in the neurohypophysis and released in response to neural impulses from the hypothalmus.

ADH acts on the kidneys, causing reabsorption of water by altering water permeability of the collecting ducts and distal tubules (Guyton 1976). The exact mechanism by which ADH exerts these identified effects on water reabsorption is postulated to be through fixed receptors and activation of the second messenger, cyclic-2',3',AMP. ADH invokes such mechanisms as disulphide-sulphydryl interchange, secretion of hyaluronidase, and stimulation of the syntheses of cyclic-3',5'-adenosine monophosphate (Dicker 1970). Dicker (1970) suggested that the sequence of events included the following:

1. Absorption of the hormone on a "receptor"
2. A possible disulphide-sulphydryl interchange
3. The stimulation of production of cyclic-3',5'-adenosine monophosphate
4. Apocrine secretion of hyaluronidase.

Dicker's description of events aligns with Ginetzinsky's (1958) hypothesis about hyaluronidase: Hyaluronidase depolymerizes the hyaluronic acid of the intercellular cement and thus, increases the permeability of the collecting duct epithelium.

The eventual outcome of the ADH effect on normal kidneys is production of smaller volumes of concentrated urine. Thirst sensation and subsequent drinking along with ADH action serve the common purpose of restoration of normal water balance in decreased hemoconcentration.

In absolute dehydration (extracellular hypovolemia), the mechanisms of water balance are more complex. The reninangiotensin hormone system and neural afferents from the great vessels of low-pressure circulation in the thorax in the left atrium and pulmonary veins are the primary mechanisms involved (Fitzsimons 1961, 1969; and Share 1969). ADH is also released because of fluid loss.

Fitzsimons (1961) first postulated the role of the reninangiotensin system in nephrectomized rats when he observed a reduction in water intake. In 1969, Fitzsimons found that decreased kidney perfusion increased drinking. The kidney juxtaglomerular apparatus (JGA) responds to decreased blood flow by liberating renin into the blood. In the blood, renin acts on a plasma substrate, angiotensinogen (Alpha-2 globulin), to release the comparatively inactive decapeptide Angiotensin I. Angiotensin I is then converted, largely in the lungs, enzymatically to the active octapeptide Angiotensin II (Ng and Vane 1968).

Angiotensin II has four functions.

1. Vasoconstriction helps to maintain normal pressure despite reduced fluid volume.
2. It compensates for sodium depletion arising from simple fluid loss by stimulating the secretion of aldosterone from the adrenal cortex. Aldosterone will, in turn, stimulate the reabsorption of sodium.
3. It triggers ADH release for increased reabsorption of water.
4. Angiotensin II induces thirst sensation and increased drinking (Epstein 1976; Epstein, Fitzsimons, and Rolls 1970; and Wong 1976).

Epstein, Fitzsimons, and Rolls (1970) proposed that the mechanism by which angiotensin induced drinking may be a result of the hormone acting on hypothalamic drinking areas. Increased drinking was demonstrated when angiotensin was injected locally in various hypothalamic drinking areas (septal, preoptic, and anterior hypothalamus). Routtenberg and Simpson (1971) have postulated that the SFO is the major site of action by dipsogenic chemical substances. The SFO lying outside the blood-brain barrier is highly responsive to angiotensin. Stimulation of the SFO by elevated blood concentrations of angiotensin provokes drinking behavior.

Epstein (1976) describes various motivational characteristics of the two types of thirst under discussion.

First, (cellular) dehydrated animals are more reluctant to drink bitter-tasting solutions than animals drinking in response to absolute (hypovolemia) dehydration.

Second, extracellular hormone (Angiotensin II) appears to provoke ingestion of salt solutions as well as water while cellular dehydration leads to the unexpected preference for pure water over salt.

Two depletional mechanisms that work together to produce thirst have been identified. They are not, however, interdependent. When the initiating stimulus is reversed by either correction or compensation, an inhibition will occur. This is accomplished by negative feedback. Stellar (1954) hypothesized that this inhibitory effect may be responsible for producing satiation.

A PHYSIOLOGICAL BASIS FOR THIRST IN THE PATIENTS WITH CHRONIC RENAL FAILURE AND A PATIENT WITH LIVER FAILURE

Several parallels can be drawn between the physiological basis for thirst and pathological states in chronic renal failure and liver failure to explain the prevalent occurrence of thirst in patients afflicted with these disease entities. From clinical descriptions of these patients, it is evident that they can be classified as being in overall positive balance; that is, fluid gain was greater than fluid loss. Positive fluid balance was demonstrated by

1. Increased weight gain
2. Increased blood pressure in relation to the fluid gain, with a reduction occurring when excess fluid was removed
3. Edema
4. Increased abdominal girth in liver failure as a result of ascites.

Even though these patients are in positive fluid balance, thirst is a prevalent clinical phenomenon. A critical analysis of the cause of thirst in these patients, in light of positive fluid balance, was warranted. The following section describes some findings that may explain thirst prevalence in the identified patient population.

Renal Failure

In renal failure, removal of nitrogenous metabolites (urea) and creatinine, both products of endogenous tissue catabolism, and normal excretion or reabsorption of electrolytes (sodium and potassium, especially) are impaired or nonfunctional (Brundage 1976; and Reed and Sheppard 1977). The end result is not only retention of fluid but also retention of solutes; a hyperosmolar state occurs. Increased osmolarity in the extracellular fluid creates an osmotic gradient inducing an intracellular to extracellular shift. Ultimately, cell dehydration occurs.

The increased osmolarity may also induce dehydration of the osmoreceptor cell in the lateral preoptic area of the hypothalamus, the subsequent release of ADH from the neurohypophysis and, the sensation of thirst.

Rise in blood tonicity obtained by injections of hypertonic urea solution is a much weaker stimulus to thirst and to ADH release than the same rise in blood tonicity obtained by injecting sodium salts. Urea, however, penetrates the blood-brain barrier poorly (Anderson, 1971). It may be that in renal failure patients, unless serum sodium is high, the stimulus strength of urea may not be enough to elicit thirst. But urea is not the only solute increasing in concentration in renal failure; other solutes include creatinine, uric acid, phosphate, potassium, sulfates, nitrates, and phenols. Furthermore, a high solute concentration of urea, along with the other solutes mentioned, is almost a constant and is relieved only temporarily by hemodialysis.

On the other hand, there is evidence that the tubules in patients with chronic renal failure show a diminished response to adequate circulating concentrations of antidiuretic hormone (Tannen, Regal, Dunn, and Schrier 1969). This diminished response to ADH appears to be related to osmotic diuresis occurring in surviving nephrons. Other factors may, however, play a role.

Tannen and colleagues (1969), in their investigation of 13 patients with chronic renal failure, report evidence of lack of response to administration of supra-maximal dose of ADH. They found that the urine of 11 patients remained hypotonic to plasma in spite of administration of high doses of ADH. They attributed lack of response to ADH to several factors:

1. Impairment of cellular response to ADH due to the presence of a uremic toxin or toxins
2. Alteration in anatomical architecture of the renal tubule or the tubular vasculature
3. Alteration of calcium homeostasis.

Wills (1978) contends that the most likely factor here is diminished cellular response to ADH.

Factors other than lack of ADH response also contribute to constant defect in chronic renal failure, that is, inability of the kidney to concentrate urine. The major factors causing impairment in urine concentration are increased filtration rate and solute load remaining in the kidneys (Tannen et al. 1969). These combined factors limit ability of the counter-current mechanism to create a hyperosmotic interstitium. Failure to create a hyperosmotic interstitium, in turn, contributes to diminished response to ADH (Tannen et al. 1969; Wills 1978; and Massary and Sellers 1976).

In light of current postulations about ADH action, it is likely that other factors play a role in target organ resistance to this hormone. Wills (1978) offers two possibilities: Interference by uremic toxins with intracellular events following ADH with dependent formation of cyclic-3',5'-AMP, and effects of intraluminal fluid flow rate on the flow of water across the luminal.

The absolute dehydration mechanism may also play a role in the manifestation of thirst in renal failure. Patients with renal failure are known to have an increased renin secretion (DeWardener 1962; and Tannen et al. 1969). This increased renin secretion may initiate absolute depletion mechanism of thirst through the renin–angiotensin hormone system. Upon transformation of Angiotensin I to Angiotensin II, the thirst center in the subfornical area of the hypothalamus is activated and increased drinking occurs.

From descriptions of patients with renal failure, several patterns as follows are apparent:

1. Where serum sodium levels were slightly below normal or within normal limits, there was still an excess in body weight, which is interpreted as excess fluid intake.
2. Any fluid can be acquired by chronic renal failure patients predialysis, in between dialysis, and postdialysis, but workers report that ice and water are the two fluids most commonly consumed.
3. When patients were hypertensive predialysis, blood pressure decreased as a result of hemodialysis.

Excess fluid intake occurred in both normal and slightly decreased serum sodium as the result of changes in the relationship between osmolality and water balance. Normally, there is a close relationship between plasma osmolality and sodium osmolality (Massary and Sellers 1976); this does not exist, however, in the uremic state. Osmolality does not relate to changes in water balance. Rather, increased concentration of urea and other metabolic by-products increase osmolality. Osmolality increase by solutes other than sodium may trigger the "cellular dehydration" thirst mechanism and thus cause increased drinking.

Patient's selection of water, in liquid or ice form, for drinking may parallel findings in animals. Animals, with relative or cellular dehydration as previously noted, are more reluctant to drink bitter-tasting solutions; they also prefer pure water over salt solutions. This selectivity may be analogous to behavioral adaptations to the physiological hyperosmolar state with the organism attempting to regulate the osmolar state by dilution (i.e., drinking pure water), especially in light of decreased response to ADH.

Also, since these patients' blood pressure decreased postdialysis, their hypertension can be labeled *salt water dependent* (Massary and Sellers 1976). This categorization implies that hypertension is well controlled by ultrafiltration of dialysis and by diet. This classification is opposed to renin–angiotensin dependent blood pressure elevation. Absolute dehydration thirst mechanisms may, therefore, not be functioning in these particular renal failure patients, in view of the fact that their blood pressures decreased with dialysis instead of remaining elevated.

Liver Failure

Both thirst mechanisms based on need may be functioning in patients with liver failure with ascites. Again, both fluid and electrolyte imbalances are apparent in this disease entity. These imbalances can be paralleled to the imbalances that have the potential of triggering the thirst sensation.

Factors in liver disease causing fluid imbalance are obstruction to flow and hypoproteinemia. Various hormone changes also contribute to the fluid imbalance as well as electrolyte imbalance.

Ascites, as accumulation of free fluid within the peritoneal cavity, results from failure of the liver to synthesize albumin. Decreased albumin, in turn, decreases plasma osmotic pressure (Daniels 1977). The development of ascites is also dependent on portal hypertension; if more fluid enters the peritoneal cavity than leaves, ascites develops. Ascites fluid is extremely rich in albumin and electrolytes absorbed from the intestine (Daniels 1977); it is, therefore, hyperosmolar. The hyperosmotic pressure created continues to draw additional body fluid. In essence, a decrease in extracellular body fluid occurs with this shift of body fluid into the peritoneal cavity. This decrease in extracellular volume, in turn, results in decreased renal perfusion, which will initiate volumetric or absolute dehydration thirst through the renin–angiotensin system.

As a result of activation of the renin–angiotensin system, systemic blood pressure is maintained, the SFO is stimulated to induce thirst and drinking behavior, aldosterone is secreted, and sodium is reabsorbed. ADH is probably released because of both angiotensin and stimulation of volume receptors in the left atrium and pulmonary veins. Increased ADH release with subsequent fluid retention, plus activation of the renin–angiotensin system and the sensation of thirst accompanied by changed drinking behavior are mechanisms patients with liver failure have operating to correct their absolute dehydration.

The hypernatremia seen in liver failure with ascites may be a stimulus for thirst sensation through the cellular or relative dehydration that results in osmoreceptors in the LPO. Stimulation of LPO receptors may account for Daniels' (1977) report of high ADH levels common in cirrhotic patients. Another triggering mechanism for thirst through the LPO is that of hyperosmolality caused by other solutes common in this disease state; among these are BUN and ammonia.

There is a strong case for a physiological basis for thirst in patients who have renal failure and patients with liver failure. Based on the physiology of thirst and the known pathophysiological basis of these two disease entities, we can postulate that both thirst mechanisms can be initiated in patients with these diseases. At least some of the clinically observed drinking behavior of this patient population are the result of true thirst, that is, dependent on body need.

THE CONTROL MECHANISMS FOR THE DEVELOPMENT OF FALSE THIRST

Thirst was also identified above as being a function of desire with the subsequent drinking being independent of the organism's hydrational state. This thirst was classified as false because it is based on desire, not need; the organism's drinking was classified as being nonregulatory. These classifications are based on the assumption that both false thirst and its associated drinking are the result of an interaction between organism and environment, whereas true thirst is the result of the interaction of the organism with its own physiological state.

The description of false thirst indicates that thirst in and of itself is not only an emergency machine that operates to defend the animal against large disorders of body water. Oatley (1973) and Collier, Hirsch, and Hamlin (1972) suggest that periodic normal drinking is based on acquired expectancies and ecological convenience. Oatley's results showed that when rats were maintained on a constant food intake, their circadian drinking rhythm was not affected. This was interpreted as indicating that drinking is not solely the result of deficits but can prevent deficits from occurring. Collier and co-workers (1972) examined the effects of a fixed daily water rotation on body weight and food intake. His findings indicate that the amount of metabolically active tissue an animal may support is determined by its water intake and is reduced when water intake is reduced. Thus, the animal is defending water balance by reducing food intake. Wong (1976) reports various studies that indicate that restriction of nonregulatory drinking water intake increases the strength of the consummatory response. The amount of water consumed is a function of the degree of water deprivation.

Stellar (1954) observed that human subjects ingest liquids in bursts and rests like the rat. He noted that as satiation developed, rests increased and bursts of drinking decreased.

Another nonregulatory drinking determinant is related to temporal effects. Wong (1976) postulates that diurnal variations in drinking occur as a result of the diurnal variation in food intake governed by a "biological clock." Under experimental conditions, a rat consumes about three quarters of its total water intake during the night. This is interpreted as reflecting the synchronization capability of the "biological clock" to the external lighting.

Holmes (1963) reported that the time of day when an individual drinks may be significantly affected by occupation or personal habits. This is clearly evident in the coffee breaks provided to employees; for many, it is the desire for a specific fluid (i.e., caffein, alcohol), and not thirst, that dictates daily drinking patterns.

Falk (1961) demonstrated that when water is concurrently available, food-deprived rats with normal water balance, fed on an intermittent schedule, will consume an excessive amount of water (schedule-induced polydipsia). The excessive drinking, Kissileff (1973) contends, is the result of frustration due to infrequent ingestion of food. Common denominators in all schedule-induced polydipsia experiments were the necessity of food deprivation and thwarting of eating. Kissileff hypothesized that emotional response as a consequence of increased levels of neurotransmitter substances accumulating in the limbic structures during periods of absence of food was a result of "frustration."

A later study (Falk 1966) demonstrated that when the reinforcement schedule was increased, a decrease in polydipsia occurred. He favored an explanation of polydipsia as a displacement behavior.

Deux (1973) reported a temperature determinant of nonregulatory drinking. He reveals that cold water satiates thirst more effectively than body-temperature water. This was demonstrated when rats were maintained on a water-rationing schedule in the continuous presence of food. Rats maintained on this water rationing not only drank less, but ate less when cold water was available than they did in the presence of warm water.

Some of these identified psychosocial determinants of thirst are apparent in patients with chronic renal failure and patients with liver failure when the therapeutic prescription is fluid restriction. These nonregulatory psychosocial determinants may initiate desire to drink, or potentiate need for drinking, especially in light of fluid restriction. Patients' desires to avoid ill effects of noncompliance with fluid restriction may be able to overcome these stimuli. An overriding of these stimuli is evident in the following changes in drinking patterns seen in hemodialysis patients: drinking more than the allowed amount the day before dialysis, consuming ice or other fluids during dialysis, and scheduling small and frequent drinks within the prescribed amount.

Not all patients are able to override the stimuli, either physiologically and/or psychosocially. Drinking, regardless of restriction, is the major noncompliant behavior in both patients with chronic renal failure and patients with liver failure. Emotional responses, like anger, anxiety, restlessness, bargaining, and manipulating, seen in these patients who are fluid restricted, may represent the "frustration" Kissileff (1973) described in rats. The parallel is drawn because, like rats, these patients are also diet restricted. However, water is not always available with patients' meals, as it was with Kissileff's rats. Instead, patients have health professionals, most often nurses, repeating the existence of and enforcing fluid restriction. Only intermittent reinforcement is given by nurses or other health professionals. This may contribute to some patients' inability to override the thirst drive.

Abusive or anger responses in liver failure patients who are fluid restricted may be interpreted in light of Falk's (1966) "displacement" concept. The angry behavior may be related to loss of control in relieving one's sensation of thirst and directed toward whoever impedes the drinking.

In summary, there is a strong psychosocial basis for the sensation of thirst in patients with renal failure as well as in patients with liver failure. Behaviors clinicians observe are not only because of the occurrence of both need and desire to drink but also the restricted fluid prescription. Whether clinicians can differentiate between true and false thirst is not the issue. Instead, the issue is how clinicians can best assist patients to relieve thirst within the therapeutic regimen of fluid restriction and to understand the reasons for their anger and inability to override it.

CONCEPTUALIZATION OF THIRST FOR NURSING PRACTICE

As an outcome of this inductive investigation of the clinical phenomenon of thirst, three schematic representations were developed. One representational model (Figure 9-1) illustrates the compilation of data collected from literature and clinical observation. It depicts the regulatory and nonregulatory mechanisms in the development of thirst and drinking, and the relationships between the triggering stimuli. The second model (Figure 9-2) illustrates the manifested responses to thirst with clinical observations, including the behaviors demonstrated by the patients. It also includes nursing implications. The third representational model (Figure 9-3) combines and amplifies the first two models. Relationships diagrammed at the left of the model are based on the premises that patients with renal failure and patients with liver failure may experience both true and false thirst; it demonstrates the behaviors of these patients in light of fluid-restriction regimens. The questions and hypotheses evolving from this framework are

1. Fluid restriction potentiates both true and false thirst.
2. In fluid restriction, false thirst potentiates the original thirst sensation caused by true body need. (False thirst potentiates true thirst.)
3. Drinking behavior is more likely to be the result of false thirst than true thirst.
4. If false thirst is satiated, true thirst may not occur even though the body is not hydrated.
5. Can IVs reduce false thirst? Is more thirst experienced by patients who are hydrated intravenously?
6. Frustration with the unmet need of thirst sensation is the major factor in noncompliance with prescribed limited fluid regimens.
7. What are the magnitudes of thirst?

Figure 9-1 Schematic Model of the Physiological and Psychosocial Aspects of Thirst

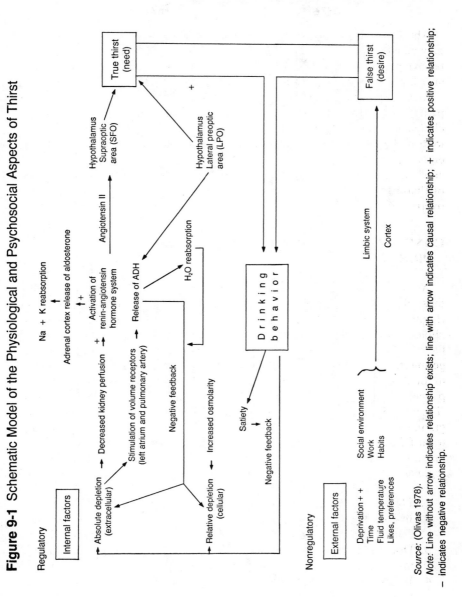

Source: (Olivas 1978).

Note: Line without arrow indicates relationship exists; line with arrow indicates causal relationship; + indicates positive relationship; − indicates negative relationship.

Figure 9-2 Schematic Representation of the Effects of Deprivation on Thirst and Drinking Behavior

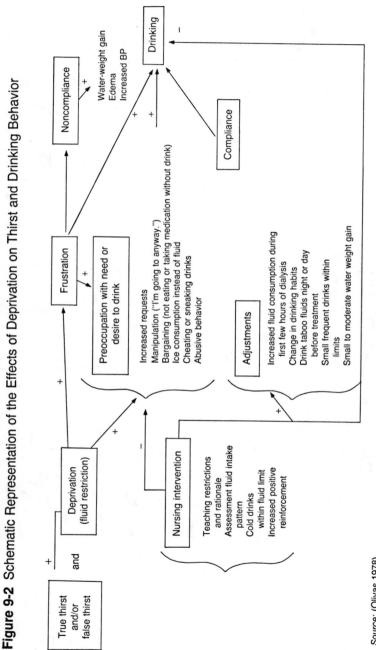

Source: (Olivas 1978).
Note: Line with arrow indicates causal relationship; line without arrow indicates relationship; + indicates positive relationship; − indicates negative relationship.

Figure 9-3 Physiological and Psychosocial Basis for Thirst and Drinking and Clinical Observations of Patients with Fluid Restriction (Figures 9-1 and 9-2 Combined and Amplified)

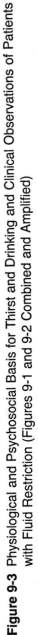
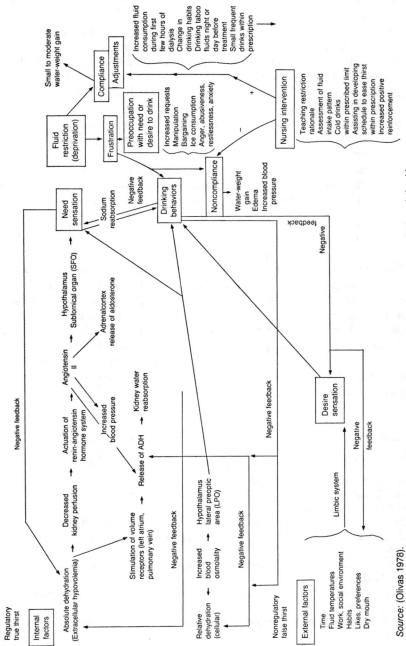

Source: (Olivas 1978).

Note: Line with arrow indicates causal relationship; + indicates positive relationship; − indicates negative relationship.

8. Cold drinks are more likely to satiate thirst than room-temperature or warm drinks.
9. Smaller amounts of cold fluids are more likely to satiate thirst than large amounts of fluids that are warm or at room temperature.
10. Fluids that are sour are more likely to satiate thirst than fluids that are sweet, salty, or bitter.
11. Pure water in fluid or ice form is more likely to relieve thirst than are other fluids.
12. Regular reinforcement of patient's compliance with limited drinking regimens is more likely to have a positive effect on compliance than verbal correction and assignment of blame.
13. Variable reinforcement of patients' compliance with limited drinking regimens, while taking longer, is more likely to have a lasting positive effect on compliance than regular reinforcement.

SUMMARY

Clarification of the clinical phenomenon, thirst, has great implications for nursing practice. This discussion has offered a rudimentary beginning for the conceptual clarification of the phenomena, focusing on patients with renal failure and liver failure on fluid restriction. In summary, if nurses are to assist these patients to cope with fluid restriction, to alleviate the discomforts associated with thirst and the inability to satisfy the need or desire to drink, the concept needs to be explored in great depths in the clinical setting. Presented here are hypotheses relevant to the concept of thirst, which can and should be tested in the clinical setting.

REFERENCES

Anderson, B. Thirst and brain control of water balance. *Am. Sci.* 58:408, Aug. 1971.

Blass, E., and Epstein, A.V. A lateral preoptic osmosensitive zone for thirst in the rat. *J. Comp. Physiol. Psychol.* 70:200–205, 1971.

Brundage, D.J. *Nursing Management of Renal Problems.* St. Louis, Mo.: Mosby, 1976.

Collier, G., Hirsch, E., and Hamlin, P.H. The ecological determinants of reinforcement in the rat. *Physiol. Behav.* 9:705–716, 1972.

Daniels, E. Chronic problems in rehabilitation of patients with Laennec's cirrhosis. *Nurs. Clin. N. Am.* 122:345, June 1977.

Denny, M.R., and Ratnor, S.C. *Comparative Psychology: Research in Animal Behavior.* Homewood, Ill.: Dorsey, 1970.

Deux, E. Thirst satiation and temperature of ingested water. *Science* 181:1166, Sept. 1973.

De Wardener, H.E. Polyuria. In D.A.K. Black (Ed.), *Renal Diseases*. Oxford, Engl.: Blackwell Scientific, 1962.

Dicker, S.E. Mechanisms of urine concentration and dilution in mammals. *Monogr. Physiol. Soc.* No. 20. London: Edward Arnold, 1970.

Epstein, A.V. The physiology of thirst. *Can. J. Physiol. Pharmacol.* 54(5):639–648, Oct. 1976.

Epstein, A.V., Fitzsimons, J.T., and Rolls, B.J. Drinking induced by injection of angiotensin into the brain of the rat. *J. Physiol.* 210:457–475, 1970.

Epstein, A.V., Kissileff, R., and Stellar, E. *Neuropsychology of Thirst: New Findings and Advances in Concepts*. New York: Wiley, 1973.

Falk, J.L. Production of polydipsia in normal rats by an intermittent food schedule. *Science* 133:195–196, 1961.

Falk, J.L. Schedule-induced polydipsia as a function of fixed interval length. *J. Exp. Anal. Behav.* 9:37–39, 1966.

Fisher, C., Ingram, W.R., and Ranson, S.W. *Diabetes Insipidus and the Neurohormonal Control of Water Balance*. Ann Arbor, Mich.: Edwards, 1938.

Fitzsimons, J.T. Drinking of rats depleted of body fluid without increase in osmotic pressure. *J. Physiol.* 159:297, 1961.

Fitzsimons, J.T. Drinking by nephrectomized rats injected with various substances. *J. Physiol.* 155:563–579, 1961.

Fitzsimons, J.T. The role of a renal thirst factor induced by extracellular stimuli. *J. Physiol.* 201:349–368, 1969.

Fitzsimons, J.T., Peters, G., and Peters-Haefeli, L. *Control Mechanisms of Drinking*. New York: Springer-Verlag, 1975.

Ginetzinsky, A.G. Role of hyaluronidase in the reabsorption of water in renal tubules: The mechanisms of action by antidiuretic hormone. *Nature* 182:1218–1219, 1958.

Gutch, C.E., and Stones, M.H. *Review of Hemodialysis for Nurses and Dialysis Personnel* (2nd ed.). St. Louis, Mo.: Mosby, 1975.

Guyton, A.C. *Textbook of Medical Physiology* (5th ed.). Philadelphia: Saunders, 1976.

Holmes, J.H. Thirst and Fluid Problems in Clinical Medicine. In J.J. Wayner (Ed.), *Thirst*. New York: Macmillan, 1963.

Kissileff, H.R. Nonhomeostatic Controls of Drinking. In A.V. Epstein, R. Kissileff, and V. Stellar (Eds.), *The Neuropsychology of Thirst*. Washington, D.C.: Winston, 1973.

Massary, S.G., and Sellers, A.L. *Clinical Aspects of Uremia and Dialysis*. Homewood, Ill.: Thomas, 1976.

Metheny, N.M., and Snively, W.D. *Nurses' Handbook of Fluid and Electrolyte Balance* (2nd ed.). Philadelphia: Lippincott, 1974.

Ng, K.K., and Vane, J.R. Fate of angiotensin I in the circulation. *Nature* 218:144–150, 1968.

Oately, K. Stimulation and Theory of Thirst. In A.V. Epstein, J.T. Kisseleff, and E. Stellar, *The Neuropsychology of Thirst*. Washington, D.C.: Winston, 1973.

Peck, J.W., and Blass, E.M. Localization of thirst and antidiuretic osmoreceptors by intracranial injection in rats. *Am. J. Physiol.* 228:1501–1509, 1975.

Reed, G.M., and Sheppard, V.F. *Regulation of Fluid and Electrolyte Balance*. Philadelphia: Saunders, 1977.

Routtenberg, A., and Simpson, J.B. Carbocol-induced drinking at ventricular and subfornical organ sites of application. *Life Sci.* 10:481–490, 1971.

Share, L. Extracellular Fluid Volume and Volume Vasopressive Secretion. In W.F. Ganong and L. Martini (Eds.), *Frontiers in Neuroendocrinology*. New York: Oxford University, 1969.

Stellar, E. The physiology of motivation. *Psychol. Rev.* 61:5–22, 1954.

Stricker, E. Extracellular fluid volume and thirst. *Am. J. Physiol.* 211:232–238, 1966.

Tannen, R.L., Regal, E.M., Dunn, M.J., and Schrier, R.W. Vasopressin-resistant hypostenuria in advanced chronic renal disease. *N. Engl. J. Med.* 280:1135–1141, 1969.

Wills, M.R. *Metabolic Consequences of Chronic Renal Failure* (2nd ed.). Baltimore, Md.: University, 1978.

Wolfe, A.V. *Thirst*. Homewood, Ill.: Thomas, 1958.

Wong, R. *Motivation: A Biobehavioral Analysis of Consummatory Activities*. New York: Macmillan, 1976.

Chapter 10

A Theoretical Model for the Study of Thirst: The Deductive Mode

Guadalupe S. Olivas

INTRODUCTION

Nursing, as an applied scientific discipline, is giving more attention to evaluation of the theory and knowledge that guide practitioners. One way to approach this evaluation is to develop and test theoretical models for nursing practice. The purpose of this chapter is to develop a theoretical model that nurses can use to study the clinical phenomenon of thirst as a behavioral adaptation process. This model represents my formalization of a *middle-range nursing theory*. Formalization of the model is guided by Gibbs's (1972) methodology of theory construction.

The model will be presented within the Gibbs frame of reference. Discussion will include identification and delineation of the two parts of a theory—the intrinsic part or empirical assertions and the extrinsic part (all additional data necessary to conduct tests of the theory). In this discussion the components—substantive terms, intrinsic statements, unit terms, and relational terms—of the proposed theoretical model will be revealed.

As defined by Gibbs, *substantive terms* are terms that designate a property or properties of one or more classes or events or things. Specific substantive terms are *constructs, concepts,* and *referentials. Intrinsic statements* are assertions about properties of an infinite class of events or things. Included in this category are axioms, postulates, propositions, transformational statements, and theorems. A *unit term* is a term that denotes a class of events or things. *Relational terms* are terms that stipulate some empirical relationship between properties denoted by substantive terms.

Delineation of the actual model will be preceded by a description of two conceptual perspectives that influenced derivation of the model. The focus includes an overview of Roy's (1976) adaptation model for nursing practice, and Wong's (1976) biobehavioral analysis of motivational processes. My conceptual synthesis of Roy's and Wong's conceptual perspectives will be described within a systems theory framework. The systems framework representation is my interpretation of the Roy–Wong perspective's potential use in clinical nursing theory development. Actual formalization of the theoretical model is accomplished by utilization of the aforementioned Gibbs structure.

DERIVATION OF THE MODEL

Roy's Adaptation Model for Nursing Practice

Roy's adaptation model for nursing practice is primarily a system's model that applies interaction concepts within the system's framework. Roy bases the model on eight basic assumptions (Roy 1974, 1976).

1. People are biopsychosocial beings.
2. People are in constant interaction with a changing environment (internal and external).
3. To cope with a changing world, people use both innate and acquired mechanisms, which are biological, psychological, and sociological in origin.
4. Health and illness are one inevitable dimension of human life.
5. To respond positively to environmental changes, people must adapt.
6. Human adaptation is a function of the stimulus to which people are exposed to and their adaptation levels. Human adaptation levels are determined by the combined effects of three classes of stimuli: (1) focal stimuli or factors immediately confronting the person, (2) contextual stimuli or all other factors present, and (3) residual stimuli or such factors as beliefs, attitudes, or traits.
7. Human adaptation levels are such that they comprise a zone that indicates the range of stimulation that will lead to a positive response.
8. People are conceptualized as having four modes of adaptation: (1) physiologic, (2) self concept, (3) role function, and (4) interdependence.

Although Roy attempts to formulate a prescriptive theory (Dickoff and James 1968) by delineating the elements of the model—values, goal, recipient, and intervention—her theory remains a grand theory. In its present stage of development, the model offers a conceptual perspective on which to base nursing practice. Using a systems theory schematic representation, interpretation of the Roy model developed for this chapter is depicted in Figure 10-1. Humankind's constant interaction with a changing environment and response to it are represented in the figure. At the left, input to the open system of humans are all environmental changes, both internal and external. The three stimuli that are

Figure 10-1 Roy's Model: An Interpretation

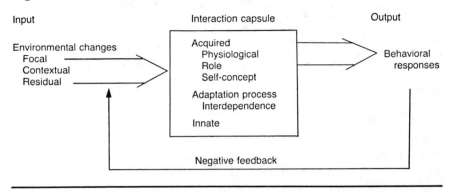

indices of environmental change (Roy, 1976) are depicted as input to the system; these stimuli act by causing tension, stress, strain, and conflict. The process of adaptation is what allows the system to regain a balance or steady state. It is the interaction of these four adaptive modes, within the innate and acquired coping mechanisms, that results in the output of the system. Output is in terms of behavioral responses that adapt to maintain the system in equilibrium. Negative feedback occurs and also becomes input into the system. The output of the system, therefore, assists and guides the system's operations.

The preceding description addresses how Roy conceptualizes human beings. Nursing is conceptualized, also, as an open system ministering to the human open system. Roy describes nursing as purposively interacting with people to assess their adaptation levels and to manipulate stimuli that are impinging on them. The ultimate aim is conservation of patient energy and achievement of a positive adaptation in all four modes. In this author's work, nursing intervention is conceptualized as having potential to be contextual stimuli. Intervention could also be directed to focal stimuli or residual stimuli. Thus, nursing intervention is conceptualized as being part of the input into the system of human beings.

Wong's Biobehavioral Analysis of Motivational Processes

Wong's (1976) biobehavioral analysis of motivational processes served as a second influence to the derivation of the model. Wong's biobehavioral approach to motivation is advocated by contemporary researchers in comparative psychology. It is based on the belief that scientific research is better suited for answering questions about the way in which events occur rather than the reasons that they occur.

Accordingly, the focus of Wong's analysis (1976) is on the interaction of biological with environmental and historical factors in the regulation of motivated behavior. He organizes his analysis around the activities rather than the processes. In this way, he attempts to analyze activities in terms of processes that have direct empirical referents.

Motivated behavior is described as activity that reflects ability of the organism to adapt to changes in its physical and social environment. For this reason, motivated behavior is characterized as being goal directed and purposive. It is guided by its consequences, related to some end point, and carried out in such a manner as to satisfy present or future biological requirements of the individual or species (Wong 1976).

Wong's (1976) analysis focuses on the behavioral manifestations of various states of the organism regarded as motivational. This approach obviates the conceptual difficulties encountered when hypothetical internal states such as hunger, thirst, curiosity, fear, or aggression are invoked to explain various forms of motivated behavior. He organizes his analysis on the activities having direct empirical referents, such as feeding, drinking, sleeping, stimulus seeking, and so forth.

In analyzing how motivated behavior occurs, Wong examines conditions that instigate and sustain various types of goal directed behavior (i.e., internal and external variables that elicit specific forms of motivated behavior). Determinant factors examined are deprivation or stimulation effects, experiential effects, temporal effects, situational effects, neural determinants and endocrine determinants. The *deprivation level* refers to duration of time in which the organism has been denied the goal–event under investigation. Stimulation, on the other hand, is exposure of the organism to the source of motivation being studied.

Experiential effects refer to effects of the organism's previous experience, with conditions similar to those under which it is being tested. *Temporal effect* refers to circadian rhythm factors.

The general context of the environmental setting in which the organism is being studied influences its behavior. Environmental cues may evoke alternative responses that differ from the responses under investigation.

There are neural structures in the brain that play vital roles in regulating motivational activities. Motivated behavior is governed by interacting neural centers. Also, motivated behavior is under control of hormonal or chemical activity. These two determinants must also be considered.

Thus, motivational acts are viewed as products of complex interactions involving the (1) internal state of the organism, (2) effects of environmental objects called *stimuli*, (3) evolution of such interaction of previous encounters with similar conditions and with other organisms, and (4) general contextual or situational setting. The basic contention is that when the complex interrelation of the factors that influence motivated behavior can be depicted, the basis for explaining this behavior is gained.

Merging Roy's and Wong's Conceptual Perspectives

Roy's (1976) grand theory of adaptation and Wong's (1976) biobehavioral analysis of motivational processes complement each other. Both address stimuli that confront the organism, adaptation process, and product of the complex interaction of all the determinant factors. Only Wong fulfills the criterion of empirical and operational adequacy; he describes hypothetical states such as hunger and thirst that represent the organism's state of adaptation. Roy conceptualizes focal, contextual, and residual stimuli as factors acting upon the organism and triggering the adaptation process, whereas Wong evaluates, operationalizes, and tests in the real world the determinant stimuli such as deprivation or stimulation and temporal and situational experiential factors. Also, Roy (1976) writes of behavioral responses while Wong both operationalizes and tests what he conceptualizes as motivated behavior. Wong (1976) analyzes specific indices of motivated behavior such as feeding and drinking.

Since fluid-restriction regimens are frequently encountered in clinical practice, with the accompanying frustrations by both patients attempting to comply and nurses attempting to enforce the regimen, development of a model to study the phenomena of thirst was undertaken for this purpose. Roy's (1976) adaptation model offers a perspective for viewing the patient. Wong's (1976) biobehavioral analysis of the motivated behavior of drinking proposes how to view the thirst mechanism and associated behavioral responses. Figure 10-2 represents the conceptual synthesis of Roy (1976) and Wong's (1976) conceptual perspectives within the schematic framework of systems theory.

Inputs to the system are both external and internal environmental changes. Environmental changes consist of a combination of focal, contextual, and residual stimuli. By creating tension, these combined stimuli act on the open system of man to create an unsteady state. The adaptation process is triggered to stimulate innate and acquired physiological and psychosocial mechanisms. The end product of this interaction with response of the organism to environment is motivated behavior. In the case of thirst, the end behavior is drinking and drink-seeking behavior. These end products serve as negative feedback to the system, thus becoming input into the system.

Formalization of this conceptual perspective within a Gibb's (1972) paradigm will move the model pictured in Figure 10-2 into a testable frame of reference.

THE MODEL: INTRINSIC AND EXTRINSIC THEORY

According to Gibbs (1972), a *theory* is a set of logically interrelated statements in the form of empirical assertions about properties of infinite classes of events or things. A *formally constructed theory* is one in which the components are

Figure 10-2 Adaptation Process of Thirst

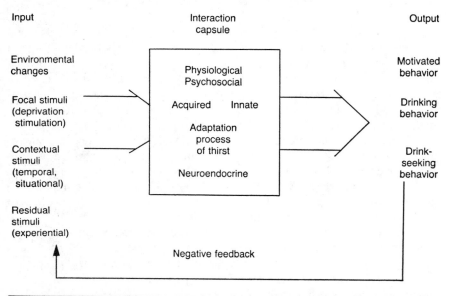

differentiated and identified systematically. The remainder of this chapter will show how to delineate the proposed theoretical model for studying thirst in clinical settings.

Identification and Definition of Substantive Terms

The constructs of the model are (1) environmental changes, (2) biopsycho-sociological adaptation process, and (3) motivated behavior. These constructs are defined as follows:

I. *Environmental changes* are alterations occurring from within and outside boundaries of the individual that act as stimuli to the individual. This definition was derived from the combined work of Roy (1976) and Wong (1976).

II. *Biopsychosocial adaptation processes* are any integrated changes in structure, function, or form of any part of the individual that produces better adjustment of the individual to the environment. This definition was also derived from the combined work of Roy (1976) and Wong (1976). Webster's dictionary, did, however, assist in its final derivation.

III. *Motivated behavior* is any goal-directed, purposive activity that reflects the ability of the individual to adapt to changes in environment (Wong 1976). Concepts in the model are degree of internal and external stimulation, thirst, and drinking behavior. They are defined as follows:

A. *Degree of internal and external stimulation* is the magnitude of alterations instigated by the combined function of focal, contextual, and residual stimuli that require adjustment.

 1. *Focal stimuli* are factors immediately confronting the individual that contribute to development of behavior.

 2. *Contextual stimuli* are other factors present that contribute to development of behavior.

 3. *Residual stimuli* are factors such as attitudes and beliefs that contribute to development of behavior. These definitions were derived from Roy (1976).

B. *Thirst* is a motivational state resulting from an interaction between physiological (absolute or relative dehydration), neuroendocrine determinants, and experiential factors, in which there is sensation of a need or desire for water, which represents attempts to adjust to changes in environment (Epstein 1976; Epstein and Kissileff 1973; Fitzsimons 1975; and Wong 1976).

C. *Drinking behavior* is goal-directed activity resulting from sensation of thirst. Thirst is displayed in two phases: (1) *appetitive phase,* which includes those activities associated with obtaining and preparing the fluid to be consumed, and (2) any activity associated with seeking fluid to be consumed as well as the consummatory phase of drinking or the actual consuming of the obtained fluid (Denny and Ratnor 1970; Wong 1976; and Fitzsimons 1975).

The referentials of the model are FCRI, BTI, PTI, DBI, and DSBI. The definitions are as follows:

FCRI is an acronym for the index of the magnitude of combined focal, contextual, and residual stimuli. FCRI is the individual score on the instrument (not yet devised). Magnitude of stimulation is to be determined by rating kind of focal, contextual, and residual stimuli. Amount of stimulation will also be determined. Among factors to be considered in determining focal stimuli are any pathology present and its associated therapeutic regimen. If fluid restriction is part of the regimen, degree of deprivation this regimen requires will be determined. Determination of contextual stimuli will be based on situational factors, that is, setting and specific nursing intervention directed toward the individual. To determine the magnitude of residual stimuli, experiential factors, drinking habits, attitudes toward existing pathology, associated therapeutic regimen, and health care beliefs must be considered (Wong 1976; and Roy 1976).

BTI is an acronym for the index of magnitude of biological thirst. A score for all biological indicators of thirst (ADH, angiotensin II, and osmolality levels) will constitute the BTI (Fitzsimons 1975; Epstein 1976; Anderson 1971; and Peck and Blass 1975).

PTI is an acronym for the index of psychosocial thirst. The PTI score will be determined by questionnaire. An attempt will be made to ascertain actual perceived sensations of thirst. Among parameters to be assessed within the PTI are presence or absence of dry mouth, desire for specific fluids, and description of the overall sensation of thirst (Wong 1976; Holmes 1963; Anderson 1971; and Fitzsimons 1961).

DBI is an acronym describing the magnitude of the drinking behavior index. The DBI is the individual's score on the instrument. To be included in this instrument are amount of fluid consumed per day, amount of each specific fluid consumed, and amount of fluid consumed when fluid temperature varies (Wong 1976; Deux 1973; Collier, Hirsh, and Hamlin 1972; and Anderson 1971).

DSBI is an acronym describing the magnitude of the drink-seeking behavior index. The DSBI is the individual's score on objective behavior demonstrated as preparation for actual consumption. Items to be included in the DSBI instrument will be both verbal and nonverbal behaviors (such as asking for fluids and evidence of anger) (Olivas 1978; and Wong 1976).

The *unit term* in this model is the individual. The *individual* is defined as any person, ill or healthy, who is interacting and responding to the environment.

Time units in this model are To, oTa, and Tn + 1. *To* represents the point in time that the individual receives the degree of internal and external stimulation. *oTa* is the point in time that physiological and psychosocial indications of adaptation occur after stimulation. *Tn + 1* represents the time that motivated behavior indicators appear and designate responses to occurrence of the sensation of thirst.

Intrinsic Statements Related to the Model

Axiom 1. Among individuals, the greater environmental changes at To, the greater the evidence of biopsychosocial adaptation process at oTa.

Axion 2. Among individuals, the greater evidence of biopsychosociological adaptation process at oTa, the greater the demonstrated response in motivated behavior at Tn + 1.

Postulate 1. Among individuals, the greater the environmental changes at To, the greater the degree of internal and external stimulation at To.

Postulate 2. Among individuals, the greater the biopsychosocial adaptation process at oTa, the greater the sensation of thirst at oTa.

Postulate 3. Among individuals, the greater the motivated behavior at Tn + 1, the greater the drinking behavior at Tn + 1.

Proposition 1. Among individuals, the greater the degree of internal and external stimulation at To, the greater the sensation of thirst at oTa.

Proposition 2. Among individuals, the greater the thirst sensation at oTa, the greater the drinking behavior at Tn + 1.

Transformational Statement 1. Among individuals, the greater the degree of internal and external stimulation at To, the greater the FCRI at To.

Transformational Statements 2 and 3. Among individuals, the greater the thirst at oTa, the greater the BTI and PTI at oTa.

Transformational Statements 4 and 5. Among individuals, the greater the drinking behavior at Tn + 1, the greater the DBI and DSBI at Tn + 1.

Theorem 1. Among individuals, the greater the FCRI at To, the greater the BTI at oTa.

Theorem 2. Among individuals, the greater the FCRI at To, the greater the PTI at oTa.

Theorem 3. Among individuals, the greater the FCRI at To, the greater the DBI at Tn + 1.

Theorem 4. Among individuals, the greater the FCRI at To, the greater the DSBI at Tn + 1.

Theorem 5. Among individuals, the greater the BTI at oTa, the greater the DBI at Tn + 1.

Theorem 6. Among individuals, the greater the BTI at oTa, the greater the DBI at Tn + 1.

Theorem 7. Among individuals, the greater the PTI at oTa, the greater the DBI at Tn + 1.

Theorem 8. Among individuals, the greater the PTI at oTa, the greater the DSBI at Tn + 1.

The schematic representation of the model appears in Figure 10-3.

Features of the Model

The proposed theoretical model has many implications for nursing. Although it appears to be a factor-relating or situation-predicting theory (Dickoff and James

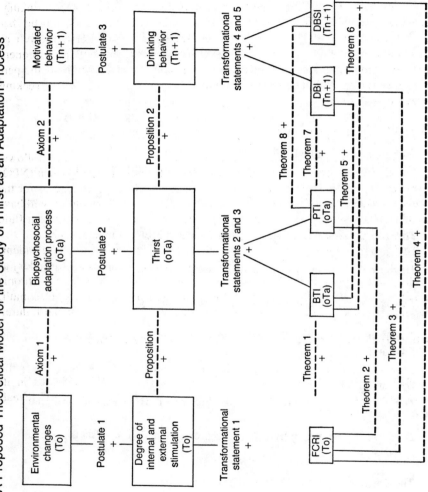

Figure 10-3 A Proposed Theoretical Model for the Study of Thirst as an Adaptation Process

1968), the model does have situation-producing or prescriptive potential. If the clinical phenomenon of thirst can be completely understood, clinicians can direct their attention to manipulating the stimuli that trigger the occurrence of thirst and drinking behavior. Nursing intervention can become a greater portion of the stimuli index in the form of contextual stimuli. In this way, nursing intervention may influence the perceived sensation of thirst and thus drinking and drinking-seeking behaviors. The model offers the potential of testing a relationship between a specific nursing intervention and the sensation of thirst, as well as drinking behavior. For example, if intervention was the scheduling of frequent fluid drinking schedules with cold fluids, it is possible to determine if the perceived sensation of thirst will differ and if drinking behavior or drinking-seeking behavior will differ.

A Walk-Through Example

An example of how the model operates at the extremes of variation follows. If an otherwise healthy individual is placed on a fluid-restricted regimen (NPO) for surgery, the individual's focal stimuli index would not be as great as for the individual with chronic renal failure, who, by virtue of the pathology, will have high focal stimulus. The chronic renal failure patient is also on a constant fluid restricted regimen, which further contributes to the focal stimuli index.

Indicators of thirst would be much higher for the chronic renal failure patient, as compared to the "healthy" surgical patient. The drinking behavior index, as well as the drink-seeking behavior index, will also be higher for the chronic renal failure patient. Nursing intervention, in the form of contextual stimuli, would need to play a greater role for the individual with chronic renal failure.

Strengths and Weaknesses of the Model According to Hardy's Criteria

The proposed theoretical model has both strengths and weaknesses in its present stage of development. Evaluation using Hardy's (1974) criteria reveals the location of strengths and weaknesses.

Meaning and logical adequacy are met by the model.

Concepts are well identified and defined.

Relationships between concepts are delineated.

The concepts and relationships are valid.

There is logic in the theoretical system.

The model has been formalized according to Gibbs's (1972) paradigm.

There are no discontinuities or discrepancies.

The theoretical model is testable.

The theory has operationally defined concepts in the form of acronyms.

The instruments need development to meet the criterion of empirical adequacy.

The relations asserted have been empirically tested by comparative psychologists. The research has, however, been in the laboratory with animals. This model is designated to be tested in clinical settings with people.

The model offers both a high degree of abstractness and contributes to the understanding of behavior.

Predictability and pragmatic adequacy can be attained once the model has been empirically tested.

REFERENCES

Anderson, B. Thirst—Brain control of water balance. *Am. Sci.* 58:408, Aug. 1971.

Collier, G., Hirsh, E., and Hamlin, D.H. The ecological determinants of reinforcement in the rat. *Physiol. Behav.* 9:705–716, 1972.

Denny, M.R., and Ratnor, S.G. *Comparative Psychology: Research in Animal Behavior*. Hinsdale, Ill.: Dorsey, 1970.

Deux, E. Thirst satiation and temperature of ingested water. *Science* 181:1166, Sept. 1973.

Dickoff, J., James, P., and Wiedenbach, E. Theory in a practice discipline. *Nurs. Res.* 17:5, Sept.–Oct. 1968.

Epstein, A.V. The physiology of thirst. *Can. J. Physiol. Pharmacol.* 54(5):639–648, Oct. 1976.

Epstein, A.V., Kissileff, R., and Stellar, E. *Neuropsychology of Thirst: New Findings and Advances in Concepts*. New York: Wiley, 1973.

Fitzsimons, J.T., Peters, G., and Peters-Haefeli, L. *Control Mechanisms of Drinking*. New York: Springer-Verlag, 1975.

Gibbs, J. *Sociological Theory Construction*. Ill.: Dryden, 1972.

Hardy, M.E. Theories: Components, development, evaluation. *Nurs. Res.* 23(2):100–105, Mar.–Apr. 1974.

Holmes, J.H. Thirst and Fluid Problems in Clinical Medicine. In M.J. Wayner (Ed.), *Thirst*. New York: Macmillan, 1963.

Olivas, G.S. Thirst Phenomenon and Fluid Restriction. In C.M. Norris. *Concept Clarification in Nursing*. Rockville, Md.: Aspen Systems Corp.,1982.

Peck, J.W., and Blass, E.M. Localization of thirst and antidiuretic osmorecepters by intracranial injection in rats. *Am. J. Physiol.* 228:1501–1509, 1975.

Riehl, J.P., and Roy, C. (Eds.). *Conceptual Models for Nursing Practice*. New York: Appleton-Century-Crofts, 1974.

Roy, C. Adaptation: A conceptual framework for nursing. *Nurs. Outlook* 18(3):42, Mar. 1970.

Roy, C. *Introduction to Nursing: An Adaptation Model*. Englewood Cliffs, N.J.: Prentice-Hall, 1976.

Webster's Third New International Dictionary of the English Language: Unabridged. Springfield, Mass.: G & C Merriam, 1967.

Wong, R. *Motivation: A Biobehavioral Analysis of Consummatory Activities*. New York: Macmillan, 1976.

Chapter 11

The Significance of Hunger to Nursing

Jacqueline Anderson

MANIFESTATIONS OF HUNGER

A twelve-year-old boy is hospitalized for abdominal pain. An emergency appendectomy is followed by an abscess and obstructed bowel requiring another surgical procedure. The boy is kept NPO from the time of hospitalization until recovery of bowel sounds following the second surgery. Subsequent to this second operation nurses' notes read, "Patient up and walking; upset behavior; pulse and respirations increased; patient consumed a pitcherful of water, vomited; patient upset by NPO order; patient hungry; patient feels 'helpless'; patient can't sleep."

The patient states, "I want to eat; my stomach hurts. It feels like I'm starving." Notes in the next few days vary from, "patient sleepy" to "patient restless," and finally, "patient very depressed, withdrawn."

What nursing interventions were offered to this hungry patient? It is recorded that, "Explanations helped the patient with his hunger and in understanding the reasons for NPO." Nurses' notes also record that the one event, which was not a purposeful intervention, that helped this boy to cope with hunger was increased activity; when he got up and walked, he seemed to feel better and to be less hungry.

There are few nursing interventions that help patients contend with enforced hunger. Explanation of the NPO order was offered and helped this hungry child, but we wonder whether the explanation included validation of the boy's behaviors and feelings by indicating that his actions and feelings were predictable and acceptable responses to hunger.

Another patient, hypertensive and on an enforced hospital diet, was described in nurses' notes as a difficult patient, hyperactive at times, lethargic at times, easily distracted except when discussing food, flat- or sullen-faced, irritable, and uncooperative. Are these characteristics typical for this patient or are they predictable behaviors of any hungry person? In our culture, obese individuals are blamed for being greedy, not really hungry, having no willpower or self-control. Nurses may unwittingly extend these societal value judgments onto patients. Nurses' notes that assess patients' eating patterns often do not identify their motives for eating. Nurses may not assess emotional factors, degree of appetite, or degree of hunger. Impugning motives, then, lays the groundwork for value judgments; it is more useful to assume the patient is hungry and proceed from there to predict and identify "hungry" behaviors. Nurses need to identify whether *behaviors* are characteristic of hunger or not. If they do this, value judgments become less common and nurses can make firmer assessments and interventions.

A group of 16 nurses interviewed for this exploratory study corroborated on the importance of hunger in nursing. Nurses indicated that both hunger and anorexia alert them to underlying malfunctions such as depression (manifested by increased or decreased hunger), hypoglycemia, diabetes, insulinoma, cancer, intestinal obstruction, pain, responses to medication and increasing obesity. Hunger, then, may have medical diagnostic potential as well as being a nursing problem requiring diagnosis and intervention.

Nurses agreed that hunger is a protective mechanism in that the brain signals the body's need for the nutrients required for functioning, maintenance, and building. They further agreed that many routine occurrences in the hospital environment create the need for nutritional vigilance. During the postpartum period, postsurgical period, posttrauma period, and during any illness, especially chronic illness, there is a crucial need for nutrients to rebuild tissue and to supply energy.

Even though hunger is perceived as protective in maintaining adequate nutrition for the body, experience reveals that patients' hunger is often subjective and not always valid. People who are undergoing stresses such as illness, injury, surgery, birth, or emotional upset may have hunger disturbances that interfere with the drive to attain the needed nutrients. There are patients who "should be hungry," but who do not, will not, or cannot eat (e.g., anorexia nervosa or depressed patients, as well as patients whose illness or injuries such as cancer or broken jaw interfere with their ability or desire to eat). Some patients experience physiological "hunger," but block mental awareness of it; others may be alert to their hunger but unwilling or unable to respond to it. One nurse said, "Patients get so worried about other things, they may forget they are hungry. This distorts their behavior and feelings." Another nurse stated, "One must identify the patient's hunger and fill that need first. It is difficult to prepare hungry patients for diagnostic procedures or to teach them self-care." Another added, "Geriatric patients often do not communicate their hunger verbally, and do not eat unless someone is alert to their nonverbal cues of hunger."

In summary, (1) certain patients (infant, child, geriatric, emotionally disturbed, very ill, or anxious) may not realize their own hunger; (2) some patients may be hungry and know that they are hungry, but for some reason, choose to suppress their desire for food; and (3) an alert nurse may identify hunger by observing patients' behaviors or appearance.

If nurses cannot depend on patients to report their hunger, clarification of the concept *hunger,* as defined by behaviors, feelings, and observable effect, is crucial to diagnosis of all a patient's nursing needs. But determining that patients are hungry is not enough; patients' hunger may be readily apparent, as when they are NPO.

On the other hand, consistently uneaten meals signals that patients are not eating, but whether hunger is present is a matter for assessment. Once hunger is identified as a problem, nurses need to be in a position to select relevant interventions from among a greater number of options. Appropriateness and number of interventions will be based on adequate comprehension of the concept hunger.

PROPERTIES OF THE PHENOMENON *HUNGER*

In studying the phenomenon hunger, the investigator perused patient charts and anecdotal notes made by nurses and interviewed and observed nine patients (three hospitalized patients and six community clients who were on diets because of obesity). After studying the data from these sources, it became clear that not all individuals experience hunger in the same way. Trends, nevertheless, could be identified.

Three apparent categories of evidence associated with or denoting hunger emerged.

One category labeled *behaviors* was identified from the sources studied. These behaviors were subdivided into three areas: preoccupation, increased activity, and emotional lability. Preoccupation behaviors included asking for food; seeking food, which at times resulted in cheating on diets; attempting to put something in the stomach to replace food (e.g., drinking a pitcherful of water, consuming more water or coffee, filling up on salad); having difficulty in concentrating because of inability to think of anything other than food; being anxious for food tray; feeling need to talk about food; fantasizing about food and eating; watching the clock until the next meal; having increased awareness of food stimuli (e.g. advertisements, sight, smell, and suggestion of food); increasing awareness that thought processes are being interrupted by ideas about food and food cravings; eating rapidly when food is obtained.

A second component of behavior category related to increased activity. Behaviors included pacing, and walking faster than usual; being restless, fidgety, wired up, or hyperactive, unable to sleep (some individuals stated that they slept more and related this to a desire to escape); eating faster; increased urination, nausea, diarrhea, or constipation.

A third subcategory of behavior is associated with emotional lability. Responses include irritability, jumpiness, impatience, moodiness, complaining, being short-tempered, feeling anxious, disagreeable, being noncaring, feeling on edge, crying easily, being angry, being frustrated, acting upset, screaming, or whining.

People also experienced and described behaviors associated with decreased energy such as being shaky, being unable to concentrate, feeling tired, moving more slowly than usual, feeling fatigued, being forgetful, being unable to think well, being weak, feeling sluggish, being sleepy, feeling lazy, being less willing to participate in self-care, being disinterested and being more passive than usual.

The second hunger category concerns what individuals who are hungry say they feel. These internal experiences also were grouped into three subcategories. The first includes feelings that may be associated with hypermotility of the gastrointestinal tract, as in *early hunger*. People say such things as "I feel my stomach growl"; "I have a noisy stomach"; "I have an upset stomach"; "I have stomach pains"; "I have hunger pains"; "I feel nauseated"; "I feel sick to my stomach"; "I feel empty"; "I crave something in my mouth"; "The bottom of my stomach feels coated with salt"; "I crave a good steak" or other particular food; "I feel a sense of urgency"; "I have increased urination"; "I have diarrhea."

The second subcategory deals with feelings stemming from emotional lability such as anxiousness, tenseness, nervousness, agitation, excitability, irritability, inability to think clearly, inability to concentrate, not in control of self, being afraid, feeling depressed, feeling frustrated, being angry, being passive, or not caring.

Another subcategory related to feelings hungry individuals complained of, seemed to come from *decreased energy*, such as faintness, nausea, shakiness, lightheadedness, inability to think clearly, like "I must have something to eat", weakness, jitteriness, fatigue, tension, dizziness, or headache. Some hungry people describe feelings and problems that are associated with decreased gastric mobility, such as constipation, flatulence, or lack of feeling in their stomachs. This last subcategory of feelings of hungry people seems to emerge from those who are more hungry or who have been deprived of food for a longer period than people in the first two subcategories.

The third category related to examination of the data about hunger is *affect* and answers the question, "What do individuals who are hungry look like?" Observations associated with food-seeking were expectant, attentive, impatient, restless, pleading look. Observations associated with increased sympathetic nervous system activity or emotional lability included anxiousness, nervousness, tension, increased perspiration, and pallor. Patients with decreased energy evidenced drawn faces (looking tired, hollow, washed out, wan), irritability, frustration, shakiness, weakness, boredom, listlessness, sagginess, lethargy, withdrawal, discomfort, and if the condition was severe, emaciation. There is also the possibility that some hungry people have no distinguishing characteristics and have no visible change in affect.

The above behaviors, feelings, and affect were categorized from empirical data gleaned from observation and interviews with patients and clients.

CLINICAL MANIFESTATIONS OF HUNGER AS COMPARED TO REPORTS ABOUT HUNGER IN THE LITERATURE

The literature reveals that many authors agree that certain behaviors and feelings are associated with hunger. Hunger may be viewed as on a continuum, that is, behavioral manifestations of initial hunger are different than when hunger is prolonged or when a state of starvation exists. The effects of hunger are progressive but behaviors and feelings overlap, regress, and fluctuate. Though individual differences are to be expected, some differences may be accounted for in relation to each person's place along the hunger continuum. Patients who are NPO may progress along the continuum fairly predictably; individuals who are on a restricted diet, however, especially if it is periodically broken, may fluctuate greatly in their position on the continuum.

The Hunger Continuum

Initial hunger. Initial hunger usually provokes release of glycogen stores, supplying increased energy. Individuals may feel excitable, energetic, nervous, and restless. Under normal conditions this energy is directed to food-seeking behavior. Very soon, people have hunger pangs, anticipatory salivation, feelings of weakness, or feelings of emptiness (Tepperman 1973). Occasionally, headache and nausea (Beland and Passos 1975, p. 770), increased taste responsiveness (Nisbett 1972), and increased gastric motility (Guyton 1976); all of these spur the search for food. In beginning hunger, activity levels increase. There is adequate energy, and there is hope of success in getting food and satisfying the hunger drive.

When food is not obtained, people become weak, irritable, withdrawn, and restless (Beland et al. 1975, p. 771). They are more prone to act fearfully because the fear threshold is lower in hunger. Hunger decreases frustration tolerance (Nisbett 1972; and Schachter, 1971). Schachter (1971) found that hypothalamus-lesioned rats displayed hyperphagia, "were easily startled, over-emotional . . . more frightened and anxious," tended to "move or scramble about in their experimental box and were more responsive to external stimuli."

As hunger progresses there is

1. Increased irritability, vindictiveness, outbursts of temper, emotional upset (crying) (Nisbett 1972).
2. Increasing apathy and decreasing activity. Here the person may have less energy and correspondingly less hope . . . thus conserves his/her energy unless prominent stimuli impinge to (a) frustrate or annoy and (b) offer hope of food.
3. Decreased interest in sex (Keys, et al. 1950).

Extreme and long-duration hunger. Leyton (1946) studied the effects of hunger on humans during famine and in concentration camps. As a captured medical officer, he observed the effects of slow starvation in German prisoner-of-war (World War II) camps in Libya, Italy, and Germany. In the classic work, *The Biology of Human Starvation,* Keys et al. (1950, pp. 783–818) explored the findings of many chroniclers of hunger, set up the Minnesota experiment that verified these reports and made significant additions to knowledge about hunger. Behavior changes noted by Keys were marked in three areas: emotionality, activity, and sex.

1. *Emotionality.* People experiencing extreme hunger become more prone to emotional upset, unusual vindictiveness, extraordinary irritability, and chronic crying (Keys et al. 1950, p. 909). It is important to note that periods of elation also occur; these are typically followed by periods of depression. This is attributed to a "starvation high." Multiphasic Personality Inventory Scales administered to humans indicated hunger's marked effects of the "neurotic triad": depression, hypochondriasis, and hysteria (Nisbett 1972). According to Halbreich (1976), there is also "impaired self-body image, impaired perception of time . . . slowing down of the inner clock . . . and change in quality and preference of taste."
2. *Activity.* Depression is accompanied by apathy, inactivity, decrease in libido, and excessive irritability (Halbreich 1976). Thus during semistarvation, humans become progressively more apathetic and inactive; it takes an effort of will to do what is necessary. Conservation of energy, fatigue, degeneration of body tissue, and decreased hope must all play a role.
3. *Sex.* Experiments of semistarved humans demonstrate nearly total destruction of sexual motivation (Keys et al. 1950). On a continuum, there is fluctuation, but a constant escalation of emotionality, accompanied by decreasing energy and loss of interest in sexual motivation.

Physical Changes Associated with Hunger

Temperature. Anecdotal notes, interviews, and chart recordings indicated that some hungry individuals said their skin felt cold; they felt more susceptible to cold and felt an increased desire for hot food. This supports Keys and colleagues (1950) who also found increased tolerance for heat:

> Tolerance to heat was increased; for example, subjects could hold hot plates without discomfort. They asked that their food, coffee, and tea be served unusually hot. Conversely, cold temperatures were poorly tolerated. Complaints of being cold or of having cold hands and feet were frequent.

Keys and co-workers (1950) also describe the following cardiovascular phenomenon:

> An outstanding constant peculiarity of severely undernourished persons is sinus bradycardia. . . . In this study the minimum heart rate was reached fairly early in starvation, when the body weight loss was only about 15 percent; thereafter the heart rate gradually rose. There is other evidence that this is a general phenomenon and that conservation of the heart by slowing its rate becomes less possible as the heart itself undergoes more profound degeneration.

They also found mild cyanosis, cold skin as indicative of reduced peripheral circulation, which is possibly an attempt of the body to conserve heat.

Edema. The six community patients in this study were on self-imposed diets. All denied evidence of edema. The hospitalized patients, however, were often noted to have edema; these patients had complicating physical problems that might account for the edema. On the other hand, the hospitalized patients who were NPO were more nutritionally deprived compared to the community-patients. In the hospital, edema was reported by health care personnel and not left up to the individual.

Keys and co-workers (1950) observed edema in many subjects:

> The edema represents a disproportion of fluid to cellular tissue which is produced by shrinkage of the cells with maintenance of an unchanged bulk of extracellular fluid. However, this must mean that the structural and elastic forces in the organs are changed.

Anecdotal notes in this study revealed that most of the subjects on unrestricted liquid intake evinced increased fluid consumption of water and, often, coffee; accompanying this was a desire for salt and spices. Polyuria and nocturia were also reported. This agrees with Keys and associates (1950).

> Polyuria is generally present, and nocturia is a frequent complaint.

The voluntary fluid intake is usually much elevated, but thirst is not often mentioned as a complaint.

Skin and hair reactions, muscle cramping, joint soreness. Often changes in skin, hair, muscle comfort, and joint ease were either not noted or were denied. However, one dieter observed weakening of fingernails; another maintained that her "skin cleared up"; a third complained of soreness in knee joints and legs. The Minnesota Experiment disclosed prolonged hunger as associated with deterioration of skin and hair, as well as feeling and acting old beyond one's years.

> Subjects experiencing prolonged hunger reported that their nails grew more slowly and that their hair was falling out . . . cuts and wounds bled less than normally and were slower to heal . . . muscle cramps and particularly muscle soreness were frequently reported. . . . jarring of knee joints . . . thinning and roughening of skin . . . complaints that the extremities went to sleep (Keys et al. 1950).

This study also supported other findings related to changes in the effects of drugs as well as the possibility of improved asthma and eczema.

> Drugs and hormones which ordinarily provoked prompt and striking effects behave as though their potency was impaired. This is seen notably with adrenalin, pilocarpine, atropine and insulin; the vasomotor effects as well as those on the glucose–glycogen system are greatly delayed and limited in magnitude. There are suggestions also that allergic and anaphylactic phenomena are repressed. In some cases eczema and asthma become less troublesome or even disappear (Keys et al. 1950).

Vision and hearing. Decreased visual or auditory acuity was denied by individuals observed or interviewed. Keys and colleagues (1950, p. 829) reported

> Standard measurements of hearing showed a slight but consistent increase in auditory acuity during the period of semi-starvation. It is difficult to determine whether the frequent complaints that ordinary sounds and noises were disturbing and annoying had a direct physiological basis in the "improved" auditory sensitivity or were primarily signs of an increased irritability.

People must not make the mistake of thinking the extremely hungry patient is not alert.

. . . his behavior is often misleading. He acts dull and insensitive; he looks and behaves as though he were unaware of or incapable of feeling many of the ordinary stimuli of sound, sight, or touch. But in fact his sensory mechanisms seem to be extraordinarily well maintained. Objective tests, as in the Minnesota Experiment, indicate that vision is resistant to deterioration in starvation and that hearing actually becomes more acute. There is some physiological basis for the old saying that "hunger sharpens the senses" (Keys et al. 1950, p. 581).

Complaints of feeling faint, weak, headachy. Individuals reported that hunger made them feel weak, dizzy, faint, shaky, headachy. These physiological reactions to hunger are commonly acknowledged.

Constipation or diarrhea. Clinically, some individuals complained of diarrhea; more often constipation was cited. Diarrhea can occur because of intervening physiological problems, and, especially in semistarvation, due to harsh or irritating foods. Constipation is more common because of decreased gastric motility and prolonged emptying time (Keys et al. 1950, pp. 592–600).

Behavioral Changes Associated with Hunger

Preoccupation with food. Most individuals interviewed demonstrated some preoccupation with food. Health care personnel who work with these people are familiar with this phenomenon. One woman, a 45-year-old asthmatic was hospitalized to lose weight. Nurses reported, "She talks constantly about eating and food. Then she goes on justifying talking about food. Food preoccupies her." The patient says, "If you'd just give me food, I'd be able to stop thinking about it." All the studies (see literature reviewed) confirm this type of behavior. People who are hungry think about food. Anecdotal notes of this study reveal that some individuals found some limited coping methods themselves. Usefulness of these mechanisms is individualized.

1. *Gum chewing.* Some people reported distraction and relief provided by gum chewing. Others felt no benefit from chewing and refused gum. Those using gum were prone to escalate chewing as hunger increased. Gum chewing may have to be restricted if patients have sore mouths or sore jaw muscles. In regard to gum chewing, it is interesting to note that one of the short-term receptors hypothesized to act in controlling hunger responses are "head receptors" (Guyton 1976, p. 975). It is proposed that after a certain amount of food passes through the mouth (with chewing, salivation, swallowing and/or tasting) the hypothalamic center is inhibited. Such inhibition has been noted even in people with esophageal fistulas, in which

food is immediately lost to the exterior, never reaching the stomach and intestines.

2. *Smoking*. Though most of the individuals studied for the purpose of clarifying hunger did not smoke, smoking is a prominent substitute for the satisfaction of eating, among both dieters and those whose food is restricted for other reasons.

3. *Activity*. Most individuals questioned indicated that an increase in activity helped them cope with their hunger. Activity functioned as a distraction in that it made patients feel better physically and psychologically and either had no effect on their hunger or decreased it (except for the woman who swam, whose hunger increased). This is in accord with Nisbett's (1972) finding. He maintains that activity itself allows the body to drop weight without having to restore its weight to the previous level. Thus, exercise does not stimulate hunger to the point of weight gain. On the contrary, "a small drop in weight occurs and the animal eats only enough to sustain itself at its new weight level. Why this occurs is a mystery." Apparently, activity aids the body to function at a lower intake level, as in the case, for example, of the 12-year-old hospitalized boy who felt better and less hungry after he got up and walked.

4. *Fantasizing*. Some of the individuals interviewed by this writer indicated that fantasizing about food was definitely helpful to them. One woman stated that devoting a special time to fantasies about restaurants and food and pleasure helped release her cravings and did not result in her breaking her diet. Some people reported that they got vicarious pleasure from watching others eat or from just smelling food. Those familiar with hungry people, with the literature of WW II concentration camps and with the professional literature know that food in every context imaginable can permeate every conversation, every activity, and all thinking.

5. *Food rituals*. Most individuals interviewed spoke of a developing need to eat more slowly, to play with their food, and to create patterns of handling and consuming the food. Nurses' notes on the asthmatic woman hospitalized to lose weight describe this typical behavior: "Given two diet gelatins at night, she assumes a ritual position on the bed; she eats very slowly, seeming to savor each bite . . . drawing it out for 15 or 20 minutes to eat one serving." Keys also notes this phenomenon.

Toying with food was mentioned by Friedrich . . . People made what under normal conditions would be weird and distasteful concoctions . . . increase in spices and salt. They played with their food for hours . . . in long, drawn-out ritual (Keys et al. 1950, Vol. II, p. 832).

Self-perception of hunger. This is an area of confusion, because it is very difficult to come to an agreement on a definition for hunger. Some individuals interviewed perceived hunger as feelings in their stomach; others had physical feelings in mouth, throat, or stomach. Some, however, expressed a much broader perception–focus, stating that they knew they were hungry when they felt weak, irritable, nervous, or restless. This confusion permeates the literature as well. Some authors make a distinction between hunger and appetite and attempt to restrict hunger to a physical sensation perceived to be in the area of the stomach. One dictionary (Tabers 1970) defines hunger as a sensation resulting from lack of food, characterized by dull or acute pain referred to the epigastrium or lower part of the chest . . . hunger pains coincide with powerful contractions of the stomach. Appetite is defined as a pleasant sensation based on previous experience, which causes one to seek food for the purpose of tasting and enjoying.

Drawing upon a selected literature review, *hunger* may be defined as a life-sustaining drive and a physiological need, characterized by pain and unpleasantness. Cognitively, there is an awareness of the need and a focusing of attention. Behaviorally, there is increased salivation, contractions of the stomach or intestines, and food-searching behavior. Hunger seems to be motivated by forces internal to the organism.

On the other hand, *appetite* is defined as a psychic desire, characterized by its pleasantness. It is conditioned by previous experience . . . and is stimulated by external sources, such as sight, smell, and taste of food, as well as by internal sources such as emotion and mood. Appetite can be present with or without hunger.

For the person who is eating regularly and is maintaining a stable weight, such a dichotomy between hunger and appetite seems accurate and useful.

Clinical Observations

In the clinical situation, however, where hungry subjects of this study could not act on their hunger and maintain a stable weight, this dichotomy between hunger and appetite seemed less useful. These people experienced a broader awareness of hunger: Their weakness, irritability, psychological cravings, mood, emotions, and the smell of food were all part of hunger for them. Hunger sensations were not limited to the stomach nor did they exclude the psyche.

The difficulty and danger of trying to distinguish hunger from appetite in the clinical situation become evident when we recognize that both are culturally laden with values. For example, people who are thin are probably hungry . . . and to be pitied, while people who are fat are not hungry; they just don't know how to control their appetite and are to be condemned.

There are many theories of obesity. It is still unclear what factors predispose to obesity. Nisbett (1972) proposed the "set point" theory. According to this theory, some individuals have a higher baseline level of adipose tissue than others. Heredity and early nutrition patterns may create a condition of hyperplasia, that is, an increase in the number of fat cells. This theory also proposes that this increased adipose tissue mass is defended by the central nervous system. Hypothalamic feeding centers adjust food intake to maintain the set point level. The extra fat cells are always waiting to be filled back up. If this theory is accurate, fat individuals are not just eating for pleasure, or appetite, but are driven by the physiological level of hunger. If these people attempt to maintain normal weight, they would be starving all the time. Patients themselves do not know the motivation for their eating behavior.

One nurse's note read, "The patient has just eaten . . . and still says she's hungry. . . . Impossible!"

Keys and co-workers (1950, Vol. II, p. 847) observed that semistarved subjects who were allowed to eat as much as they wanted often ate to the point where stomach distention made continuing impossible, yet they reported that they were still hungry. For example, he speaks of the rehabilitating individual, "No. 20 who stuffs himself until he is bursting at the seams, to the point of being nearly sick, and still he felt hungry." Perhaps here long-term regulators that have been long deprived are dominant over the short-term regulators that should be telling the individual that the stomach is full and can hold no more. The body as a whole is crying to be filled up *now*!*

The simplest definition of hunger is by Orbach (1978, p. 108), "The word 'hunger' usually connotes the desire to eat. The body is depleted and needs nourishment. In its extreme form, hunger becomes starvation."

Assertion and control as a coping mechanism against hunger. Some interviewed individuals said that talking helped them cope with their hunger as did asserting themselves and feeling more in control. Keys and others (1950, p. 835) stress the need of hungry individuals to talk, to control the manner of intake of whatever food is allowed, and to avoid social contact (i.e., control their environment). Orbach (1978) also identifies the relationship between assertion and hunger.

Decreased energy. Some individuals, especially the community-health dieters interviewed, said their energy increased; this usually was nervous energy, however. As previously noted in the initial stages of hunger, people often experience increased energy and restlessness, which under normal conditions is directed to food-hunting behavior. If food-seeking is not allowed, as in dieting

---

*For a review of long- and short-term regulators, see Guyton (pp. 972–976). Some hypothesized examples of long-term regulation are hypothalamus, higher centers (amygdala and cortical areas of the limbic system); glucostatic theory; amino acid concentration theory; lipostatic theory; body temperature. Some hypothesized short-term regulators are gastrointestinal distention, head distention, head receptors, habit, and emotions.

or NPO, this energy often takes the form of restlessness, nervousness, increased physical activity, and/or irritable response.

Some of the individuals studied, especially inpatients, exhibited lethargic, apathetic, depressed behavior. Unlike community clients, these hospitalized patients had no diversions, no activities, and no responsibilities toward which to direct their behavior. The community clients all commented that they "kept busy"; the more they did this, the better they coped with their hunger and the better they felt. Perhaps the possibility for distraction and directed activity is one reason they did not become as lethargic as some of the hospitalized patients.

The 12-year-old hospitalized boy, NPO for 2 weeks, indicated that getting up to walk helped him to cope as noted previously. Nonetheless, it must be noted that the hospitalized patients usually had physiological problems beyond weight loss that might account for increased lethargy and exhaustion. These patients also demonstrate mood swings. Keys and colleagues (1950) note this fluctuation of energy and mood as follows:

> Some spells of elation occurred. . . . Feeling "high" was sometimes attributed by the men to a "quickening" effect of starvation or to success in adjusting to the semi-starvation diet. These feelings of well-being and exhilaration lasted from a few hours to several days but were inevitably followed by "low" periods. . . . Personal appearance and grooming began to deteriorate as the stress progressed.

Increased emotional lability. Some people were unable to control their moods.

> The even-temperedness, patience and tolerance . . . gave way . . . irritability increased to the point that it became an individual and group problem. Although the men were well aware of their hyperirritability, they were not altogether able to control their emotionally charged responses. Outbursts of temper and periods of sulking and pique were not uncommon (Keys et al. 1950).

These same investigators noted unusual vindictiveness and chronic crying. Their findings were supported by the work of Halbreich (1976).

Schachter (1972) reports hungry people as more responsive to external stimuli and prone to being easily frustrated, frightened, and annoyed.

Self-perception of hunger. Some of the patients investigated, though deprived of food for some time, refused food and expressed no hunger.

Individuals during rehabilitation or semistarvation often experienced more severe awareness of stomach hunger than did those persons in complete starvation.

Sex. Most of the individuals interviewed indicated decreased interest in sex, which supports Keys's and co-workers' (1950) findings that

> Sexual feelings and expression declined in the Minnesota Experiment until by the end of the semi-starvation period they were virtually extinguished in all but a few subjects.

Biologically, this decreased interest in sex may be an adaptive measure to protect the individual's well-being through energy conservation. Decreased sex impulse is accompanied by decreased sociability in general.

HUNGER AND VALUES

Hunger is a positive, protective mechanism. Hunger drives the organism to eat and to live. The mechanism can be distorted by emotional or physiological processes; it can be abnormally increased to the point of obesity or abnormally decreased, as in anorexia, to the point of starvation. Western culture judges hunger to be bad and generally encourages people to avoid it—indeed, to avoid any painful state—at the first sign of discomfort. This may help explain our proclivity to conclude that obesity is caused by appetite rather than hunger. If obese people were perceived as really hungry, whether for food, self-confidence, or love, we could not make them into scapegoats; their need would be real and their condition painful.

In considering the evolutionary relationship of hunger, emotion, and our state of civilization, hunger that was once protective has sometimes become distorted. Life may have once been such that triggering emotions triggered hunger, which was protective. If we became angered, frustrated, or threatened, we would need increased sustenance to flee or fight. Eating responsiveness before or after the triggering emotional event was crucial to survival. Today, we have fewer opportunities to respond in an active way to our emotions. We are taught to suppress anger, fright, or excitement. It is impolite to yell and jump around; it is not acceptable to run away or to attack someone. Thus, emotional drives that are paired with hunger and with the need to increase energy are no longer protective; they may, in fact, be damaging. The individual becomes fat and overlays all the negative emotions associated with the state of obesity in our society on top of other emotions he or she is already having difficulty handling. We wonder whether the following thesis might be valid.

Considering the laws of survival of the fittest, and the historical need for increased energy for flight or fight, the individual who most closely pairs emotion with an eating response would be most likely to survive. Considering today's lack of need for energy for flight or fight, the individual who disassociates emotion and a hunger response will be most likely to survive.

HUNGER AND NURSING

The first nursing task in caring for people who are hungry and on weight-reducing regimens is to clarify our feelings about obesity. Whether nurses do this through examination of the personal threat fat poses or whether they accept the hyperplastic theory that eliminates individual responsibility makes no difference as long as blame and condemnation are eliminated in the approach to these people. Nursing care needs to be predicated on the assumption of hunger and not rampant appetite or lack of self-control.

Complete lack of hunger may portend severe physiological or psychological deterioration; affected individuals may require immediate and massive intervention. Nurses may be the ones to recommend that patients be put on hyperalimentation. Such therapy is now safe and effective and may get a patient over a critical period to the point where natural hunger again takes over.

Many things influence an individual's self-perception and expression of that perception as hunger. Nurses need to look beyond the expression and/or perception of hunger and recognize hunger by behavioral signs.

Hungry people are more responsive to external stimuli and would be susceptible to increased anxiety related to nursing events. Teaching needs to be carried out in an environment of controlled and reduced stimuli to minimize the possibility of frustration. Activity must be adjusted to each person's capacities and preferences.

There is a tendency toward increased emotional lability-like loss of self-control, anger, irritability, demandingness, weeping, sullenness, depression, or withdrawn behavior. Hungry people may also be vindictive. If nurses are not committed to maintaining an environment in which these behaviors can occur without being judgmental or moralizing, the dynamics of interpersonal interaction can become hostile and destructive. Nurses can anticipate a hungry patient's emotionality and not react personally. Rather, nurses need to conserve and redirect the patients' energy. They need to explain patients' behaviors to them and reassure them that it is normal for the situation. Further, nurses need to communicate understanding and acceptance of labile behaviors.

Energy levels in hungry patients fluctuate suddenly and drastically. Also, patients may exhibit drastic mood swings. Sudden change in mood and increased energy are not necessarily signs of better coping or improved health; they usually portend a low period.

It is important to recognize that certain behaviors accompany the deenergized state. Anecdotal notes indicate that nurses are judgmentally negative and irritated by the hungry individual's untidy appearance, rumpled bed, and messy hair. Nurses note that hungry patients take no responsibility for their own care. These are typical characteristics of hungry individuals; for them, it takes an effort to do what is necessary. The body fights to conserve energy.

RELIEF OF DISCOMFORTS

Discomforts of hunger are often relieved by increased activity. People who get up and walk or who have something to do feel better. Discomfort is also eased, even in children, by understanding the reasons why food is withheld and what would happen if food were eaten. They need to understand their hunger for salt. Patients who are hungry, whether self-imposed or medically imposed, need reassurance that their polyuria, nocturia, and increased fluid intake are normal and to be expected. They need to be taught how to assess themselves for edema and to be monitored for it by professional personnel. If there is marked increase in salt use, electrolytes may need to be checked. Many individuals have a tendency to drastically increase coffee and tea intake during hunger. These drinks serve to increase fluid (i.e., fill the empty stomach), to warm, and to provide pep due to caffeine content. Some individuals may suffer physiological disturbances, however, from a high intake of coffee and will need guidance to be moderate and to find alternative fluids.

Hungry individuals, fat or thin, beg for, hoard, and steal food. This is typical behavior and is not to be condemned. It is useless to castigate these people and tell them to stop thinking about food. It is better to sympathize with their discomfort and offer options for relief that have been generally identified as useful such as activity, occupational therapy, diversion, chewing gum, or fluids if allowed. Nurses need to be able to support relatives and friends to resist the imploring of a hungry person so they can be supporting and comforting themselves. While smoking is identified as useful coping behavior, nurses need to use it as a last resort, recognizing that for the smoker, giving up smoking and tolerating hunger over a long period of time causes almost unbearable stress.

Hungry people, as already noted, are preoccupied with food; they talk about it, cook it, remember good meals and holidays, make menus, watch others eat, savor smells from the kitchen, read cookbooks, and read recipe sections of magazines and food ads. Nurses tend to recognize this as a universal coping strategy of hungry people. These people need free expression, acceptance, and even encouragement for their talk about food. This may become annoying and boring to nurses, who nonetheless need to resist shaming and squelching this predictable behavior.

Hungry people also toy with food and may develop rituals to prolong eating, such as chewing each mouthful a hundred times, playing with the food and mixing it up, taking only so much on the fork at a time, sucking food in minute amounts off the end of a spoon. Nurses who work with these people need to be able to tolerate all manner of eating patterns and be able to allow the time required for ritual eating. If the nurse cannot accept some of the bizarre coping used by hungry people, both nursing care and client progress is jeopardized.

When hungry people are again allowed to eat, nurses need to guard against overeating to the point of nausea and vomiting. They also need to anticipate and explain that even with overeating and stuffing, these people still feel hungry.

People who are hungry may feel quite helpless. If they can assert themselves and feel in control of their situation, they are more comfortable. They need to be able to plan and control the food intake they are allowed: when, where, and how to eat or drink the quantity allowed and how it should be apportioned. They need to be able to control who they see and for how long and to avoid visitations if they want to. On the other hand, nurses need to be mindful that hungry patients may, in some areas, be too depleted in energy to desire control and may prefer that the nurse carry the burden. However, in areas where the patient needs to control, this may be a powerful coping strategy. Nurses must be sensitive to such contradictions and ready to relinquish or maintain control in accord with patients' needs.

As hunger increases and is prolonged, nurses need to watch for tolerance to cold and provide warm clothing and bedding. If food or drink is allowed, hungry people may prefer it hot because it is warming and thus comforting. Patients' increased tolerance to heat warns nurses to watch for burning and to check for lower hemoglobin levels.

Since people may not observe or may even deny the presence of edema, nurses need to be alert to this complication in food-deprived people. Weight monitoring must be done with cognizance of possible edema. This is important also during rehabilitation (patients off NPO and eating). Gains in weight during this time may be false affirmations of improvement, for most weight gain may be due to the effect of edema. The fact that patients are rehabilitating and eating does not mean that they cannot be, or are not, hungry. Similarly, initial weight gain may not mean recovery, but may be edema.

Hungry patients also require meticulous skin care. Nurses must recognize that this applies to all individuals, and not just the person who has traveled through the continuum to the stage of emaciation. Healing, loss of hair, roughening, and thinning of skin need to be looked for in all hungry patients. Patients with muscle cramps, soreness in joints and muscles, and "sleepy" limbs may need reassurance, and certainly require comfort measures. Hot baths, warm sponging, rub downs, and/or changes in bedding may be of some benefit.

Hungry people who are lethargic and hallucinate or whose fear susceptibility is increased, need nurses who are not only careful of their attitudes and actions, but who can shield them from stimuli that may be perceived as sudden, frustrating, or hostile. Inappropriate or unexplained comments or glances may cause terror in such a patient.

Hungry people may be more prone to accidents. Both hospital and community nurses must alert these people and their families to possible delays in movement. Rushing them may cause both frustration and injury. Perhaps individuals who are at home who feel hyperactive and anxious are in the most danger. Nurses need to caution these individuals that their feelings may belie their physiological incapacity: Reaction time may be slowed, kitchen knives may slip, car accidents can occur, and falling is a hazard.

Lack of or delayed physiological reactivity to drugs and hormones (e.g., insulin, pilocarpine, and atropine) and lack of response to Mantoux and Pirquet's tests is critical knowledge for nurses who must identify new standards of assessment and evaluation based on concentrated dosages, delayed reactions, and loss of utility in the case of some agents.

Individuals who were interviewed at home tended to resort to laxatives to increase bowel action, as noted. Nurses need to look for this tendency; affected individuals should be reassured that decreased frequency of bowel movements is normal and to be expected. If there is difficulty with hard stools, dietary modification, if any food or liquids are being consumed, should be investigated first. If a laxative must be used, the nurse needs to be alert to the individual's choice of laxative, for the body is already suffering tremendously increased stress. It may be that oil retention, tap water, or saline enemas are less stressful for energy and less stressful to the maintenance of fluid and electrolyte balance than many so-called laxatives. Hospital nurses also need to be alert to patients' comfort in this regard. Hungry patients are more prone to focus on their body functions, yet, they do not have the energy or psychological resources to be wasted on unnecessary concerns.

Nurses need to recognize that hunger is *painful* and that undistracted, clock-watching, waiting hunger is torture. When a hungry patient pleads, demands, or acts out for the nurses' attention "for no apparent reason" or "just to talk about food again," the fact of his or her undistracted hunger pain is a quite sufficient reason. The patient is calling attention to the failure of nursing intervention to provide distraction, to create and support hunger coping behaviors.

Patient and nurse need to work together to choose hunger coping mechanisms that work for that patient. The nurse needs to accept, interpret (both to him- or herself and to the patient), and to respond to the patient's assertive behavior whether it is demand for attention, for talk of food, for comfort, or for reassurance.

There are a myriad of nursing measures that must be explored if hungry patients are to be effectively cared for by hospital, clinic, and community health nurses.

MODELS OF HUNGER

Nurses who wish to pursue studies of hunger need to develop their hypotheses out of a conceptualization of the phenomenon. Three primitive models (Figures 11-1, 11-2, and 11-3) are used in this chapter to elucidate the author's conceptualization. From these models, the propositions and following hypotheses emerged:

1. An increase in activity level decreases hunger in the diet-restricted hospitalized patient.
2. Increased fluid intake helps a patient cope with hunger.
3. Hungry patients find hot foods and liquids more comforting than cold food and liquids.
4. Hungry patients require more bedding and clothing for comfort than do nonhungry patients.
5. Extremely hungry patients develop rituals of eating and eat very slowly.
6. Hungry patients often feel constipated.
7. Hot-water bottles applied to body surfaces may decrease a patient's perception of hunger.
8. Hungry patients are more prone to accidents than other patients.
9. Hungry patients who become elated will subsequently experience depression.
10. Explaining the concept of hunger and anticipating with the patient the behaviors that may be experienced help the patient cope with hunger.
11. A person's inability to perceive hunger is a negative prodromal sign.
12. People who are hungry sleep less.
13. Relaxation techniques aid in coping with hunger.
14. Gum, ice chewing, or other chewing activity helps alleviate hunger.
15. Talking and other oral activity alleviates hunger.
16. Controlling the time and the way in which one eats aids in coping with hunger.
17. People who cope effectively with their hunger heal faster.

REFERENCES

Beland, I.L., and Passos, J.Y. *Clinical Nursing: Pathophysiological and Psychosocial Approaches.* New York: Macmillan, 1975.

Guyton, A.C. *Textbook of Medical Physiology.* Philadelphia: Saunders, 1976.

Hagen, R.L. Theories of Obesity: Is There Any Hope for Order? In W.S. Martin, and J.P. Forety, (Eds.), *Obesity: Behavioral Approaches to Dietary Management.* New York: Bunner, Mazel, 1976.

Halbreich, U. Obesity: Some psychological considerations. *Confin. Psychiatr.* 19:46–56, 1976.

Hoshaw, D.O. *Nursing Care of the Patient with Medical–Surgical Disorders.* In H. Moidel, G. Sorensen, E.S. Giblin, and M. Kaufmann (Eds.), *Nursing Care of the Patient with Medical-Surgical Disorders.* New York: McGraw-Hill, 1971.

Keys, A., Brozek, J., Henschel, A., Mickelsen, O., and Taylor, H.L. *The Biology of Human Starvation.* Minneapolis: University of Minnesota Press, 1950. Vol. I and II.

Leyton, G.B. Effects of slow starvation. *Lancet* 251(2):73–79, July 20, 1946.

Linton, P.H., Conely, M., Kuechenmeister, C., and McClusky, H. Satiety and obesity *Am. J. Clin. Nutr.* 25:368–370, Apr. 1972.

Nisbett, R.E. Hunger, obesity and the ventromedial hypothalamus. *Psychol. Rev.* 70:433–453, Nov. 1972.

Norris, C.M. Restlessness: A nursing phenomenon in search of meaning. *Nurs. Outlook* 23:103–107, Feb. 1975.

Orbach, S. *Fat Is a Feminist Issue*. New York: Paddington, 1978.

Schachter, S. Some extraordinary facts about obese humans and rats. *Am. Psychol.* 26:129–143, Feb. 1971.

Tabers Cyclopedic Medical Dictionary. Philadelphia: Davis, 1970.

Tepperman, J. *Metabolic and Endocrine Physiology* (3rd ed.). Palo Alto, Calif.: Year Book, 1973.

Figure 11-1 Model for Hunger Continuum

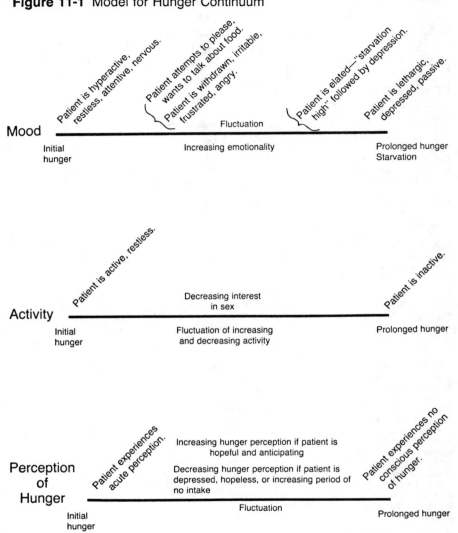

Figure 11-2 Model for Perception of Hunger

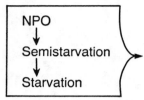

Aspects of hunger perception

Behaviors	. Feelings	Affect
Preoccupation with food: asks for food, has difficulty concentrating, fantasizes about food, has overwhelming desire to talk about food, stuffs self if food is available, watches clock, shows increased awareness of food stimuli and suggestion, experiences cravings	*Hypermotility of GI:* stomach pain or growling, nausea, emptiness, oral cravings, increased urination, diarrhea	*Food-seeking:* pleading look on face, attention, impatience, restlessness
Increased activity: restlessness, pacing, hyperactivity, nervousness, decreased sleep, increased urination, diarrhea	*Emotional lability:* tension, hyperactivity, agitation, irritability, lack of control, anger, depression, frustration, lack of caring, passivity	*Emotional lability:* frown, sullenness, mad upset, nonsmiling face, inappropriate laughter, anxiousness, tension
Decreased energy: shakiness, weakness, slow movement, sluggishness, passivity, laziness, decreased interest in sex or social interaction, decreased interest in participating in own care, no interest in doing much, no interest in socializing (except to discuss own problems or food, decreased concentration, fatigue, depression	*Decreased energy:* faintness, dizziness, nauseousness, jittery feeling, light-headedness, inability to think, need for something to eat, dizziness headache	*Decreased energy:* paleness, drawn face, listlessness, lethargy, boredom, tension, withdrawal, emaciation
Emotional lability: irritability, jumpiness, bad mood, elation, depression, impatience, nervousness, fear, easy frustration, noncooperation, difference from usual, tension, lack of care, anger, upset, tendency to cry	*Decreased GI motility:* constipation, flatulence, decreased perception of stomach hunger	*Increased sympathetic nervous system:* restlessness, nervousness, shaking, tension, increased perspiration and/or pallor, nervousness

Figure 11-3 Model for Hunger Interventions

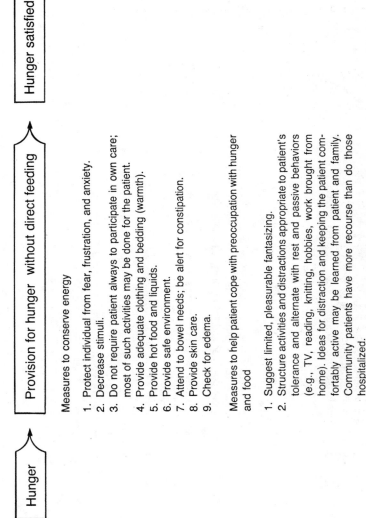

Hunger → Provision for hunger without direct feeding → Hunger satisfied

Measures to conserve energy

1. Protect individual from fear, frustration, and anxiety.
2. Decrease stimuli.
3. Do not require patient always to participate in own care; most of such activities may be done for the patient.
4. Provide adequate clothing and bedding (warmth).
5. Provide hot food and liquids.
6. Provide safe environment.
7. Attend to bowel needs; be alert for constipation.
8. Provide skin care.
9. Check for edema.

Measures to help patient cope with preoccupation with hunger and food

1. Suggest limited, pleasurable fantasizing.
2. Structure activities and distractions appropriate to patient's tolerance and alternate with rest and passive behaviors (e.g., TV, reading, knitting, hobbies, work brought from home). Ideas for distraction and keeping the patient comfortably active may be learned from patient and family. Community patients have more recourse than do those hospitalized.
3. Provide periods of undivided attention to patient's need to talk, to verbalize about food and discomforts.

Figure 11-3   Continued

4. Try relaxation techniques.
5. Try periods of activity, such as walking.
6. Offer ice or gum to patient during specified times of heightened need (e.g., at normal "meal hours").
7. Provide hot baths, skin care, hot-water bottle.

Measures to help patient to cope by increasing knowledge and feelings of control

1. Explain concept of hunger to patient—what patient may be experiencing, recognition that this is expected, normal, and appropriate behavior and will be accepted and not condemned.
2. Explain to patient that nurse and patient will work together to intervene in above behaviors in an attempt to help the patient to cope.
3. Plan distractions with patient, activities, rest periods, times when allowed food is to be offered.
4. Give patient control of times and ways patient eats.
5. Allow patient to talk.
6. Allow patient food rituals and a structured environment.

Chapter 12

Shivering and Surface Cooling

June C. Abbey

Human shivering occurs in response to exposure to cold or during serious illness accompanied by fever. Shivering can also follow administration of certain anesthetics (Hunter 1979, p. 588). Whether drug-related shivering is actually in response to a fall in temperature or to the pharmaceutical agent used continues to be debated (Bay et al. 1968). Postpartum shivering in certain patients creates discomfort shortly after parturition. In everyday conversation, a shiver is clearly differentiated through both context and use from shivering, by such expressions as, "a shiver of delight," "a shiver of dread," or "the shiver of someone walking over my grave." Such occurrences are singular, transient, superficial, and unaccompanied by physical discomfort. Shivering, in contrast, is by definition a course-generalized, protracted series of muscular reactions of involuntary, periodic contractions by voluntary (skeletal) muscles (Chatonnet and Minaire 1966). The causes for the discomfort associated with shivering remain speculative because in the healthy subject there is no pain. Still, no one likes to shiver; the process elicits a feeling of tenseness, dread, and loss of control even if only experienced for a short time. When continued over a protracted period, fatigue, exhaustion, and muscular pain result. Shivering is a massive total body response.

Shivering in a clinical situation demands the nurse's attention on a number of levels. Psychological discomfort, dread, helplessness, and loss of control are examples. Cardiovascular and pulmonary reserves can be embarrassed in already physiologically compromised patients. Shivering requires a nursing intervention and action, whether simply reporting the phenomenon, or restoring lost heat, modifying the rate of heat loss, interfering with the process of physiological determination of heat loss, or giving drugs to prevent the response.

DEGREES OF SHIVERING

The clear description of the progression of shivering involved in reporting permits the recognition of stages or levels. Considerable work has been done to establish grades of shivering. Girling and Topliff (1966, p. 45), in order to study the effects of breathing different percentages of oxygen on the onset of shivering, developed degrees as follows: $1° =$ slight bursts; $2° =$ moderate bursts; $3° =$ moderate and continuous with severe bursts; $4° =$ severe and continuous shivering. Daniels and Baker (1961, pp. 421–422) were interested in comparing the amount of body fat and metabolic rate with shivering. Their rating scale was: $0 =$ no evidence, $+ =$ evidence of increase in muscle tone that was scattered or consisted of localized tremors, $+ + =$ more severe tremors involving more of the body and generally continuous, $+ + + =$ generalized severe signs without teeth chattering, $+ + + + =$ generalized rigors with teeth chattering.

Obviously, differentiation of degrees is possible, but can these gradations also be put into levels of progression? What if one wanted to intervene, subvert, or modify the actual rate of heat loss? or the physiological interpretation of heat loss? What, if any, modifications can be made with these measurement classifications that presages clinical nursing intervention?

Scientific interest in shivering relates closely to the development of knowledge in the area of body temperature and control. Burton and colleagues (1935) carefully describe shivering as being ushered in by a generalized feeling of coldness, tenseness, and some stiffness followed by irregular bursts of muscle groups. Early in cooling, the Burton investigators found that the muscular contractions could be controlled by the subject by either relaxing or bracing the muscles. Later in the cooling process, however, the subject, although still able to perform voluntary movement, cannot control or prevent shivering (Burton et al. 1935). Twenty years later, Burton (1955) found that *amplitude* of the bursts of muscular contractions increased during inspiration and decreased during expiration. He felt that this was due to spinal reflexes related to the activity of the diaphragm. Stuart and co-workers (1963) later studied the *frequency* of the bursts as contrasted to amplitude. Frequency appears to remain unchanged.

In 1937, Denny-Brown and associates reported that the initial shivering contraction first appears in the masseters "as a twitch" then moves to the pectoral or neck regions (p. 233). Horvath and others (1956) conclude that the last muscle groups to be involved are those of the arms and legs. The findings of Petajan and Williams (1972) both agree and disagree with Horvath and workers (1956). Petajan and Williams (1972) unequivocally found that both preshivering and shivering first appear in the extensor and proximal muscles on the upper arms and trunk.

Clinical nursing observations corroborate that muscle contractions of the trunk precede the onset of shivering. Hickey (1965) voices the clinical stance when she says, "Close observations of the patient's chest can alert the nurse when visible shivering is about to begin. Just before its onset, the chest quivers or the muscles show a ripple-like movement (Hickey 1965, p. 120)."

The relevance to clinical care and the development of a measurement tool of stages or levels rests on the following factors:

1. Shivering begins in the masseters (Denny-Brown 1937).
2. Shivering then moves to the trunk (Petajan and Williams 1972; Denny-Brown 1937; and Hickey 1965).
3. Clinical nursing can and does use trunk observations (Hickey 1965).
4. Shivering continues on to involve long muscle groups (Horvath 1956).
5. Teeth chattering is the final involvement (Girling and Topliff 1966; and Daniels and Baker 1961).

If the levels can then be formulated into replicable, identifiable stages of shivering, then clinical decisions and actions can be instituted that would prevent or lessen the advance of shivering. Clark and Darron (1967, p. 454), when working on cats, noted that ". . . minimal shivering could be detected more accurately manually than with the electromyogram." Using palpation for masseter twitch would therefore be as accurate and certainly more acceptable in the clinical arena to determine masseter twitch. Both palpation and electromyograms for pectoral "quiver" would then demonstrate the degree of reliability. This, plus inter-rater reliability testing for masseter-twitch identification, could substantiate essentially five measurements of shivering as follows: 0 = no evidence; 1 = palpable evidence of increased muscle tone in the masseters; 2 = palpable evidence of increased muscle tone in the pectorals; 3 = general continuous shivering without teeth chattering; and 4 = general continuous shivering with teeth chattering. The five-point (degree) scale on testing with a research team and clinical nurses clearly delineated between the stages, thus making it possible to study any one of the levels of shivering (Abbey and Close 1979). The pectoral quivers described by Hickey (1965) were thus second-degree shivers, which then became the indicator in some hospital settings for administration by the nurse of drugs that would decrease or prevent shivering (Stevens 1972, p. 41).

EFFECTS OF SHIVERING

The response to cold with a rapid temperature shift can cause massive regulatory response because, as Brown and Brengelmann (1965) point out, "in extreme shivering, the metabolic rate can reach 250 Kcal per hour per meter squared, a rate equivalent to heavy exercise (p. 1046)." Spurr and associates (1956) measured the oxygen uptake of nude men who shivered when exposed to low temperatures; they found the oxygen consumption of these men to be 300 to 400 percent greater than that of men in the control group. Dill and Forbes (1941) found that lightly sedated patients, upon cooling, used more oxygen because of shivering and voluntary motion. Stone and colleagues (1956) studied men who were lightly anesthetized so that shivering would not be curtailed; at 28°C these subjects used twice the amount of oxygen as at 37°C. Even in cold-acclimatized subjects, the pattern of increase in oxygen consumption parallels that of the degree of shivering (Budd and Warhoft 1966). In the clinical situation, according to Boba (1960), "[while] the oxygen requirement of the shivering hypothermic animal at normal temperature may be three to four times greater than that of the resting animal, [it may be] as much as eight times greater than the non-shivering hypothermic animal at the same temperature (p. 15)." Boba feels that the relationship holds with patients and that, if shivering is prevented, the temperature decay curve becomes linear and there is no increase in oxygen consumption.

Two aspects of muscular activity in shivering need to be considered: (1) the amount of oxygen needed and (2) the fate of the by-products. Oxygen delivery depends on the efficient functioning of the respiratory system. There must be patent airways and adequate chest movement, as well as sufficient diffusion of oxygen and carbon dioxide. While the gaseous exchange is a passive force, breathing is work. Hyperventilation itself contributes to the rise in oxygen consumption. Hyperventilation, a respiratory rate of 44 or more breaths per minute, also causes excessive heat loss to the central core (Cooper et al. 1964; and Cooper and Kenyon 1967).

It is now recognized that oxidation of fat is essential to supplying energy for the sustained muscular activity involved in shivering (Alexander 1979, p. 99). The proportion of fat to carbohydrate used varies widely. Work done on animals indicates that glucose supplies 70 percent of the metabolic energy for a human leg during shivering (Alexander 1979, p. 99).

In the case of fasting, however, data indicates fat to be the sole source of energy (Himms-Hagen 1972). Although much more is known about substrate energy use for exercise than for the shivering muscle, there is no logical reason to expect differences in the basic mechanism (Himms-Hagen 1976; and Chatonnet and Minaire 1966). The availability of fatty acids and glucose appears to be the major determinant of the rate of oxidation (Himms-Hagen 1976). The likelihood of differences in metabolic conversions between species presents an inherent problem in generalizing animal findings to humans in substrate energy support for shivering.

The efficacy of shivering in protecting the body from total heat loss is estimated to be about 11 percent (Hovarth et al. 1956). Due to the vasodilatation from increased blood flow to the muscles, shivering leads to an increased core loss and, hence, it is only a short-term compensatory mechanism, not an efficient method for maintaining body temperature (Burton and Bazett 1936).

Both pulse rate and arterial blood pressure rise as a result of shivering, and therefore pulse rate is often used as a guide to the onset of shivering (Dundee and King 1959). A rise in pulse rate, however, is not diagnostic, because the cardiovascular system interrelates with many other phenomena. Bigelow and associates (1950) were the first to show that shivering causes a rise in venous pressure. Rosomoff (1956) corroborated this finding and extended it to include a marked elevation in cerebrospinal fluid pressure, an effect that negates the purpose of hypothermia in the neurological patient.

It has been Boba's (1960) experience that patients may shiver without any apparent untoward alteration of glucose level or plasma acidity. The by-products of shivering that would be of particular concern are ketone bodies and lactic acid. At a normal temperature—37°C—lactic acid contributes to the rebuilding of glycogen stores. Two investigators (Blair 1969; and Fisher 1955) have found hypoglycemia under conditions of starvation or shivering. But the literature is unclear about the exact conditions of shivering, particularly at which level of hypothermia hypoglycemia accompanies the phenomenon. In true hypothermia, where core temperature is 30.5°–35°C (Hickey 1965, p. 116), the natural tendency is toward acidosis. Rosenfeld (1963) agrees but adds that, "metabolic acidosis is of negligible significance provided shivering is completely abolished and that tissue anoxia is avoided (p. 680)." Shivering accelerates the production and accumulation of lactic acid in the blood during hypothermia (Boba 1960; and Rosenfeld 1963). Acidotic shock, which occurs most often during the rewarming of the hypothermic patient, is the result of the rapid release of accumulated fixed acids by shivering (Boba 1960; and Bellinger et al. 1961).

The effects of shivering, then, are the nursing concerns. Other than for a very effective short-term means of raising the body temperature in response to cold, shivering overall is fatiguing, increases cerebral spinal fluid pressure, consumes energy stores, requires marked increases in oxygen consumption and circulatory support, and creates an elevation in workload as the patient mobilizes to meet the demands of the shivering process. Fullblown, level 4 shivering with teeth chattering can totally involve the subject, both psychologically and physiologically.

Stages or levels of shivering suggest an orderly progression in intensity and the orderly progression introduces concepts of control and regulation. This, in turn, fosters the idea of timely interruption, or intervention, to change the order and thereby modify the control or divert the regulation. The question then becomes, "What is known and conjectured about regulating shivering?"

REGULATION OF SHIVERING

In thermoregulation, vasoconstriction (vasomotor) and shivering (musculature) are the effectors of heat production. The center for heat maintenance has long been known in the preoptic regions of the hypothalamus. Recently, it was reported that Takata and Murakami (Ogata and Murakami 1972) discovered through electrical stimulation that the posterior hypothalamus includes a shivering center, the descending pathway of which controls shivering development, a shivering inhibition center, which with electrical stimulation reduces shivering intensity, and "another area that has nothing to do with shivering (p. 64)." From their results it appears that the shivering center is activated by thermoreceptors in the skin, especially cold receptors, or is inhibited by warm receptors. Further research by these investigators has revealed that local temperature changes in the anterior hypothalamus also contribute to the activity level of the shivering center. This research suggests that shivering is a function of both preoptic hypothalamic and ambient temperatures acting conjointly with the primary motor center of the dorsal hypothalamus. It is also likely, the investigators say, "that the activity of the shivering center is proportional to the product of skin temperature and preoptic temperature (p. 62)." The investigators suggest that a hierarchical arrangement of thermoregulatory responses exists: a vasomotor first defense, followed by a change in skin temperature within a given range, then shivering to maintain body temperature.

These findings are compatible with the studies of patients with spinal cord transection made by Downey and associates (1969) and by Johnson and Spalding (1966) and with the work in intact and spinal animals by Thauer (1970)—studies that conclude that deep central sensors exist and that they interrelate with peripheral skin thermoreceptors. The results clearly demonstrate why "shivering can proceed in the decerebrate" (Hemingway 1963; and Perkins 1965) and therefore would not be of great use to the nurse as a determinant of the degree of cortical involvement in early head trauma.

The feelings of tenseness and dread associated with shivering, even before the level 1 masseter twitch, probably result from the intense vasoconstriction of the skin of the entire body when the core temperature becomes less than 37°C. Vasoconstriction can also be elicited by stimuli other than cold, such as psychological flight or shock, hemorrhage, or trauma. It is therefore, in itself, not indicative of impending shivering but does in fact conserve body heat. By shunting the blood from the body surface to the deeper structures, less heat is lost. At the same time, however, skin temperature sensors (receptors) register a cooler skin because of the decrease in perfusion and the loss of the corresponding heat of the blood. The preoptic area then, acting conjointly with signals from the skin and spinal cord, decreases its control over the posterior hypothalamus and if the temperatures continue to fall, shivering begins.

Brenglemann and co-workers (1973) postulate that vasomotor control in man is correlated with body core temperature and *rate of change* of skin temperature but not with skin temperature per se. Research does however, lead us to conclude that ". . . the nature of temperature regulation in man during cooling is fundamentally different from that during warming; proportional control seems to operate during warming, but not cooling (Mitchell 1977, p. 20)." Iggo (1969) further substantiates this with his work, which demonstrates that cold receptors (sensors) produce a transient burst of impulses with a frequency that correlates first with the *rate of fall* in temperature and then stabilizes at a steady discharge in which frequency relates to the absolute temperature.

Two investigators, Simon (1972) and Nutik (1973), propose that the brain does not receive separate information from central and peripheral cold sensors (receptors) but rather, the inputs act convergently with cold signals coming from the skin and spinal cord (Simon 1972) and from the skin and hypothalamus (Nutik 1973). This then could be integration. Shivering can be induced by cooling the medulla oblongata in animals that have had the hypothalamus destroyed (Lin and Chai 1974). Shivering can also be induced by cooling the spinal cords of animals with disconnection of the spinal cord from the brain (Kosaka and Simon 1968). Cutaneous vessels normally constrict in animals exposed to cold. The reaction is disrupted if the posterior hypothalamus nervous tissue is destroyed.

A cohesive summary of factors isolated from the foregoing discussion reveals the following:

1. A shivering center exists that acts with: (1) a descending pathway for shivering development control and (2) a shivering inhibition center (Okata and Murakami 1972).
2. Peripheral skin receptors and deep central centers interact (Downey et al. 1969; Johnson and Spalding 1966; and Thauer 1970). Research has been done on both humans and animals.
3. Relationships exist between skin and the spinal cord (Simon 1972) and skin and the hypothalamus (Nutik 1973).
4. Vasomotor reaction is disrupted if the posterior hypothalamus is destroyed (Kosaka and Simon 1972).
5. Rate of change of skin temperature, warming (Brenglemann 1973) and cooling (Iggo 1969), affect vasomotor control and neuron firing.
6. Both heat loss or maintenance centers and heat gain centers interact in the hypothalamus.
7. Shivering can proceed in the decerebrate exclusive of the hypothalamus (Hemingway 1963; and Perkins 1965).

The questions that derive from this summary are not as numerous as we might expect because of the focus or constraints imposed by nursing. The subjects for testing out any questions, or hypotheses, will be human, probably patients. The measurements and observations will need to be noninvasive, benign, and painless. Any planned intervention (independent variable) must meet with the same constraints. To lessen shivering would be beneficial. The questions therefore at this stage of speculation still involve the existing knowledge about shivering and thermoregulation. The questions then revolve around the responses and the nature of mediation. Are these reflexes mediated? Does the mediation result from integration? Can parts of the input for integration be manipulated in the clinical arena by nurses to curtail shivering? How do we get at the input?

Inherent throughout the development and in presentation of the research findings is the basic concept of interrelatedness, or order, of mediation, of control, and of response to change. The formulation clearly involves a pattern of input-comparison-output-feedback through input and adjustment through output. Shivering, in this instance, is the output that shows the capacity for adjustment by delineated levels of activity. Shivering can therefore be a measurable dependent variable if the nursing intervention can modify either the center, or centers, of comparison or the input. Other than through drugs, the hypothalamus and the spinal cord are immune to nursing measures. The skin, however, is not, and thus skin, which appears to be a focal point in thermoregulation and shivering investigations, becomes the focus for nursing. The skin and its temperature sensors (receptors) form the last essential component to the paradigm and the input sensors for feedback loops, the object for first review and then later nursing action.

RECEPTORS (SENSORS) AND CENTERS

Some confusion can occur when using the terms *receptor, sensors,* and *centers,* particularly when discussing the central areas for control or reception. For clarity, sensors and receptors are used interchangeably throughout this discussion to indicate sensing or input with some referent range, as with phasic, or a point, as with static, to refer to the hypothalamus. Although the hypothalamus is most often assigned the role of integrator of thermal sensor input because it contains recognized neurons sensitive to local changes as well as to changes in temperature in other body regions (Boulant and Hardy 1974), many authorities argue against a set point (Houdas and Guieu 1975) or the negative feedback (adjustment) model (Huckaba and Downey 1973). Clinical studies involving human beings by Cooper and colleagues (1965) and Cabanac and Massonet (1974) support the hypothalamic thermoregulatory set point theory. Bligh (1973) goes even further and presents models generally based on the concept that the hypothalamus is the sole regulator. A more conservative approach is presented by Kluger (1979) who states that, "Integration of thermal information in vertebrates is thought to occur in the hypothalamus with some integrative abilities residing in other central nervous areas (p. 211)." Neuropharmacological studies also implicate the hypothalamus, but then offer the question of whether the drugs affect the hypothalamus as a sensor or as "the hypothetical thermoregulatory integrator (Kluger 1979, p. 212)."

For the purposes of this discussion, the hypothalamus is regarded as a center of integration, and, because of the preoptic interrelationship with the posterior–

dorsal shivering center of Takata and Murakami (Ogata and Murakami 1972) as the primary location of both thermal and shivering control and regulation. Secondary centers are acknowledged to be in the spinal cord. As previously mentioned, the hypothalamus, as a sensor, when subjected to the constraints of the nursing stance, can only be affected by drugs. By contrast, however, as an integrator with temperature and shivering centers, the hypothalamus processes input from both central (spinal and abdominal or deep organ) and peripheral (skin) sensors. Skin sensors are available to nursing actions and hypothalamus integration, thus the control of shivering enters the province of nursing.

The logical extension of concentrating on skin sensors excludes internal or central disturbances that might cause shivering, such as those that accompany open-heart surgery and extracorporeal circulation, or even the shivering that accompanies hyperpyrexia and fever. Only when shivering is due to peripheral and skin exposure to cold can a strictly nursing action be appropriate to the argument. Loss of heat to the skin sensors elicits vasoconstriction for heat conservation.

To regulate the core temperature through a negative feedback loop, the body requires a system of sensors, comparison to a reference level, activation of effectors for correction of the assessed difference, and the resensing by the system of the modification. Since the range of optimal function is narrow—36.4 to 37.5°C—both the sensing and correcting systems must be rapid in response and relatively automatic. Cornew and associates (1967) conclude that fine control of temperature is achieved by regulating the size of the blood vessels of the periphery and that, however the vascular responses are controlled, they are essentially instantaneous.

EXPOSURE TO COLD

A threat of reduction of core temperature meets formidable resistance (Burton and Edholm 1955). The homeotherm first initiates insulative defenses when blood is diverted by vasoconstriction to the deeper layers of the body, thus insulating the main bloodstream from the cooling surface or agent. Euler (1961) states that, in response to cold, cutaneous blood flow—and thereby conductance of the peripheral tissue—decreases to such a very low level that "a third to one-half of the body mass can be excluded from the effective temperature regulation (p. 366)." Hardy (1961), in his extensive review of temperature regulation, takes exception to this figure and states that, "although vasoconstriction does not enhance body insulation by an order of 10 in man upon cold exposure, it does assist in maintaining a degree of thermal insulation (p. 531)." Aschoff and Heise (1972) conclude that the variability of conductance is largely caused by the variability of blood flow. The blood flow of the extremities, they say, fluctuates considerably with the variability increasing from proximal to distal parts. Since the hands and feet are the most distal, they can have an extremely steep decrease of conductance, accompanied by a marked decrease in heat loss despite an increasing heat gradient. The high surface-to-volume ratio of the extremities causes them to act as heat-radiating vanes, and a steep conductance gradient therefore presents an efficient system of heat loss.

Sensor Characteristics

What elicits the vasomotor response? Hensel (1970) has done considerable work in the area of receptors (i.e., in the "nerve endings that are highly selective to temperature stimuli" located in the skin) and concludes the following:

1. They have a static sensitivity to constant temperature.
2. They show a dynamic sensitivity to temperature changes, with a positive temperature coefficient for warm receptors and a negative coefficient for cold receptors.
3. They are not excited by mechanical stimuli within reasonable limits of intensity.

Warm receptors fire with a transient increase to sudden warming and with an inhibition of response to cooling, while cold receptors respond with the opposite pattern. Both cold and warm receptors discharge continuously and increase their respective frequency according to the direction and extent of the temperature change. The rate of change markedly affects the dynamic sensitivity and the maximum frequency of cold receptors. *Dynamic sensitivity* (impulses/sec/C°) is defined as the change in frequency when a temperature change of 1°C occurs. With sudden cooling, the maximum frequency of cold fibers can reach 150 impulses per second, or ten times greater than the stationary (static) maximum.

According to Dykes (1975), sensors convey information through two codes: (1) there is a frequency code for rapid or phasic change, and (2) there is a patterning code for absolute skin temperature between 20°C and 37°C. Hardy (1970) believes that the sensors "lead" the body temperature change; hence, their effect will be anticipatory and related to the rate of skin temperature fall. His subjects experienced a large drop in skin temperature, accompanied by a decided decrease in heart rate suggestive of vasoconstriction. Iggo (1969) says that thermoreceptors are characteristically more sensitive to a given range midway between their limits of sensitivity, with decremental function to each side of the range, and he states unequivocally that, "there are cutaneous and lingual temperature detectors which have a high selective sensitivity or specificity (p. 406)." External body surface and tongue temperature information is probably dependent to a large extent on these thermosensors.

Central versus Peripheral Thermoreceptors

There has been considerable discussion about the relative roles of the central and skin thermosensor systems in thermoregulation. Initially, Burton and Edholm (1955) proposed that the skin receptors accounted for most of the then-known facts and theories. But Benzinger (1963) propounded a theory of central dominance when skin temperature exceeds 33°C and said that skin temperatures of less than 33°C modify the central regulatory system. The work of Barbout (1921) had demonstrated the existence of thermoreceptive centers in the brain, and Magoun and associates (1938) located these structures in the preoptic and supraoptic regions of the hypothalamus. During the past 15 years, the relative roles of central and peripheral thermoreceptors (sensors) have been the focus of study (Hammel 1968; and Hardy 1961). Thauer (1970) found that thermosensitive structures, both cold and warm, exist in the spinal cord and that these sensors transmit afferent impulses to supraspinal centers. Thermal response seems to be a summation or integration of all of the various sensor interaction, with the rate of change of cutaneous sensors being an important component of sensation. The experiments of Brown and Brengelmann (1970) indicate that, with "fluctuation of skin temperature between 29.5°C [and] 31.5°C, mean metabolic rate will rise even if the mean value of skin temperature remains at 30.5°C (p. 699)."

Clinically, oxygen consumption increases during the initial part of surface cooling before the core temperature changes become evident. It is interesting to note that in core-cooled or anesthetized experimental animals, an increased oxygen consumption is much less. Popovik and Popovik (1974) report that the amount of oxygen consumed "depends not only on the temperature of the internal vital organs, or hypothalamus, but also on the temperature of the skin (p. 171)." Such an increase in oxygen consumption evidences a concomitant increase in metabolism. It therefore follows that to increase markedly the metabolic rate—and hence body heat—in response to cold, increased muscular activity or shivering is necessary.

Exposure to cold—despite vasoconstriction, the insulative responses of shunting and countercurrent (Keatinge 1969), and minimal heat loss from the limbs—results in loss of core temperature, because no physiological control protects the trunk from simple conductive heat loss from the deep organs to the body surface and thence to the cooling surface (Cannon and Keatinge 1960). Cabanac (1975) states that "the tonus of visceral and cutaneous beds appear to respond oppositely to the same stimulus" and that "skin vasoconstriction as a cold defense reaction and skin vasodilation as a warm defense reaction [are] compensated by simultaneous opposite responses in the thermal core (p. 418)." All of these factors contribute to heat loss. Carlson and associates (1958), Pugh and co-workers (1960), and Keatinge (1969) all report that heat loss in cold water is in a reciprocal relationship to the thickness of subcutaneous fat. In their studies, both fat and

234 CONCEPT CLARIFICATION IN NURSING

thin men increased their metabolic rates in water of less than 33°C. This occurred apparently in response to skin cold thermoreceptors (Keatinge 1969).

Nonshivering thermogenesis, although rapid in onset, appears to be a response to long-term exposure in which there is a catecholamine-mediated type of heat production (Bruck and Wennenberg 1970). That is, there is an increase in metabolism and oxygen consumption without concurrent shivering (Adolph 1972).

The characteristics relative to formulation of a model of shivering that will support a nursing intervention to either prevent or decrease the shivering response to cold in the foregoing exposition are functions of blood flow and vasoconstriction, the surface-to-volume ratio of the extremities and sensor responses. These are summarized, as follows:

1. Variability of blood flow determines variability conductance (Ashoff and Heise 1972).
2. Extremity blood-flow variability increases in fluctuation from proximal to distal parts (Ashoff and Heise 1972).
3. The hands and feet are most distal and they have greatest heat conductance.
4. Extremities have a high surface-to-volume ratio, causing them to act as radiating vanes. The steep heat conductance gradient and large surface area promote rapid heat loss.
5. The rate of temperature change markedly affects rate of firing (input) of sensors (Brenglemann et al. 1973).
6. Sensors "lead body temperature change" (Hardy 1970).
7. Sensors have static sensitivity to temperature changes, show dynamic sensitivity to dynamic change, and are unaffected by reasonable mechanical stimuli (Hensel 1970).
8. No physiological control protects the trunk from simple conductive heat loss (Cannon and Keatinge 1960).
9. Nonshivering thermogenesis is a response to long-term exposure (Bruck and Wennenberg 1970).

MODIFICATION OF SHIVERING

The model for shivering control would of necessity fit within an overall model of normothermic regulation (Figure 12-1). The pathway whereby nursing can affect the central comparator and integrator is through the peripheral skin sensors prior to the integration. The skin sensors are both phasic and static and do not respond to moderate mechanical stimulation. The questions then become "Where on the skin could nursing affect the sensors most? Where is the greatest lability? the largest heat loss? and the steepest conductance gradient?"

Observation of the constraints of clinical nursing practice dictates that action be noninvasive, painless, and benign. Whereas the administration of a drug to

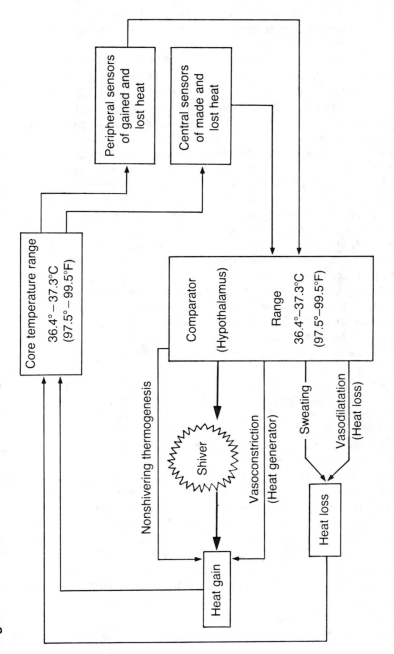

Figure 12-1   Overview of Normothermic Regulation

decrease shivering clearly lies within nursing practice, selecting and prescribing does not. This option is therefore considered to be outside of the province of nursing. Another aspect of the action is that it must withstand testing, be replicable in clinical practice, and, preferably, be economical.

From the foregoing, the nursing plan would (1) lessen the slope of the conductance of the skin, (2) concentrate efforts on the areas of greatest lability, heat loss, and conductance, and (3) use skin areas most available to the practicing nurse. The extremities fit the requirements of the plan. All that remains is to determine what the action will be, where shivering presents a problem to nursing, and when patients are deliberately exposed to cold. Open-heart patients being warmed after extracorporeal circulation are excluded from discussion because the deep sensors rather than the skin would be the active thermoreceptors.

Surface cooling in the clinical setting is used to combat hyperpyrexia or excessive fever. At such times, the patient is placed on a mattress that contains coils of circulating, cooling fluid attached to an electrical pump and reservoir that remove the heat picked up by the liquid from the patient through conductance. With the heat loss, the patients usually experience 3- or 4-degree shivering. Neurological patients with increased intracranial pressure often run high temperatures because of the irritation and ischemia to neurological tissue. Surface cooling (hypothermia) is used to combat temperature elevation and its concomitant effect on vital signs and physiological workload. Shivering, in these cases, adds an additional burden and increases cerebral spinal fluid pressure. Drugs, usually the phenothiazines, given to control or prevent shivering, frequently cause a serious drop in blood pressure. Occasionally, blood dyscrasias or hepatic difficulties occur.

A population for testing the model of manipulating the sensor input is therefore available. Shivering creates a real problem to hypothermia patients and to the nurses, who are concerned for the patient's well-being. The question remains, "What will be the nursing action?"

The simple answer is, "to protect the extremities from the cold, which will decrease the conductance slope, lessen heat loss, and reduce lability." Clinical concerns of intravenous and arterial lines require that the method be noncomplicated, provide ease of extremity observation, and permit replacement if soiled or wet. The action, or intervention, is to wrap the extremities in bath towels. If, however, the towels decrease heat conductance and heat exchange to hypothermia mattress, what will maintain the continued overall core heat loss to the body? The trunk has no physiological mechanisms to protect itself from conductance heat loss, hence it is posited that heat loss will continue.

A clinical study was done to test the hypothesis of possible shivering response modification (Abbey, 1976).* The research involved acutely ill subjects ($N = 35$)

---

*Grant No. NU-44083, Division of Nursing, Bureau of Health, Manpower Education, DHEW.

undergoing therapeutic surface-cooling hypothermia. Depending on the under-lying physical diagnoses—either of a neurological or a nonneurological hyper-pyrexia—two groups of subjects ($N = 25$, $N = 10$, respectively) were randomly assigned to experimental and control groups. The four extremities of the exper-imental subjects were wrapped with three thicknesses of terrycloth toweling before being placed on hypothermia. The wrapping extended from the elbows over the fingers and from the knees over the toes. The control subjects remained unwrapped. A standard hypothermia procedure was used for both groups. Patient measurements included three temperatures (rectal, auditory canal, and lateral thigh), an electromyogram, and an EKG. Other measurements were made of the blanket gauge, the coolant temperature, and the blanket probe temperature. Telemetry was used for the patient measurements with pre- and post-calibration, indicating accuracy at $\pm 0.1°C$. Nursing observations included vital signs, levels of consciousness, pupil size, mental state, and skin color. Statistical analysis included Chi-square and Fisher's tests. Pearson correlations were used between dependent variables.

The treatment was statistically significant in decreasing overall shivering ($p = 0.02$). The experimental neurological subjects showed a significant de-crease in shivering incidence. The results were confounded in hyperpyrexic subjects by the use of acetaminophen. Those hyperpyrexic subjects receiving acetaminophen four to six hours prior to application of the hypothermia blanket also showed a decrease in shivering ($p = 0.03$) over the control subjects. Neu-rological subjects did not receive acetaminophen. Four stages of shivering as follows were successfully defined: 1 = masseter tensing; 2 = pectoral muscle tensing; 3 = frank shivering without teeth chattering; 4 = frank shivering with teeth chattering. No one temperature site predicted shivering in this study.

The instrumentation, despite initial difficulties, proved a successful innovation for collecting multiple physiological measurements over time in an acute-care setting using critically ill subjects. Out of approximately 140 hours of monitoring, less than four percent were lost to the study as missed data.

The hypothesis that the shivering process can be modified by a nursing in-tervention that changes the gradient of sensory input was predicated on the ability to discern changes. In the process of clearly delineating the phenomenon to be changed, shivering, the ordering of progression became apparent. The possibility of a center of temperature regulation seemed logical and probable. The inves-tigations of others provided explanation, support, and boundaries for an approach or design for the study. The study confirmed the hypothesis for one group of patients, namely the neurological subject, but also opened up an entirely new avenue for thinking and further exploration when acetaminophen appeared to successfully decrease shivering in patients with high fevers from infections.

First, isolating the phenomenon to a decrease of shivering in hyperpyrexic patients when acetaminophen was administered 4 to 6 hours prior to hypothermia but not closer to or during surface cooling, was startling. The drug supposedly: (1) had no effect on shivering, (2) was an antipyretic, and (3) detoxified within a 4-hour period. In these cases, acetaminophen was not an effective antipyretic. The patients still had dangerously high fevers that required surface cooling; if acetaminophen was given 4 to 6 hours prior to cooling, shivering was prevented.

A review of the literature revealed Feldberg's (1975) work on the effect of prostaglandins (PGEs) and the anterior thermoregulatory areas of the hypothalamus. Two stages of prostaglandin activity are involved: (1) synthesis, such that a sufficient amount is made and (2) release, such that a sufficient amount is available for reaction. Vane (1971) has shown that antipyretics decrease synthesis. We could therefore speculate that acetaminophen reduced synthesis and that the shivering center also could be stimulated by PGEs. Thus, if PGEs were decreased, shivering would also be lessened.

One possible population for testing out the speculation would be postpartum women who suffer from shivering. The idea remains merely a speculation because the necessary review of research findings, isolation of contributing factors, and delineation and description of the process has not been done. Surface cooling is not involved and thus the existing paradigm for a nursing intervention is not appropriate.

My approach to shivering modification hinged on discovering the order, recognizing the constraints of nursing, and coupling the available work, study, and findings of others. Truly a series of concepts, strung together into a pattern of application, organized for the moment, and generalized to the future are needed to guide nurses in further study and treatment of patients with shivering and surface cooling.

REFERENCES

Abbey, J.C. A Study of Control of Shivering during Hypothermia. In *Hypothermia Study: Terminal Report*. Grant No. NU-00483, Division of Nursing, Bureau of Health, Manpower Education, U.S. Department of Health, Education, and Welfare. Apr. 1, 1974–Oct. 15, 1976.

Abbey, J.C., and Close, L. A study of control of shivering during hypothermia. Presented at the 12th Annual Communicating Nursing Research Conference, WICHEN/WSRN. Abstract published in *Proceedings*. Denver, Col.: May 2–5, 1979.

Adolph, E.F. Physiological Adaptation in Infant Animals. In S. Itoh, K. Ogata, and H. Yoshimura (Eds.), *Advances in Climatic Physiology*. New York: Springer-Verlag, 1972. Pp. 159–171.

Alexander, G. Cold Thermogenesis. In D. Robertshaw (Ed.), *International Review of Physiology Environmental Physiology, III*. Baltimore, Md.: University Park Press, 1979. Vol. 20, pp. 46–155.

Aschoff, J., and Heise, A. Thermal Conductance in Man. In S. Itoh, K. Ogaga, H. Yoshimura (Eds.), *Advances in Climatic Physiology*. New York: Springer-Verlag, 1972. Pp. 334–348.

Barbour, H.G. The heat-regulating mechanism of the body. *Physiol. Rev.* 1(2):295–326, Apr. 1921.

Bay, J., Nunn, J.F., and Prys-Roberts, C. Factors influencing arterial Po_2 during recovery from anaesthesia. *Br. J. Anaesth.* 40:398–407, 1968.

Benzinger, T.A. Peripheral cold and central warm receptions, main origins of human thermal discomfort. In Proceedings of the National Academy of Sciences, USA, Washington, D.C. 49:832–839, June 1963.

Bigelow, W.G., Mustard, W.T., and Evans, J.G. Some physiologic concepts of hypothermia and their applications to cardiac surgery. *J. Thorac. Surg.* 28(5):463–480, Nov. 1954.

Blair, E. Generalized hypothermia. *Fed. Proc.* 28(4):1456–1462, Jul.–Aug. 1969.

Bligh, J. *Temperature Regulation in Mammals and Other Vertebrates.* New York: Elsevier-North Holland, 1973.

Boba, A. *Hypothermia for the Neurosurgical Patient.* Springfield, Ill.: Thomas, 1960.

Boulant, J.A., and Hardy, J.D. The effect of spinal and skin temperatures on the firing rate and thermosensitivity of preoptic neurons. *J. Physiol.* (Lond.) 240(3):639–660, Aug. 1974.

Brenglemann, G.L., Wyss, C., and Rowell, L.B. Control of skin forearm blood flow during periods of steadily increasing skin temperature. *J. Appl. Physiol.* 35(1):77–84, Jul. 1973.

Brown, A.C., and Brengelmann, G. Energy Metabolism. In T.C. Ruch and H.D. Patton (Eds.), *Physiology and Biophysics.* Philadelphia: Saunders, 1965. Pp. 1030–1049.

Bruch, K., and Wunnenberk, W. Masked Control of Two Effector Systems: Nonshivering and shivering thermogenesis. In J.D. Hardy, A.O. Gagge, and J.A.J. Stolivijk (Eds.), *Physiological and Behavioral Temperature Regulation.* Springfield, Ill.: Thomas, 1970. Pp. 562–580.

Budd, C.M., and Warhoft, N. Body temperature, shivering blood pressure and heart rate during a standard cold stress in Australia and Antarctica. *J. Physiol.* (Lond.) 186(1):216–222, Sept. 1966.

Burton, A.C., and Bazett, H.C. Study of average temperature of tissues, of exchanges of heat and vasomotor responses in man by means of bath calorimeter. *Am. J. Physiol.* 117:36–54, Sept. 1935.

Burton, A.C., and Edholm, O.G. *Man in a Cold Environment.* London: Edward Arnold, 1955.

Cabanac, M. Temperature Regulation. In J. Comroe, R.R. Sonneuschein, and I.S. Edelman (Eds.), *Annual Review of Physiology* (37). Palo Alto: California Annual Reviews, 1975. Pp. 415–439.

Cabanac, M., and Massenet, B. Temperature regulation during fever: Change of set point or change of gain? A tentative answer for a behavioral study in man. *J. Physiol.* (Lond.) 238(3):561–568, May 1974.

Cannon, P., and Keatinge, W.P. The metabolic rate and heat loss of fat in thin men in heat balance in cold and warm water. *J. Physiol.* (Lond.) 154(2):329–344, Dec. 1960.

Carlson, L.D., Hsieh, A.C.L., Fullington, F., and Elane, R.W. Immersion in cold water and total body insulation. *J. Aviat. Med.* 29(2):145–152, Feb. 1958.

Chatonnet, J., and Minaire, Y. Comparison of energy expenditure during exercise and cold exposure in the dog. *Fed. Proc.* 25(4):1348–1350, Jul.–Aug. 1966.

Clark, G., and Darron, G.H. The spinal pathway for shivering. *Exp. Neurol.* 18:453–458, Aug. 1967.

Cooper, K.E., and Kenyon, J.R. A comparison of temperatures measured in the rectum, esophagus, and on the surface of the aorta during hypothermia in man. *Br. J. Surg.* 44(188):616–619, May 1967.

Cooper, K.E., Cranston, W.I., and Snell, E.S. The temperature in the external auditory meatus as an index of central temperature changes. *J. Appl. Physiol.* 19(5):1032–1035, Sept. 1964.

Cornew, R.W., Hauk, J.C., and Stark, L. Firm control in human temperature regulation system. *J. Theor. Biol.* 16(3):406–426, Sept. 1967.

Daniels, F., Jr., and Baker, P.T. Relationship between body fat and shivering in air at 15°C. *J. Appl. Physiol.* 16(3):421–425, May 1961.

Denny-Brown, D., Gaylor, J.B., and Uprus, V. Note on the nature of the motor discharge in shivering. *Brain* 58(2):233–237, June 1937.

Dill, D.B., and Forbes, W.H. Respiratory and metabolic effects of hypothermia. *Am. J. Physiol.* 132(3):685–697, Apr. 1941.

Downey, J.A., Miller, J.M., and Darling, R.C. Thermoregulatory responses to deep and superficial cooling in spinal man. *J. Appl. Physiol.* 27(2):209–212, Aug. 1969.

Dundee, J.W., and King, R. Clinical aspects of induced hypothermia. *Br. J. Anaesth.* 31:106–133, Mar. 1959.

Dykes, R.W. Coding of steady and transient temperatures by cutaneous "cold" fibers serving the hand of monkeys. *Brain Res.* 98(3):485–500, Nov. 21, 1975.

Euler, C. von. Physiology and pharmacology of temperature regulation. *Pharmacol. Rev.* 13:361–398, Sept. 1961.

Feldberg, W. The Ferrier Lecture, 1974: Body temperature and fever: changes in our views during the last decade. *Proc. R. Soc. Lond.* [Biol.] 191(1103):199–229, Nov. 18, 1975.

Fisher, B. Experimental evaluation of prolonged hypothermia. *Arch. Surg.* 71(3):431–448, Sept. 1955.

Girling, F., and Topliff, E.D.L. The effect of breathing 15%, 21%, and 100% oxygen on the shivering responses of nude human subjects at 10°C. *Can. J. Physiol. Pharmacol.* 44:495–499, May 1966.

Glickman, N., Mitchell, H.H., Keeton, R.N., and Lambert, E.H. Shivering and heat production in men exposed to intense cold. *J. Appl. Physiol.* 22(1):1–8, Jan. 1967.

Hammel, N.T. Regulation of internal body temperature. *Ann. Rev. Physiol.* 30:641–670, 1968.

Hardy, J.D. Physiology of temperature regulation. *Physiol. Rev.* 41(3):521–606, July 1961.

Hardy, J.D. Thermal Comfort: Skin Temperature and Physiological Regulation. In J.D. Hardy, A.P. Gagge, and J.A.J. Stolwijk (Eds.), *Physiological and Behavioral Temperature Regulation.* Springfield, Ill.: Thomas, 1970. Pp. 856–873.

Hemingway, A. Shivering. *Physiol. Rev.* 43(3):397–422, Jul. 1963.

Hensel, H. Temperature Receptors in the Skin. In J.D. Hardy, A.P. Gagge, and J.A.J. Stolwijk (Eds.), *Physiological and Behavioral Temperature Regulation.* Springfield, Ill.: Thomas, 1970. Pp. 856–873.

Hickey, M.C. Hypothermia. *Am. J. Nurs.* 65(1):116–122, Jan. 1965.

Himmis-Hagen, J. Lipid metabolism during cold exposure and during cold-acclimation. *Lipids* 7(5):310–323, July 1972.

Himms-Hagen, J . Cellular thermogenesis. *Ann. Rev. Physiol.* 38:315–351, 1976.

Houday, Y., and Guieu, J.D. Physical Models of Thermoregulation. In P. Lomax, E. Schonbaum, and J. Jacobs (Eds.), *Temperature Regulation and Drug Action.* Basel: S. Karger, 1975. Pp. 11–21.

Hovarth, S.M., Spurr, G.B., Hull, B.K., and Hamilton, L.H. Metabolic cost of shivering. *J. Appl. Physiol.* 8:595–602, May 1956.

Huckaba, C.E., and Downey, J.E. Overview of Human Regulation. In A.S. Iberall and A.C. Guyton (Eds.), *Regulation and Control of Physiological Systems.* Pittsburgh: ISA, 1973. Pp. 212–216.

Hunter, A.P. Body Temperature during General Anaesthesia. In P. Lomax and E. Schonbaum (Eds.), *Body Temperature: Regulation, Drug Effects and Therapeutic Implications.* New York: Marcel Dekker, 1979. Pp. 587–593.

Iggo, A. Cutaneous thermoreceptors in primates and subprimates. *J. Physiol.* (Lond.) 200(2):403–430, Feb. 1969.

Johnson, R.H., and Spalding, J.M.K. The role of central temperature receptor in man. *J. Physiol.* (Lond.) 184(3):773–780, June 1966.

Keatinge, W.R. *Survival in Cold Water.* Oxford and Edinburgh: Blackwell Scientific, 1969.

Kluger, M.J. Temperature Regulation, Fever, and Disease. In D. Robertshaw (Ed.), *International Review of Physiology: Environmental Physiology III* (20). Baltimore: University Park Press, 1979. Pp. 209–251.

Kosaka, M., and Simon, E. The central nervous spinal mechanism of cold shivering. *Pfluegers Arch.* 302:357–373, 1968.

Lin, M.T., and Chai, C.Y. Independence of spinal cord and medulla oblongata on thermal activity. *Am. J. Physiol.* 226(5):1066–1072, May 1974.

Magoun, H.W., Harrison, F., Brobeck, J.R., and Hanson, S.W. Activation of heat loss mechanisms by local heating of the brain. *J. Neurophysiol.* 1(2):101–114, March 1938.

Mitchell, D. Physical Basis of Thermoregulation. In D. Robertshaw (Ed.), *International Review of Physiology: Environmental Physiology II*, Volume 15. Baltimore: University Press, 1977. Pp. 1–27.

Nutik, S. Convergence of cutaneous and preoptic region thermal afferent on posterior hypothalamic neurones. *J. Neurophysiol.* 36(1):250–257, Jan. 1973.

Ogata, K., and Murakami, N. Neural Factors Affecting the Regulatory Responses of Body Temperature. S. Itoh, K. Ogata, and H. Yoshimura (Eds.), *In Advances in Climatic Physiology.* New York: Springer-Verlag, 1972. Pp. 50–67.

Perkins, J.F., Jr. The role of proprioceptors in shivering. *Am. J. Physiol. Med.* 145:264–271, Dec. 1965.

Petajan, J.N., and Williams, D.D. Behavior of single motor units during pre-shivering tone and shivering tremor. *Am. J. Physiol. Med.* 51(1):16–22, Feb. 1972.

Popovik, V., and Popovik, P. *Hypothermia in Biology and Medicine.* New York: Grune & Stratton, 1974.

Pugh, L.G.C., Edholm, O.G., Fox, F.H., Wolff, H.F., Hervey, G.R., Hammond, W.H., Tanner, J.M., and Whitehouse, R.H. A physiological study of channel swimming. *Clin. Sci.* 19(2):257–273, May 1960.

Rosenfeld, J.B. Acid–base and electrolyte disturbances in hypothermia. *Am. J. Cardiol.* 12:678–682, Nov. 1963.

Rosomoff, H.L. Effects of hypothermia on physiology of nervous system. *Surgery* 40:328–336, Aug. 1956.

Simon, E. Temperature signals from skin and spinal cord converge on spine–thalamic neurons. *Pfluegers Arch.* 337(4):323–332, 1972.

Spurr, G.B., Hutt, B.K., and Horvath, S.M. Shivering, oxygen consumption, and body temperature in acute exposure of men to two different cold environments. *J. Appl. Physiol.* 11(1):58–64, Jul. 1957.

Stevens, V. Clinical hypothermia: Some nursing concepts. *J. Neurosurg. Nurs.* 4(1):33–43, Jul. 1972.

Stone, H.H., Donnelly, C., and Frosbese, A.S. Effect of lowered body temperature on cerebral hemodynamics and metabolism of man. *Surg. Gynecol. Obstet.* 103:313–317, Sept. 1956.

Stuart, D.G., Eldred, E., Hemingway, A., and Kawamura, Y. Neural Regulation of the Rhythm of Shivering. In C.M. Herzfield and J.D. Hardy (Eds.), *Temperature, Its Measurement in Science and Industry.* New York: Van Nostrand Reinhold, 1963. Vol. 3, pp. 545–557.

Thauer, R. Thermosensitivity of the Spinal Cord. In J.D. Hardy, A.P. Gagge, and J.A.J. Stolwijk (Eds.), *Physiological and Behavioral Temperature Regulation.* Springfield, Ill.: Thomas, 1970. Pp. 472–491.

Vane, J.R. Inhibition of prostaglandin synthesis as a mechanism of action for aspirin-like drugs. *Nature New Biol.* 231:232–235, June 23, 1971.

Chapter 13

Shivering: Postpartum

Mary Ann Schroeder

For over 7,000 years, people caring for the sick have been concerned about patient comfort related to body temperature. Translations from the papyri of Egypt admonish health care givers in the temples to keep the patient's head cool. Only 40 years ago, nurses were still taught the principle that a major key to patient comfort was in keeping the feet warm and the head cool.

Antibiotics, central heating systems, and the general use of air-conditioning have decreased the occurrence of elevated body temperatures, almost eliminated shaking chills, and produced a temperate, comfortable environment. Despite the fact that some chilling, shivering, shaking, and shuddering still occur in patients, the once-pervasive and important area of comfort through warming and cooling techniques emerged with low- or no-priority ratings for clinical nursing.

Technical modalities of medical care, unresolved problems, and adjustments made in environmental control to save energy may bring the issues of chilling and overheating into focus again. One unresolved problem observed by nurses is the shivering of women in the immediate postpartum period.

DEFINING SHIVERING

The sensation of shivering is a phenomenon that virtually everyone has experienced at some time. The concept of *shivering* has been rather narrowly limited to the physiological domain in which it has been defined as a thermoregulatory mechanism, the function of which is to maintain body temperature. Physiologists have described the shivering response by identifying those muscles of the body that exhibit rhythmic contraction. They have manipulated the ambient temperature to induce a shivering response and have identified the receptors, neural pathways, and control mechanisms for initiating and resolving shivering.

Using a conceptual approach to describing and explaining behavior, we need to discover whether there are correlates that may serve to describe, explain, and possibly predict incidences of shivering caused by factors other than a thermo-regulatory response.

A typical response to the question, "When do you shiver?" is, of course, "when I'm cold." But is this true for the postpartum women who experience shaking following delivery? In studies, the proportion of women who experienced shaking seemed to be greater than 50 percent of those observed during my investigation. Shaking occurs approximately 10 minutes after the birth of the infant and lasts for about 15 to 20 minutes. This phenomenon has been labelled the *postpartum chill* and also is called postpartum shivering (Clapp and Abrams 1976; and Jaameri, Jahkola, and Perttu 1966).

Since the etiology of postpartum shivering is unknown, we can speculate about whether this observed phenomenon was really shivering or whether stimuli other than cool temperatures initiated shivering. Conversations with colleagues, friends, and associates revealed that shivering was not associated uniquely with a feeling of coldness. Various kinds of shivering, including nervous shivering, cold shivering, shivering associated with an intensely pleasant emotional experience, and shivering associated with a fear-producing experience, were described. All of these experiences initiated shivering responses, which varied as a function of the experience.

These findings raise a question about the validity of defining shivering within the narrow confines of a physiological model. A typical definition of shivering advocated by physiologists is that offered by Jensen (1976, p. 1002), who defines shivering as the involuntary rhythmic contraction of skeletal muscles that serves as a physiological mechanism to increase heat production in very cold environments. Numerous animal studies, as well as those conducted on humans, have elicited a shivering response when temperatures were decreased to approximately 34°C rectally (Hemingway 1963). Neurosurgical patients on hypothermia blankets elicited a shivering response when body temperature was maintained at 30°C (Abbey 1973).

Physiologists define involuntary rhythmic contraction of skeletal muscles as shivering. Do informants describe shivering in the same manner? Physiologists also describe the intensity of this involuntary contraction in degrees ranging from 1 (slight) to 4 (tremor). Do informants define a violent shiver as shivering? To refine the definition of the phenomenon of shivering, I decided to interview shivering victims.

RESEARCH METHOD AND RESULTS

Using an inductive approach, information was elicited that served to describe, explain, and predict shivering under selected conditions. As indicated previously, physiologists have hypothesized stimuli that incite shivering, have identified the feedback mechanisms regulating and controlling temperature, and have manipulated the temperature of the environment in order to elicit thresholds for the shivering response. No report in the literature was found that investigated shivering associated with variables other than temperature.

For my study, an informal survey of nursing colleagues was used to describe the phenomenon. The following questions were asked: What is shivering? Are there different kinds of shivering? Are there different causes of shivering? What are the means that relieve shivering? These data would facilitate clarification of the concept of shivering by describing, explaining, and predicting the phenomenon. In addition, this clarification would be applicable in the settings where people experience shivering.

First, some decisions need to be explicit about methods of collecting data to define a concept. There are two possible approaches: (1) ask a random sample about experiences with shivering or (2) delimit a specific sample population and collect data in a bounded area. In this study, the sample population was limited to postpartum women who had delivered a baby within 1 week of data collecting. The rationale for this sample selection was as follows:

1. A hunch that the shivering observed in the postpartum woman was different from shivering observed under other circumstances
2. A desire to compare this shivering with other kinds of shivering
3. A need for more adequate descriptions of shivering in women who had recently delivered
4. Little about postpartum shivering appears in the literature
5. The etiology of shivering is unknown.

Selection of this sample restricts the generalizability of findings but facilitates development of substantive knowledge.

Interviews were conducted with 16 postpartum women who had had live births within 1 week of data collection. Four of the women had delivered at home. Six open-ended questions guided the conduct of the semistructured interview. These questions sought information about (1) the incidence of postpartum shivering, (2) a description of this shivering, (3) the effectiveness of nursing interventions in controlling shivering, and (4) a comparison of postpartum shivering with other kinds of shivering.

Two predominant themes emerged: (1) the word *shivering* is culturally associated with being cold and (2) postpartum shivering is not really a shivering, but a shaking. Women tended to describe their postpartum as well as their predelivery shivering as a "shaking." "I shiver when I'm cold . . ." "I shook following delivery of my baby." The word *shaking* was used by all women who had experienced a postpartum shiver; this term may more adequately describe the intensity of the muscle activity. Shaking prior to delivery was confined largely to the large muscles of the thighs, while in the immediate postpartum period the shaking occurred systemically. This was described by statements such as, "I shook all over," and "My whole body was shaking." Women reported that the shaking following delivery began as a shivering noted in the muscles of the face or by the chattering of the teeth. It appears, therefore, that *shaking* could be defined as a more violent form of muscle activity than that experienced when shivering.

Categories of Postpartum Shivering

The verbal responses of these postpartum women to the open-ended questions were arbitrarily grouped into seven categories as follows to encompass a possible taxonomy of shivering: types of shivering, stimuli initiating shivering, types of coldness, onset, location, powerlessness, comfort measures thought to alleviate shivering. Further refinement of these categories will be undertaken as further studies are done.

Types of shivering refers to the mothers' perceptions of different kinds of shivering: (1) cold shivering or (2) noncold shivering. These two types of shivering were described in terms of the named causative stimuli; therefore, it was necessary to merge the two categories of types of shivering and stimuli. Cold shivering was described as occurring in response to a cool or cold environment with a feeling of coldness produced by this environment. "The delivery room was cold and this caused the shaking." "I felt cool." One woman described cold as being "inside" or "outside." The postpartum feeling of coldness was an "inside" one, which was not relieved by warm blankets, while an "outside" cold as experienced from a cold environment was relieved by applying a warm coat or a blanket over the body.

Women identified the feeling of cold as a stimulus to invoke shivering. Cold seemed to initiate the shivering response but did not perpetuate this activity. "I was shivering, but I wasn't cold." This represents a distinct difference between shivering experienced when coming in from the cold and postpartum shivering or shaking. Typically, when a person warms up, the shivering stops; this is not the case in postpartum shivering.

Noncold shivering was traced to such stimuli as trauma, fear, fever, fatigue, tension, hunger, or a release of energy. Responses included, "The trauma of the delivery or of the cesarean section created a shock to my body." "I was nervous and this caused me to shake." "I was tired and weak." The property of "release of energy" was expressed to describe the shaking both postpartum and predelivery. Release of energy in the predelivery state is in the form of muscle tenseness and, as a result, energy is being transmitted to the environment as, for example, when the woman is holding onto the bed rail tightly. This action would provoke a noncold shivering and it could be postulated that the pain-fear-tension syndrome advocated by Dr. Dick Read is the initiator of this behavior. Energy is being released into the environment through the bed rail. Release of energy in the postdelivery stage is more in the context of energy being released in the form of heat to the surrounding environment. The new mother is transferred from the delivery room table to the recovery room stretcher and the drapes are removed. Heat is lost to the immediate surroundings.

The three categories of onset, location, and powerlessness have been merged here in the interest of economy in description. These categories tend to form a composite during the various stages of labor and following delivery.

The *onset of shivering* refers to that moment at which shivering during or after delivery was first perceived by the mother. Women reported that shaking occurred either during the second stage of labor, the third stage of labor, the fourth stage of labor, or in both the second and fourth stages of labor. Prior to delivery, this shaking was controllable and located primarily in the thighs. Following delivery, shaking occurred over the entire body. This shaking was involuntary and uncontrollable. Women reported that prior to delivery, shaking could be controlled by relaxation techniques. Following delivery, however, relaxation techniques were ineffective in bringing the shaking under control.

Powerlessness refers to the degree to which the woman felt she was able to control shaking either before or after delivery. Women expressed a physical powerlessness as well as a cognitive or psychological powerlessness. *Cognitive powerlessness* refers to their perceived inability to escape from the situation. This feeling was verbalized by such statements as, "I felt as if I would jump out of my skin" and "I thought I would go nuts." Powerlessness, therefore, could be operationalized in terms of the two dimensions of physical and cognitive or psychological control.

Comfort measures to alleviate shaking pertain to those nursing interventions that mothers perceive as relieving postpartum shaking. Women expressed the feeling that nursing measures such as the application of warm blankets to alleviate shaking following delivery was comforting but did not eliminate shivering. Shivering associated with an outer chilling such as that experienced when coming in from a cold outer environment was alleviated by securing warm blankets or warm clothing.

UNIQUE CHARACTERISTICS OF POSTPARTUM SHIVERING

It seems, therefore, that the experience of shivering during the childbearing process could be differentiated from other kinds of shivering with respect to the initial stimulus—a cold room or a cold feeling as well as fear and tension during the predelivery period. The intensity of the experience is greater than that experienced when shivering from the cold and, therefore, this shivering is really shaking more than shivering. Furthermore, shivering following delivery was thought to be uncontrollable, annoying, and fatiguing. The following propositions could be generated from the data:

1. Postpartum shaking is initiated by a cold feeling that could be generated from within oneself or from the external environment, by fatigue, by trauma, by nervousness, or by a release of energy.
2. The initial stimulus, the cool feeling, or cool environment does not perpetuate the shivering once it is initiated. Women reported that following delivery they were shaking but were not cold.
3. Postpartum shaking is involuntary and uncontrollable, but predelivery shivering can be controlled through mechanisms such as relaxation techniques.
4. Warm blankets help to comfort but do not relieve postpartum shaking.
5. The initial perception of muscle activity is described as a shivering sensation but as this muscle activity is intensified, this experience is described as a shaking rather than a shivering.
6. Shaking in the postpartum period is more uncomfortable than that experienced when shivering from the cold because of: (1) the increased magnitude or intensity, and (2) the lack of available mechanisms to relieve the shaking experience.

Table 13-1 A Typology of Shivering during the Childbearing Process

Onset Stage	Type	Stimulus	Location	Control Measures	Comfort Measures
Second stage of labor	Noncold	Fear Tension Nervousness Release of energy	Thighs	Relaxation	Touch
Third stage of labor	Cold	Release of energy	Thighs		
Fourth stage of labor (postpartum period)	Cold	Cold environment Cold feeling Fatigue Release of energy	All over	(Uncontrollable)	Warm blankets

CONCLUSION

In summary, these data indicate that postpartum shivering is unique and different from other types of shivering. The etiology is unknown and this is an area for further investigation. The stimulus for postpartum shivering may be a temperature imbalance due to the rapid loss of weight and heat following delivery. Heat loss results not only from the expulsion of the infant, but also from the delivery of the placenta and loss of fluid. Postpartum women are not necessarily cold when they shiver and their reaction is not radically different from the nervous shiver, the fear shiver, or the pleasurable emotional shivering experience. Postpartum shivering is uncontrollable and of a longer duration than other types of shivering. Shivering from a fearful scene is, for example, fleeting.

The purpose of this investigation was to clarify the concept of shivering experienced during childbearing. Dickoff and James would classify this level of theory development at the *naming stage*. The next step to be undertaken is *explaining the concept*. This will require further study to delineate a profile of those women who shivered following delivery and those who did not experience the phenomenon.

This study has, then, developed a definition of shivering in postpartum women and has renamed the experience *postpartum shaking*. Based on the descriptions of postpartum women, it can be defined as the occurrence of intense muscular activity involving the entire body; it is characterized by its uncontrollable nature and uncomfortable quality, and it occurs approximately 10 minutes following delivery and lasts for approximately 10 to 15 minutes.

REFERENCES

Abbey, J., Andrews, C., Avigliano, K., Blossom, R., Bunke, B., Engberg, N., Halliburton, P., and Peterson, J. A pilot study: The control of shivering during hypothermia by a clinical nursing measure. *J. Neurosurg. Nurs.* 5:78–88, 1973.

Clapp, J., and Abram, R. The postpartum chill. *Isr. J. Med. Sci.* 12:1131–1133, 1976.

Dickoff, J., James, P., and Wiedenbach, E. Theory in a practice discipline: Part I. Practice oriented theory. *Nurs. Res.* 17:415–435, 1968.

Hemingway, A. Shivering. *Physiol. Rev.* 43:357–418, 1963.

Jaameri, K.E., Jahkola, A., and Perttu, J. On shivering in association with normal delivery. *Acta Obstet. Gynecol. Scand.* 45:383–388, 1966.

Jensen, D. *The Principles of Physiology.* New York: Appleton-Century-Crofts, 1976. P. 1002.

Chapter 14

Fatigue

Laura K. Hart and Mildred I. Freel

Fatigue, a multifaceted, diverse concept, originated as a lay term to label states of self-realized human inadequacy symptomatized by discomfort and productive incapacity as well as feelings of weakness and futility. Study of the phenomenon has interested many different groups. Understanding fatigue is, for example, of practical concern to industry, as its management and decrement pays off in increased profits. A second group, researchers in aerospace medicine, is extremely interested in the effects of fatigue because safe, efficient, and effective functioning of pilots and crew members depends on understanding the effects of this phenomenon. A third group, with long-standing interest in fatigue is involved in the pursuit of athletic prowess, where winners are those who become fatigued last.

The medical field's interest in the phenomenon is stimulated by the fact that fatigue is probably the most prevalent symptom and often the first indication of both physical and mental illness (MacBryde 1970). Patients so accept that fatigue accompanies illness that they often do not mention it unless they are asked. At least 50 percent of patients seen by internists, however, complain of this symptom (Burkhardt 1956). When patients voluntarily complain of fatigue, it is either very prominent or impeding an important aspect of their lives.

PROBLEMS IN DEFINITION

Although several disciplines have done concentrated study, the complex phenomenon of fatigue is still not well understood nor clearly delineated. Lay origins of the term may partially account for fatigue being divergently used when referring to objective work decrement, subjective appraisal of bodily feelings, and physiological changes in activity of bodily mechanisms. Such a broad spectrum of use suggests the difficulty in arriving at a practical and inclusive definition, especially since the term has roots reaching into physiology, pathology, and psychology. Each discipline places its own parameters on the concept and uses its special focus for interpretation. Physiologists often consider fatigue as simply a decrease in physical performance. Pathologists view it as a prime indicator of neuromuscular or metabolic disorders.

Psychologists, on the other hand, consider it a condition affecting the whole organism, which includes decreased motivation as well as deterioration of mental and physical activities. This diversity yields at least two definitions. *Fatigue* can be described as a subjective sense of weariness or tiredness resulting from exertion or stress or as a condition of impaired efficiency, resulting from prolonged mental and/or physical activity or from an attitude of boredom or from disgust with monotonous work (Schreuder 1966).

FATIGUE, TIREDNESS, AND EXHAUSTION

Grandjean (1970), a prominent current worker in industrial fatigue, further delineates fatigue as one phase on the continuum of experiences persons encounter as they move from a subjective state of feeling tired to a state of complete exhaustion. *Tiredness,* a part of normal, healthful living, is a state in which a person feels a generalized lessening of strength and energy. Such tiredness can easily be dispelled by sleep and rest or by increasing nourishment and/or fluid intake. *Exhaustion,* at the end of the fatigue continuum, occurs when the expenditures of the body's energy reserves exceed its ability to replenish these reserves, forcing the body to stop functioning. Subjective feeling of general fatigue is defined by Grandjean (1970) as a nonspecific state indicative of a decreased level of vitality, which has the protective function of forcing the body to avoid further stress, thus allowing recovery to take place.

FATIGUE CATEGORIES

The impact of rest upon ability to recover differentiates acute from chronic fatigue. *Acute fatigue* quickly responds to rest or sleep while chronic fatigue is little changed by either. *Chronic fatigue* is more likely to be temporarily decreased by an increase in activity, change in activity, or diversion. While acute fatigue is seen as produced by hard physical or mental work, chronic fatigue is frequently attributed to a psychological or psychiatric problem base (McFarland 1953). Fatigue of psychic origin often relates to overstress, unresolved conflicts, losses, and depression and disappears when the conflict is resolved. In addition, chronic fatigue is frequently cumulative and is characterized by boredom, loss of incentive, and progressive anxiety (MacBryde 1970).

Another useful delineation of fatigue is to categorize it into local muscle, general muscle, and generalized fatigue. *Local-muscle fatigue* is a singular entity occurring after use of a local muscle group. This condition may be due to a malfunction in impulse transmission (Nachmanson 1960; and Pringle 1960) or due to a change in muscle itself, such as the depletion of its glycogen stores (Bergstrom and Hultman 1967; and Hermannsen, Hultman, and Saltin 1967). In general-muscle fatigue, muscle exertion may be one of the main variables, but its production is primarily due to failure of circulatory and metabolic adaptations rather than to local-muscle failure (Christenson 1962). When the adapting mechanisms of increased cardiac output, shunting of blood to working tissues, and increased efficiency in oxygen transport begin to reach their upper limits, general-muscular fatigue becomes evident.

A much broader phenomenon appears operative with generalized fatigue. This state, resulting in a decrement in performance, does not necessarily involve failure of muscular contraction nor exhaustion of circulation or metabolic supply. Miller (1963) suggested that the generalized fatigue state may be the result of a mild midbrain dysfunction. By 1968, advances in neurophysiological evidence led Grandjean (1968) to suggest the most likely site of central control of this generalized fatigue state as the reticular formation of the midbrain and medulla, since this area of the brain relates to consciousness and unconsciousness, arousal and depression, and sleep and wakefulness. When general fatigue is viewed as the opposite of arousal, multiple connections of this part of the brain to higher and lower centers might explain the many modifications seen in general-fatigue symptoms.

PHYSIOLOGY

Neurophysiology experiments reviewed by Grandjean (1970) suggest that cortical inhibition results from two different causes: (1) Cortical activity may be reduced by increased activity of the inhibitory system, which appears to be regulated through humoral factors. (2) The raphe system located in the midline of the brain stem appears to affect feelings of fatigue through secretion and accumulation of serotonin. Grandjean (1970) labels this process the *active inhibitory system*. Fatigue occurs in this situation because initial stimulation of the reticular activating system is lacking. When these inhibitory systems dominate, the organism is in a state of fatigue; if the activating system prevails, the organism is ready to increase performance and feels fresh and full of initiative. In light of present neurophysiological knowledge, generalized fatigue could be considered a central nervous system state controlled by antagonistic activity of inhibitory and activating systems of the brain stem. These regulating or adaptive systems are susceptible to reaction to stimuli from the surrounding environment, to stimuli from the conscious part of the brain, and to humoral factors originating within the organism.

In medical and general thinking, fatigue is frequently regarded as something to be avoided entirely. Avoidance of fatigue may not, however, be entirely desirable if it is viewed in relation to the process of adaptation. The disagreeable sensations referred to as fatigue may be essential indicators that physiological equilibrium somewhere in the body is breaking down (Dill 1967). Fatigue is not an index of breakdown of physiological adaptations; rather, it is an index of early stress on adaptative mechanisms. Total avoidance of fatigue could eventually lead to loss of neuromuscular function and circulatory adaptability as a result of disuse. Thus, fatigue could be defined as a defense mechanism, a protective phenomenon, that helps maintain physiological equilibrium by stimulating a desire for work decrements or stress avoidance when the response to stress reaches a level of discomfort (Bartley 1965, 1967, 1976).

When fatigue involves decrease or impairment in enthusiasm for work and/ or a lowering in efficiency, the following objective and subjective signs and symptoms are exhibited:

1. Decreased attention
2. Slowed and impaired perception
3. Impaired thinking
4. Decreased motivation
5. Decreased performance in physical and mental activities (Grandjean 1969).

INTERVENING VARIABLES

Predisposing and underlying physiological impairments that may precipitate fatigue cannot be viewed as synonymous with fatigue. Precipitating physical and mental stress that cause symptoms of the impairment should be viewed as distinctly separate from fatigue and its symptoms (Darling 1971). In fact, no direct correlation has been found between the signs and the amount of physical or mental stress and the resultant amount of fatigue (Bartley 1965). This, no doubt, occurs because individuals react differently depending on treatment, ability to perform a task, adaptability, and physical and mental fitness.

While it would appear that signs and symptoms associated with stress should afford a good measure of the body's capacity from the standpoint of fatigue and efficiency, their practical usefulness is limited because of the inability to gauge an individual's dynamic compensatory mechanisms (Luongo 1964). It has often been noted that fatigue and expenditure of energy, in terms of caloric output, are totally unrelated. Also, fatigue and impairment or decrement of performance are not necessarily proportional since in an emergency, the well-motivated, competent person will excrete enough adrenalin to compensate for subjective feelings of tiredness or weariness. On the other hand, at times, very pleasurable activities can be carried on continuously without feelings of fatigue (Schreuder 1966). Since fatigue is on a continuum, mental and/or physical activity can be sustained or resumed in spite of fatigue. Perseverance at a task depends on interest and determination. Pleasure and satisfaction often reduce the impact of fatigue while disinterest increases it. Motivation is a very influential factor.

The presence of pathological conditions can also alter the "logical" relationship between stress and fatigue. Activities, which in healthy individuals do not produce the usual signs of stress, may quickly precipitate signs and symptoms of fatigue in individuals afflicted with pathological conditions. In healthy individuals, activities that would precipitate only symptoms of local-muscle fatigue may so stress the ill person that general-muscle fatigue or even a state of generalized fatigue occurs.

SIGNS AND SYMPTOMS

Associating any consistent, overt physical behavior with fatigue, especially in clinical situations where underlying disease or pathology plays a part, is especially difficult. In general, patients who complain of fatigue tend to appear worn, wan, lethargic, slowed down, and lacking in energy. The face sags, the body slumps, and the voice may be dull and expressionless. No specific circulatory or respiratory changes are consistently evident (Astrand 1960). Patients who complain of fatigue use such terms as weary, all in, tired, worn out, pooped, listless, no pep, no interest, no energy to carry on, and a strong desire to stop, rest, lie down, or to sleep in describing this subjective experience.

Predicting the occurrence of fatigue is difficult because the major component of this phenomenon relates to subjective feelings, which may show little or no correlation between amount of stress, signs of stress, and occurrence of the state of fatigue. Measuring generalized fatigue quantitatively is a complex process because stress symptoms are often concurrent with the symptoms of fatigue. Symptoms of stress such as increased body temperature, heart rate, hemoglobin, negative nitrogen and potassium balance, emotional lability, perspiration, and paleness may or may not be present during states of fatigue.

Identifying symptoms specifically related to fatigue was undertaken in 1967 by the Industrial Fatigue Research Committee of the Japanese Association of Industrial Health (Yoshitake 1971). The results of this work was a 30-item fatigue symptom checklist containing three dimensions or categories.

1. The first symptom dimension was described as a dull, sleepy factor, representing general feelings of incongruity in the body. Symptoms in this category included heaviness in the head, tiredness in body, tired legs,

yawning, brain hot and/or muddled, drowsiness, eyestrain, rigid and/or clumsy moving, unsteadiness while standing, and desire to lie down. The last three symptoms are actually more indicative of exhaustion than just a dull or drowsy factor.

2. The second dimension pertaining to a decline in motivation to work was composed of mental symptoms that appear to lack a physical basis. Symptoms included were difficulty in thinking, weariness while talking, nervousness, inability to concentrate, loss of interest in thinking, forgetfulness, lack of self-confidence, inability to straighten up in posture, anxious, and lack of patience.

3. The third dimension pertained to projections of fatigue to specific parts of the body or feelings of incongruity in specific body parts. Included in this dimension were headache, stiff shoulders, pain in waist, constrained breathing, thirst, husky voice, dizziness, eyelid spasms, tremor in limbs, and feeling ill. The last four symptoms of this dimension may represent dysfunction of the autonomic nervous system with the others being primarily specific sensory projections.

When Yoshitake (1971) investigated the relationship of these symptoms to levels of fatigue among bank and broadcasting workers, he found the more numerous the symptoms the greater was the level of fatigue. In this healthy-worker group, specific feelings of incongruity had the greatest relationship to levels of fatigue. However, while specific feelings had the greatest impact, feelings of general incongruity were almost always present in states of fatigue regardless of work type. Also, in only rare instances did mental symptoms exist without accompanying physical symptoms.

Kashiwagi (1971) attempted to construct a fatigue rating scale based on this checklist that would allow an objective judgment of fatigue through evaluation of a person's appearance. He interpreted the Japanese fatigue symptom checklist's three dimensions as relating to: (1) weakened activation (dull, sleepy factor), (2) weakened motivation (mental symptoms), and (3) physical disintegration (specific feelings). Since he perceived the physical disintegration category as symptoms specific to specific types of work and the other two dimensions common to all kinds of work, he utilized only the first two dimensions. He used the following objective symptoms to indicate weakened activation: tired walk, unsteady voice, absentmindedness, hollow-cheeked, avoidance of conversation, sulky face, spiritless eyes, irritability, listlessness, and dull face. The weakened motivation symptoms were: making many misstatements, avoiding other's eyes, being difficult to speak to, sluggishness, restlessness, anxiety, pale face, stiff face, trembling fingers, and inability to concentrate or listen. He found that the component of weakened activation played the most important role in effectively being able to objectively evaluate changes in the level of a person's fatigue.

FATIGUE SYMPTOMS IN ILLNESS

While the specific symptoms just discussed have been found to provide fairly effective indicators of fatigue in a healthy person, it seems that in a disease state the specific precipitating pathology provides an additional symptom dimension needed to assist in clinical monitoring of fatigue. These symptoms should be as specific to the pathology present as the symptom dimension of incongruity in specific body parts is to specific types of work performed. For example, when working with a patient who has multiple sclerosis it has been clinically observed that an early indicator of progressing fatigue is increase in rate of speech and rise in voice pitch. Patients who are undergoing radiation therapy will frequently complain of feeling they must lie down about 30–60 minutes after treatment. Preoperative cardiac bypass patients often complain they are too tired to even talk. Unfortunately, nursing as yet has not documented which fatigue symptoms are specific to pathology conditions.

FEELINGS OF FATIGUE

While symptoms of fatigue are a basis for expressing the feeling of fatigue, they are not exactly the same thing. That is, symptoms of fatigue are expressions of specific complaints, while the feeling of fatigue is a feeling of overall unpleasantness. This feeling tone can be quantified by identifying the level, intensity, degree, or point on a continuum between refreshed and exhaustion felt by an individual. Pearson and Byar (1956) developed a fatigue feeling self-rating scale designed to measure and provide a quantifying score of how a person perceived his or her fatigue at the time of measurement. This 10-item adjective list defined the fatigue level continuum in short, easily understood phrases: extremely peppy, very lively, very refreshed, quite refreshed, somewhat refreshed, slightly pooped, fairly well pooped, petered out, extremely tired, and ready to drop. Each adjective is scored in relationship to whether the person at that time felt better than, the same as, or worse than that specific feeling. Weighting the "better than's" as one, same as as two, and worse than as three provides a score that increases as fatigue levels increase.

GENERAL-MUSCLE FATIGUE ASSESSMENT

Measurement of the subjective nature of fatigue is primarily based on self-estimation of the state of fatigue and prediction of continued ability. Objective fatigue measures that can help estimate certain tolerances are also available. For example, if decisions about possible tolerance of general-muscle activity are to be made, the physiological measure of heart rate provides a measure on which to base comparisons of fatigue states. Activity levels depend on work capacity of the heart and skeletal muscles. The circulatory strain encountered often is the most limiting factor (Muller 1962). Heart rate provides a better expression of the demands made by an activity (Asmussen, Klausen, and Puolsen 1960), and is in better agreement with subjective estimates of fatigue (Suggs and Splinter 1961) as well as objective ratings of effort (Borg 1962) than are actual oxygen requirements. The heart rate is also more sensitive than oxygen consumption to the environmental stresses of heat and humidity (Brouha, Maxfield, Smith, and Stopps 1963), static loads, awkward postures (Scholtz 1957), and poorly spaced rest pauses (Muller 1953). Implications of such an objective measure are shown in industrial fatigue studies where it has been found that activity levels that elevate heart rate to 110 beats per minute for leg work and 99 beats per minute for arm work is the maximum allowable to be in keeping with good labor management (Brouha 1960; Snook and Irvine 1969; Suggs et al. 1961; and Wells, Balke, and VanFonssan 1957). That is, to keep workers working at these levels is to keep the fatigue state at a level having least impact on production. It is also suggested that at least 15 percent of working time should be devoted to rest pauses; a ratio of 20 to 30 percent is often necessary with strenuous types of activity. Since heart rate recovery is greatest at the beginning of a rest period, several short pauses are more advantageous than one long rest period. Heavier work requires evenly distributed rest periods (Astrand 1960; Bergstrom and Hultman 1966; and Grandjean 1969). Industry has found that environmental conditions conducive to either overheating or chilling will precipitate fatigue more quickly (Bergstrom et al. 1966; and Kumudavalli and Swami 1967). Type of diet and spacing of nutritional intake also affects the ability of workers to maintain their maximum production (Bergstrom et al. 1966; and Hermannsen et al. 1967).

FATIGUE ANTECEDENTS

Fatigue studies done so far show how other disciplines have delineated many of the fatigue responses that occur in healthy individuals in a variety of situations. Health fields, however, have done very little work in delineating fatigue experiences or management protocols of the fatigue that patients experience. This seems peculiar since in many pathological conditions fatigue is a major complaint or symptom of the patient's disease and/or side effect of treatment regimes.

Usually antecedent conditions associated with precipitation of fatigue in healthy people are stresses or energy demands that exceed the body's psychic, cardiovascular, or metabolic capacity, where there are deficient nutrient supplies, and/or when deficient motivational levels occur. When pathological conditions exist, fatigue is more complex. For people with disease, fatigue is also precipitated by conditions such as a deficient utilization of nutrient supplies, neuromuscular defects, and alterations in body metabolic functioning such as occur with inadequate endocrine or hormonal levels and elevation of toxins.

Knowledge of causes or antecedents of fatigue may be helpful to the physician who is primarily concerned with eliminating or neutralizing effects of the antecedent condition. The nurse, however, is more concerned with:

1. Delineating activity tolerances and determining the impact of environmental and nutritional regimens on fatigued patients' experience
2. Developing an activity–rest program that keeps patients in energy balance
3. Providing activities that stimulate, involve, and keep patients' physical movement, affective responses, thinking processes, and social interaction in balance
4. Recognizing manifestations of the need for rest and the need for activity
5. Intervening to prevent patients from becoming overfatigued.

As fatigue increases, clients' ability to make sound judgments decreases so the nurse often finds limit setting a major part of fatigue intervention.

CONCLUSION

In summary, fatigue can be conceptualized as a state of increased discomfort and decreased efficiency resulting from expenditure of energy reserve. Peoples' energy and their expenditure of it are not in balance as a result of stress that may be physiological, psychological, or pathophysiological in nature. The stress may precipitate either local-muscle fatigue, general-muscle fatigue, generalized state of fatigue, or a combination of the three. Fatigue may also be an acute or chronic experience characterized by ineffective task performance, self-assured inadequacy, aversion to activity, tiredness or a sense of weariness, feelings of body discomfort, and attempts to terminate the feelings of discomfort. Etiology of fatigue appears to be the body's inability to maintain a state of equilibrium when faced with a stressor that taxes its homeostatic mechanisms (Bartley 1965, 1967, 1976; and Grandjean 1968, 1969, 1970).

While the occurrence of fatigue is expected to accompany and, at times, be a precursor to most pathological conditions, few attempts have been made to describe the phenomenon, its expected duration, or its course as it relates to pathological change. Since fatigue is one common harbinger of the presence of illness and disease progression, its identification is important in clinical monitoring of patients. In addition, the sensitivity of fatigue states to changes in illness as well as to the impact of other stresses on the patient make fatigue a prime indicator to use in the evaluation of the effect of interventions. The challenge of delineating the characteristics of this phenomenon as it relates to pathological changes persists.

REFERENCES

Asmussen, E., Klausen, K., and Puolsen, E. *The Determination of the Energy Requirements of Practical Work from Pulse Rate and Ergometer Test*. Copenhagen: Communications, Testing and Observation Institute, Danish National Association for Infantile Paralysis, 1960.

Astrand, I. Aerobic work capacity in men and women with special reference to age. *Acta Physiol. Scand*, 49 (Suppl. 169): 79–86, 1960.

Bartley, S.H. *Fatigue: Mechanism and Management*. Springfield, Ill.: Thomas, 1965.

Bartley, S.H. *The Human Organism as a Person*. Philadelphia: Chilton, 1967.

Bartley, S.H. What Do We Call Fatigue? In E. Simonson and P. Weiser (Eds.), *Psychological Aspects and Physiological Correlates of Work and Fatigue*. Springfield, Ill.: Thomas, 1976.

Bergstrom, J., and Hultman, E. The effect of exercise on muscle glycogen and electrolytes in normals. *Scand. J. Clin. Lab. Invest*. 18:16–20, 1966.

Bergstrom, J., and Hultman, E. A study of the glycogen metabolism during exercise in man. *Scand. J. Clin. Lab. Invest*. 18:16–20, 1967.

Borg, G.A.V. *Physical Performance and Perceived Exertion*. Copenhagen: Ejnor Munksgäard, 1962.

Brouha, L. *Physiology in Industry*. New York: Pergamon Press, 1960.

Brouha, L., Maxfield, M.E., Smith, P.E., and Stopps, G.J. Discrepancy between heart rate and oxygen consumption during work in the warmth. *J. Appl. Physiol*. 18:1095–1098, 1963.

Burkhardt, E.A. Fatigue—diagnosis and treatment. *N.Y. State J. Med*. 56:62–67, 1956.

Christensen, E.H. Muscular Work and Fatigue. In K. Rodahl and S.M. Horvath (Eds.), *Muscle as a Tissue*. New York: McGraw-Hill, 1962.

Darling, R. Fatigue. In J.A. Downey and R. Darling (Eds.), *Physiological Basis of Rehabilitation Medicine*. Philadelphia: Saunders, 1971.

Dill, D.B. The Harvard fatigue laboratory: Its development, contributions, and demise. *Circ. Res*. 20 (Suppl. 1): 161–170, 1967.

Ettema, J.H., and Zielhuis, R.L. Physiological parameters of mental load. *Ergonomics* 14:137–144, 1971.

Fox, E.L., Robinson, S., and Wiegman, D.L. Metabolic energy sources during continuous and interval running. *J. Appl. Physiol*. 27:174–178, 1969.

Grandjean, E.P. Fatigue: Its physiological and psychological significance. *Ergonomics* 11:427–436, 1968.

Grandjean, E. *Fitting the Task to the Man—An Ergonomic Approach*. London: Taylor and Francis, 1969.

Grandjean, E.P. Fatigue. *Am. Ind. Hyg. Assoc. J*. 31:401–411, 1970.

Hermannsen, L., Hultman, E., and Saltin, B. Muscle glycogen during prolonged severe exercise. *Acta Physiol. Scand*. 71:129–139, 1967.

Kashiwagi, S. Psychological ratings of human fatigue. *Ergonomics* 14:17–21, 1971.

Kumudavalli, I., and Swami, K.S. Effects of a temperature on the physiology of muscular fatigue. *Indian J. Exp. Biol*. 5:162–164, 1967.

Luongo, E.P. Work and physiology in health and disease. *J. A. M. A.* 188:27–32, 1964.

MacBryde, C.M. *Signs and Symptoms*. Philadelphia: Lippincott, 1970.

McFarland, R.A. *Human Factors in Air Transportation*. New York: McGraw-Hill, 1953.

Miller, W.H. Fatigue—Some special effects and tests. *J. Aviation Med.* 7:161–165, 1936.

Muller, E.A. The physiological basis of rest pauses in heavy work. *Q. J. Exp. Physiol.* 38:205–215, 1953.

Muller, E.A. Occupational work capacity. *Ergonomics* 5:445–452, 1962.

Nachmanson, D. *Structure and Function of Muscle*, II. New York: Academic, 1960.

Pearson, P.G., and Byars, G.E. *The Development and Validation of a Checklist for Measuring Subjective Fatigue*. (Report No. 56-115). Randolph A.F.B., Tx.: School of Aviation Medicine, U.S.A.F., Dec. 1956.

Pringle, J.W. *Models and Analogues in Biology*. Cambridge: University Press, 1960.

Scholz, H. Changing physical demand of foundry worker in the production of medium weight castings. *Ergonomics* 1:30–38, 1957.

Schreuder, O.B. Medical aspects of aircraft pilot fatigue with special reference to the commercial jet pilot. *Aerospace Med.* 37 (Sect. 2): 1–44, 1966.

Snook, S.H., and Irvine, C.H. Psychophysical studies of physiological fatigue criteria. *Hum. Factors* 2:291–299, 1969.

Suggs, C.W., and Splinter, W.E. Effect of environment on the allowable workload of man. *Trans. Am. Soc. Agricultural Engineers* 4:48–54, 1961.

Suggs, C.W., and Splinter, W.E. Some physiological responses of man to workload and environment. *J. Appl. Physiol.* 16:413–420, 1961.

Wells, J.A., Balke, B., and Van Fonssan, D.D. Lactic acid accumulations during work. *J. Appl. Physiol.* 10:51–55, 1957.

Yoshitake, H. Relations between the symptoms and the feeling of fatigue. *Ergonomics* 14:175–186, 1971.

Chapter 15

Tiredness and Fatigue

Mary L. Morris

INTRODUCTION

There are subtle nuances between a healthy tiredness and a gradual slowing down due to aging and between the insidious warning of a premyocardial infarction with concomitant increase in need for sleep and the monotonous tedium of repetitive assembly line jobs that make sleep an escape. Expenditure of energy in anxiety states and expenditure in survival of a serious physical illness produce end results that appear very similar. The resultant state from these events and from other stressful life experiences is labeled *fatigue*.

The problem for nurses lies in assessing, sorting, and classifying clues and discerning those that are attributable to normal stresses from those that are prodromal or early manifestations of serious physical or emotional problems. The fatigued state, whatever its underlying mechanism, culminates in energy or alertness depletion and inability to continue the normal level of activity. A wide variety of events leads to the development of fatigue, and nurses confronted with lethargic individuals have to identify realistic criteria for recovery. This includes identifying positive physical, social, and cultural resources available to construct support systems. People are helped to define and redefine goals that can be attained as they move toward a higher level of physical or emotional well-being. Recovery states will vary with individuals; there is no easy formula for relieving fatigue.

This chapter explores normal, acceptable tiredness as well as states of fatigue, proposes some concepts related to these states, and develops a framework within which to approach nursing intervention.

HEALTH AND FATIGUE

A systemic study of fatigue is almost as difficult as the assessment of its causes. The usual health continuum identifies some generally accepted characteristics of health or describes what healthy people can do. Using these as criteria provides one means of considering deviations from "normal." In a healthy state, individuals are able to do their chosen work without excessive stress or strain, to exert themselves physically without exhaustion, and to feel refreshed after rest and relaxation. Healthy individuals also identify and attain a satisfying number of realistic goals and enjoy the company of other people as well as periods of solitude (Montag and Swenson 1959). While not inclusive, these criteria cover important areas of daily activity that result in a feeling of well-being—one goal of health.

The activity of the human organism is rhythmical and geared toward the maintenance of a dynamic, healthy equilibrium. Well-documented processes such as circadian rhythms, cardiac work–rest cycles, humoral and neural balances, and compensatory mechanisms all contribute to maintaining this dynamic equilibrium. The body is not only rhythmical in function but is always, in health, maintained in a state of watchfulness. A state of slight muscle contraction, the ease with which flight–fight forces are initiated, and the so-called conservation–withdrawal process, which warns of impending energy depletion are normal reactions that enable the organism to maintain a balanced state in spite of constant bombardment from internal and external stimuli. It is this ability to adapt that enables individuals to continue to function when situations fluctuate (MacBryde and Blacklow 1970).

Bafitis and Sargent (1977) defined *human adaption capacity* as the individual's ability to cope successfully with the stresses of life—a capacity that encompasses the morphological, biological, chemical, physiological, and psychological processes that, singly or in combination, bring about coping responses. They further noted that the height of adaptive capacity is that period of minimum mortality occurring during a period of maximum adaptive capacity and at the same time the organs and systems needed to deal with the stress are at their peak level of development. Peak years were identified in relation to seasonal mortality rates of different age groups and the years of maximum ability to engage in physical work. Variability of function was noted, especially in declining endurance beginning soon after reaching peak attainment. Bafitis and Sargent (1977) suggested that health was better defined in functional terms using adaptive capacity as one criterion.

HEALTH CONTINUUM

On any given day, in any situation there will be people at high levels of health mingling with the near ill and the overtly ill. On hospital units, there will be seriously depleted people struggling to survive, people who have successfully fought off critical conditions and exhibit evidence of "battle fatigue," those on the road to recovery, and those simply "tired" from yet unidentified causes. Personnel exhibit varying degrees of wellness as do families of patients and visitors coming to hospitals. All individuals exhibit clues to their state of well-being.

Nixon and Bethell (1974) propose a conceptual framework of human behavior arranged in the natural order of passage from health to breakdown. This concept was engendered by Starling's Law of the Heart, which states that the energy of the heart, other things being equal, depends on the stretch of muscle fibers. When stretch increases, heart performance increases. However, if the fibers become overstretched, deterioration and breakdown occur. The peak of the curve or performance produced by a given stretch varies and is affected by age, degree of freshness of the person, and neurohumoral influences brought to bear (Nixon 1976). The Nixon curve of human function is described as comparable to Starling's Law based on performance plotted against arousal. In health, increasing arousal results in increasing performance. In fatigue, performance falls off and in exhaustion, if arousal persists, deterioration, breakdown, and ill health result (Nixon 1976).

In health, people feel well, are relaxed in manner, engage in recreation, and reject pressures that could cause ill health. Others see them as healthy, adaptive, approachable, capable of rapid flexible thought, and vigorous enough for sustained activity. Arousal brings peak performance and both are realistic in degree. The term *acceptable fatigue* includes recognition of tiredness and steps taken to overcome it as soon as possible. Performance is increased with arousal but requires a greater expenditure of energy. Sleep, self-discipline, and mild stimulants such as the caffeine in coffee, competition, and similar energizing forces enable the person to sustain performance. These people are perceived as healthily tired; their tiredness does not make them anxious (Nixon 1976).

ILLNESS CONTINUUM

Fatigue leading to exhaustion and breakdown occurs when people reject maintaining a reasonable balance between high endeavor and rest. Faced with periods of unusually heavy work, these susceptible individuals make no effort to prepare to sustain themselves during times of stress; they become increasingly unable to distinguish essentials from trivia. Increased arousal results in a greater gap between actual and intended performance since people's capacity to perform worsens. Personal relationships deteriorate as fatigued people become irritable, unable to produce, and resentful. Many fatigued persons function at this level for long periods of time. Unless relief is found, however, a breakdown due to complete exhaustion triggered by an aggregate of completely overwhelming adverse circumstances will eventually occur (Nixon 1976).

FATIGUE CONCEPTUALLY DEFINED

Fatigue is sometimes used synonymously with feelings of anxiety, uncertainty, depletion, nervousness, and tension. While these factors may be components, fatigue describes "a feeling of inability to mobilize the energy to carry on . . . is associated with (feelings of) depression, helplessness, hopelessness and apathy" (MacBryde and Blacklow 1970, p. 632). These feelings may stem from physical incapacities, environmental deprivation, or psychological failure. Other terms associated with fatigue and connoting a sense of exhaustion include *lassitude, weariness,* and *weakness.* There is also inability to continue in whatever situations people find themselves.

PROBLEMS OF FATIGUE

Specific Vulnerable Groups

The health of its people is considered to be the most valuable economic resource of a nation. What are the effects of fatigue on health and economy? How common is the state of fatigue, or inability to continue? Is a particular population vulnerable to fatigue? Who is most vulnerable to fatigue? Hargreaves (1977) described a "fatigue syndrome" associated with moving to a new town. Young married women were affected predominantly and evidenced tiredness, irritability, tearful episodes, muscular aches, loss of ability to concentrate, and other similar problems. None had a history of mental illness nor reported loss of appetite or sleep disturbances. Hargreaves (1977) reasoned that increased physical work, loss of known community with its patterns of behaving, and emotional upheaval of moving had depleted the energy resources of these women. A regimen of extra rest (12 hours daily) with very small doses of antidepressants and tranquilizers for a 3-week period resulted in complete recovery. The key to recovery was rest, but attaining it required assistance from spouses and others sharing the physical work load. The greatest barrier was the acceptance of this regimen by the women since their self-images were affected by being unable to cope with what is considered a normal task—moving. Women who did not acknowledge fatigue as a problem and accept the prescribed therapy experienced a worsening of the situation and symptoms, and, in some instances, became depressed (Hargreaves 1977).

Fatigue as an early and insidious symptom of impending MI has been demonstrated retrospectively. Electrocardiology and angina pectoris as indicators of an impending MI have not always been reliable predictors. Unusual fatigue was reported in 77 percent of a study population following an acute MI. The time from onset of fatigue to development of the infarction varied from 6 weeks to a year or more. Seventy-two percent of this group reported excessive sleepiness during the same period. In similar studies, people were slower to recognize the presence of fatigue in themselves than were their families. A slowing down in gardening activities, sleeping during television programs, and similar instances were recalled although there was some denial that this was meaningful by almost all the victims interviewed (Nixon and Bethell 1974).

The magnitude of fatigue can be documented by problems related to trying to determine its underlying causes. Monotonous work, repetitive noises, and bombardment by external stimuli contribute to fatigue. A small group of persons who for years complained of muscular pain and fatigue, attended medical clinics, and had neurological and psychiatric work-ups with no evidence of myopathy were studied by means of an exercise routine. They were found to have significantly higher concentrations of blood lactates and pyruvates compared to normal volunteers. Since the levels of glucose and plasma free fatty acids were similar in both groups, Rennie and co-workers (1973) concluded that the fatigued subjects suffered from a decreased amount of available muscle glycogen. While there seemed to be no organic base for their disability and only some evidence of "neurotic symptoms," researchers concluded that people presenting with muscle fatigue should be assessed for metabolic disturbances (Rennie et al. 1973).

The above illustrations involve different populations, scope of involvement, and expected outcomes. However, certain describable threads appear in common (Bafitis and Sargent 1977). The people involved were unable to continue at their usual level of activity (Carver, Coleman, and Glass 1976). Exhaustion appeared to be the result of exertion beyond the individual's capacity to recover within a normal length of time, the subjects had experienced stressful situations, and all had had to acknowledge the need for help either on their own initiative or by becoming overtly ill. In two groups, it was demonstrated that without help the conditions worsened. The following generalizations about fatigue emerge:

1. Fatigue can be emotionally engendered and result in psychological and physiological manifestations.
2. Fatigue can be physiologically engendered with both psychological and physiological symptoms.
3. Fatigue can be a warning signal of approaching health disaster.
4. Fatigue can be relieved by prescribed rest. (The prescription for rest is not limited to physical inactivity; hence there is need for diagnosis of cause.)

HEALTH SERVICE PROVIDERS' OUTLOOK ON FATIGUE

Fatigue is probably the most prevalent symptom of illness, both mental and physical. The anticipation of fatigue tends to reduce its importance to care providers and often to the patient, who hesitates to report anything so common.

Inherent in the problem is the failure of health care providers to determine if action can be taken to prevent or alleviate fatigue or if there is a cluster of recognizable clues that could be used to predict who is most likely to experience fatigue. The challenge of coping with fatigue is further compounded by the orientation of health care personnel, which can be either strongly psychological or strongly physiological. The medical service to which the person is assigned affects the importance attached to lassitude; its importance on a psychiatric unit mig. All of these obstacles to managing fatigue are usually more unconscious than conscious but have to be recognized as barriers in order to deal with them. To assess the presence and level of fatigue in a subject requires that the health provider—in this case, the nurse—knows what to look for objectively, what to ask about, and understands the physical diseases preceded or accompanied by fatigue and the psychological components of the state. In addition, a data base is needed. Nurses need to examine the "who's"—who epidemiologically, realistically, and conceptually is most likely to become fatigued. Then nurses, with an adequate data base, can devise, implement, and test nursing measures to prevent, predict, and/or relieve the problem.

Clinical Description

Fatigued, people look tired, wan, and lethargic. They describe feelings of "having no pep," "all in," and "tired and worn out." There is a strong desire for sleep and rest and an all-pervasive feeling of being no longer able to mobilize the energy to continue the usual activities of daily life. Fatigue is experienced as lassitude, muscular pain, mental depletion, or in varying combinations and degrees of these. The difference between what is termed normal tiredness and what is abnormal can be elicited when usual modes of recovery are no longer effective; for example, a night's sleep does not restore vigor or, at least, requires extended sleep time to do so. Physiological fatigue may yield to sleep with people awakening refreshed only to find that energy is short-lived and their endurance fades early in the day. Fatigue produced by primarily psychological factors (e.g., as in depression) is unrelieved by sleep. People awaken tired but may feel better as the day progresses with something near an acceptable energy level achieved late in the day. Few specific signs, for example, circulatory or respiratory changes, can be detected until the individual is near exhaustion. Objectively, these people exhibit sagging face and body, lack of interest in surroundings, and dull voice tones (Harrison 1977).

There are, however, some identifiable effects on normal persons experiencing fatigue. These are in the form of (1) biochemical and physiological changes in body organs, (2) overt disorder in behavior (e.g., a reduced output of work known as "work decrement"), and (3) expressed dissatisfaction and a subjective feeling of tiredness (MacBryde and Blacklow 1970). Biochemically, continuous muscular work results in a depletion of muscle glycogen and a buildup of lactic acid and other metabolites that tend to diminish the strength of muscle contraction. With extremes of work, muscle fiber necrosis occurs with an increase in the levels of serum enzymes such as creatinine phosphokinase. Muscles may be sore and swollen. If contractions are continued, the result is tremulous inept movements. These extremes in work are accompanied by increases in blood pressure, respiration, and other metabolic changes geared to try to meet arousal stimuli and maintain muscle efficiency (Harrison 1977).

Behavioral changes resulting in work decrement encompass many factors that are not clearly understood. Industrial researchers have demonstrated that fatigue decreases productivity. Motivation, individual differences in body build, personality traits, and energy potential have strong influences on the work output of manual and clerical workers. Physiologically, if a worker is exposed to the same inundation of stimuli as the brain—monotonous noise, meaningless routine, or demands for increased production—the same damping of the transmission of signals through synapses aimed at reducing stimuli to a bearable level might play a part. In decremental conduction, through the synapses, signals become progressively weaker during long periods of excitation so that reverberatory feedback is blocked. After an adequate period of rest, conduction resumes and stimuli are no longer blocked (Guyton 1976). Since exhaustion of energy at the cellular level will be the absolute determinant that further performance is impossible, it appears reasonable to expect that some neural feedback and regulating mechanisms can be available to the total organism. The physiological state that attempts to guard against absolute fatigue includes a general decrease in motor activities, metabolic adaptation, and cardiovascular output and inhibition of all sympathetic and some parasympathetic activities (MacBryde and Blacklow 1970). The body seems to withdraw and tries to utilize its fuels carefully. Thus behavioral observation of decreased productivity can be associated with fatigue—whatever the cause—and seen as symptomatic of bodily changes. Analyses of ways to build up endurance through muscle training and reward system have produced limited data to attest to presence of metabolic and neural process activities that guard against overstressing (DeLateur, Lehman, and Gasconi 1976). If overstressing is monotonous (e.g., noise or boredom), it supports the contention that a decrease in synaptic conduction might result in work decrease.

Subjective feelings of fatigue in the normal person were discussed earlier but are restated here to round out the description. The weariness and the individual's inability to deal with complex problems, arrive at decisions, and make mental associations all produce a state of unhappiness that is especially noticeable in the formerly alert and astute individual. The phrase, "too tired to think," sums up these feelings.

The foregoing seems somewhat belabored but the juncture where normal becomes abnormal fatigue is difficult to pinpoint. The paired control systems of flight–fight and conservation–withdrawal as described by MacBryde and Black-low (1970) pictures continued vigilance on the one hand and some mechanism that replenishes and resembles sleep–wakefulness cycle on the other. In addition, when flight–fight becomes ineffective, conservation–withdrawal takes over. Exhaustion is not a normal conservation–withdrawal, but is an end result of over-stressing the conservation–withdrawal system also (MacBryde and Blacklow 1970).

THE WHO'S OF FATIGUE

As we move along the health and illness continua it is evident that many conditions are common in both, with degree being the dividing point. The nurse is confronted with the task of pulling together signs, symptoms, objective evidence, and epidemiological data to identify those persons most likely to suffer from fatigue: those for whom it is an integral part of the disease process, those for whom it is a warning sign, and those for whom prevention is important. From the material presented so far, some further generalizations as follows can be made regarding the state of fatigue:

1. Fatigue appears to be a protective mechanism.
2. Fatigue exists at normal and abnormal levels.
3. Fatigue can be used positively in helping individuals define or redefine goals.
4. Fatigue can be assessed by nurses in terms of probable causes.
5. Fatigue is the end result of excessive energy consumption.
6. Fatigue, other things being equal, yields to prescribed rest based on identification of the source of excessive energy consumption.
7. Action to relieve, prevent, or predict fatigue is a nursing function that can be assumed independently and collaboratively with other health providers.

Whom Do Nurses Observe for Signs of Fatigue?

Who is epidemiologically vulnerable to fatigue? This group includes the entire age spectrum. Human adaptability capacity shows that mortality in children rises during the winter, especially in ages 0–4 years; children and infants show a marked intolerance to cold. Older people show the same intolerance to heat; for example, 70 percent of all heat-stroke victims are over 60 years of age (Bafitis and Sargent 1977). The very young and the very old demonstrate the need for energy conservation normally in the extension of their sleep requirements. While patterns vary in the two extremes, the increased need for rest is observable.

In the elderly, the decline in physical activity requires maximal oxygen intake even though mechanical efficiency is not reduced. Aging decrements can be delayed through a physical fitness program (Bafitis and Sargent 1977). Another group who are epidemiological targets are the very ill. The consumption of energy and humoral agents used in the body's response to insult may leave the person exhausted and unable to fight further or in a depleted state that prolongs convalescence. Persons transferred from the overstressed environment of the ICU to a less acute unit find themselves labile physically and emotionally. Observers saw many patients who found it difficult to reconcile the physicians' and nurses' cheery assurances that they are "just fine" with the overpowering lassitude they felt. During this postcritical period the health team, relieved to have brought another patient through a life-threatening situation, moves on to another dramatic fight and the patient is left to shift for him- or herself to a greater degree than is manageable. The patient may be more vulnerable to additional injury at this period than at any other time in the illness since he or she does not understand what is happening and what to expect next. Transition from critical care to general care areas demands a level of expertise in nursing far greater than understanding monitors and other technological aids. We need to determine these areas of expertise and test them in the clinical area.

Who is realistically vulnerable to fatigue? This may be an unlikely term, and the separation of patients epidemiologically and realistically is an arbitrary one. Aside from the previously discussed prodromal signs, such as in heart disease, there are many physical illnesses that are accompanied or signalled by fatigue. These include mitral stenosis, endocrine disorders, nutritional deficiencies, severe anemia, neoplasia, neuromuscular defects, and liver disease. Liver disease produces a type of lassitude that is distinctive; it results in a complete demobilization of resources to engage in physical activity. Affected patients lie in one position for extended periods before getting up enough energy to reposition themselves. On the other hand, the fatigue of heart disease may be related to exertion or position. Another group of patients suffer fatigue due to physical overload; this group includes the very obese, whose excess pounds tire them. This author heard a physician suggest to a group of obese patients that they tie several 5-pounds bags of sugar to their clothing and then engage in their usual activity in order to determine energy needs for carrying excess weight. This physical-overload group can include victims of arthritis, amputation, stroke, and other crippling conditions in which the weight of a body part is unable to carry its own load or where use of an appliance to become mobile makes excessive energy demands. There is no intent to underestimate the toll that the briefly mentioned illnesses can extract whenever energy demands increase. The problem for nurses is to look specifically at the presenting condition. When treating an exhausted patient, the nurse considers whether the cardiac output is reduced so that needs for oxygenated blood cannot be met except with greatly diminished activity or whether the lethargic patient, recovering from a severe bout of pneumonia, is resting to marshal energy for the work of convalescence.

One person who realistically may come to the fatigued state is the hardworking, aggressive achiever—the Type A personality. Not only is such a person coronary-prone, he or she suppresses symptoms of fatigue and persists in working near capacity, denying tiredness (Carver, Coleman, and Glass 1976). Infections, serious and extensive surgery, and similar conditions can demonstrate a depleted person ready for complications.

Realistically, the depressed person is a fatigued individual; energy is expended in mental anguish. Depletion of resources of home, family, job, health, or whatever helped sustain in the past leaves the person in a state from apathy and a sense of heaviness to developing one of the major affective disorders. Feelings of worthlessness and complete debility can accompany physical illness. Physical illness brings emotional problems into focus (MacBryde and Blacklow 1970). Affected persons require expertise in assessment as great or greater than for the conditions discussed previously. Identification of the variables critical to diagnosing fatigue in depression is needed as well as projection and testing of nursing interventions.

Conceptually, who is vulnerable to fatigue? Fatigue is a counter-balance to flight–fight or passivity replacing aggressiveness. One conceptually vulnerable group has had more life changes than most organisms can tolerate well. Study and documentation of the effects certain strong emotional and physical events, both positive and negative, have on individuals is well known. The occurrence of single or multiple illnesses following aggregates of loss of family, job, or money or after winning honors, promotions, and so forth has been documented. The endurance of any particular organism is limited and a recovery period after illness is mandatory. Otherwise, the person becomes host to invading viruses or other microorganisms.

Anxiety is both forerunner of and concomitant with fatigue. Anxiety prepares us for danger, when the anxious state is relieved or the source of anxiety resolved, a conservation–withdrawal process results. When anxiety is not resolved, the ability to continue unrelieved can be tolerated for only a limited period. Then the organism demobilizes and the usual conservation–withdrawal mechanism of restoration fails to resolve the problems of restoration, and exhaustion occurs. Anxiety yields to what may be depression.

In both of these groups—persons who have undergone change or loss and persons who have suffered prolonged anxiety—we find not only vulnerable patients but vulnerable families. It has been a recurrent experience of nurses to watch a family member sustain the patient through severe trauma or lengthy illness and then succumb to a personal illness. Support persons could possibly be protected from fatigue by a system of predictors and preventive activity.

NURSING CONCEPTS AND THE FATIGUED PATIENT

This chapter is focused largely on physiologically engendered acute illnesses and on care given in large secondary-care institutions. Given the wan, listless patient lying passively in a hospital bed, what then? Conceptually, if the fatigued state is the result of a depletion of cellular fuel that has occurred because the patient has answered threatening stimuli to his or her full capacity and beyond and if restorative powers are exhausted, then rest should be restorative. Unfortunately, it is not that simple. It is therefore proposed here that positive energy conservation plus positive energy use can add up to energy restoration or a formula of $EC^+ + EU^+ = ER^+$ and that there are three nursing concepts to cope with fatigue: energy conservation, energy utilization, and energy restoration.

Energy conservation (positive) is determination of the state of depletion and the probable factors producing it. In energy conservation all activities of the patient that demand fuel will be weighed against the negative problems of promoting an inappropriately dependent patient. Some aspects of daily self-care are needlessly tiring; for example, a self-administered bath using a basin is less efficient than a quick shower. A shower requires less effort, refreshes and does not threaten the individual's lack of participation in personal care. Diagnostic procedures are often very demanding on the patient's fuel reserves. Preparation for gastrointestinal procedures in themselves are strenuous. The patient who has had no rest because of laxatives and enemas may arrive for radiology examination sleepless and weak. Anxiety accompanying the unknown, related to both diagnostic procedures and the outcomes, takes a toll. Elevated temperatures, decreased cardiac output, and severe anemia exert demands for common daily activities that appear insurmountable to the patient. Rest does not comprise merely lying in bed; it includes an environment in which the person can relax, mentally and physically, and can profit from the opportunity to replenish his or her energy supply. Nurses may have to learn more about dependence in order to establish a healthy dependent relationship in which nurse and patient can collaboratively move toward independence.

Energy use (positive) is somewhat an extension of or the natural outcome of energy conservation. While conserving resources, it is equally important to determine what strengths the patient brings to the situation and to build on these. Muscle retraining and strengthening can be done through short walks with goals extended as the patient's endurance increases. Teaching individuals to note the first symptoms of overtaxation must be accompanied by giving positive feedback for symptom recognition. Retraining in breathing for an emphysema patient will help promote maximum exhalation; determination of those activities that will probably never be tolerated again and substitution of other more suitable endeavors are moves toward positive energy utilization.

I recall a young nurse who had been diagnosed as having early rheumatoid arthritis; a day's work on a hospital unit resulted in limping and pain. A regimen worked out for her that included swimming daily, resting one hour every day, and avoiding some activities such as vacuuming the house, has resulted in minimal pain and little evidence of joint changes. As a graduate student, she accepted the fact that toward the end of the semester she became more tired even though she tried to pace her work. Therefore, she finished assignments as quickly as possible to avoid the "logjam" most students experience near the end of the term. What energy she had was used toward positive gains; this even included occasional ski trips.

Energy restoration (positive) refers to the point when the goal of restoration is reached and the fuel to do work is replenished. For this to be a positive attainment requires that certain changes occur along the way that will enable the individual to maintain the new level of wellness. The nurse, as the promoter of an environment in which recovery can occur, is the prime person to assist the patient in planning for continued health. This involves the assistance and understanding of friends and family as well as the patient. First, there must be recognition that a problem existed and determination of how it came about. Unless this occurs, a repetition of the fatigued state is almost assured. Second, a realistic setting of goals and the defining of how these may be attained must be made. The young married women moving into new situations and the tired professional ready for a strenuous vacation, for example, will need to accept the fact that periods of excessive activity must be prepared for by accruing energy supplies prior to the strenuous event. Third, the acceptance of fatigue is a normal component of living within acceptable limits and to overextend is less healthy than to acknowledge limitations. Fourth, follow-up through feedback from the nurse can promote the positive reinforcement that will enable the person to remain in a healthy state.

CONCLUSION

The origin of fatigue is seldom purely psychological or physiological. I have made no attempt to differentiate between the sources or the symptoms produced. Fatigue has been discussed in its varied manifestations—from normal, acceptable fatigue to the state of exhaustion. Some generalizations have been made related to this state and three concepts of nursing intervention, which might enable the person to recover, have been proposed. Nurses must diligently pursue clues that can predict fatigue so that it may be managed effectively.

REFERENCES

Bafitis, H., and Sargent, F. Human physiological adaptability through the life sequence. *Gerontol.* 32(4):402–410, Jul. 1977.

Carver, C.S., Coleman, A., and Glass, C. The coronary prone behavior pattern and the suppression of fatigue on a treadmill test. *J. Pers. Soc. Psychol.* 33(4):460–466, Apr. 1976.

DeLateur, J., Lehman, F., and Gasconi, R. Mechanical work and fatigue: Their roles in the development of muscle work capacity. *Arch. Phys. Med. Rehabil.* 57:319–324, Jul. 1976.

Guyton, C. *Textbook of Medical Physiology* (5th ed.). Philadelphia: Saunders, 1976.

Hargreaves, M. The fatigue syndrome. *Practitioner* 218:841–843, June 1977.

Harrison's *Principles of Internal Medicine* (8th ed.). New York: McGraw-Hill, 1977.

Harvey, A., McGehee, Johns, J., Owens, H., and Ross, S. *The Principles and Practice of Medicine* (19th ed.). New York: Appleton-Century-Crofts, 1976.

Klumpp, G. Some thoughts on fatigue in older patient. *Med. Times* 104(10):87–93, Oct. 1976.

Krupp, A., and Chatton, J. *Current Medical Diagnosis and Treatment 1976.* Los Altos, Calif.: Large Medical, 1976.

Levi, L. *Stress: Sources, Management and Prevention.* New York: Liveright, 1967.

Looney, M., and Metcalf, S. The fatigue factors in drug addiction: Insufficient motivation for treatment. *Hosp. Community Psychiatry* 24(8):528–530, Aug. 1974.

MacBryde, C., and Blacklow, R.S. *Signs and Symptoms* (5th ed.). Philadelphia: Lippincott, 1970. P. 632.

Marsden, C.D., Meadows, J.C., and Merton, P.A. Fatigue in human muscles in relation to the number and frequency of motor impulses. *J. Physiol.* 258:94–95, June 1976.

Mills, I. The disease of failure of coping. *Practitioner* 217:529–538, Oct. 1976.

Montag, M., and Swenson, P. *Fundamentals of Nursing Care* (5th ed.). Philadelphia: Saunders, 1959.

Newbold, G.F. Prolintane in debility and fatigue. *Practitioner* 213:868–870, Dec. 1974.

Nixon, G.F., and Bethell, H.J.N. Preinfarction ill health. *Am. J. Cardiol.* 33:446–449, Jul. 1974.

Nixon, P.G.E. The human function curve. *Practitioner* 217:765–770, Nov. 1976.

Rennie, M.J., Johnson, R.H., Park, D.M., and Sularman, W.R. Inappropriate fatigue during exercise associated with high blood lactates. *Clin. Sci.* 45(1):5, Jul. 1973.

Selye, H. *The Stress of Life.* New York: McGraw-Hill, 1956.

Selye, H. *Stress without Distress.* Philadelphia: Lippincott, 1974.

Shands, H.C., and Finesinger, J.C. A note on the significance of fatigue. *Psychosom. Med.* 14:309, 1952.

Theorell, T., Lind, E., Froberg, J., Karlson, C.G., and Levi, L. Life changes, catecholamine excretion and related biochemical changes. *Psychosom. Med.* 34(6):505–516, Nov.–Dec. 1977.

Weinberg, E.G., and Tuchanda, M. Allergies tension—fatigue syndrome. *Ann. Allergy* 314(4):209–211, Apr. 1973.

Chapter 16

Fatigue and the Postsurgical Patient

Debra Rhoten

INTRODUCTION

American society values energy and productivity, praises high levels of energy, and perceives energetic people as "go getters." Even if energetic people do not get things done, they personify the Protestant ethic of the virtue in work. People without energy are described disapprovingly as slow, sluggish, or lazy. Television commercials reinforce this value promising that, "Coke adds life," or that "Geritol will energize tired blood." If energy and vitality are positive values, fatigued people whose feelings and sensations are diametrically opposed to the pole of energy are to some extent devalued.

Connotatively, fatigue is a negative and undesirable condition that interferes with optimal functioning. Denotatively, fatigue is a positive condition that serves an important function in the homeostatic processes of the body. Exercise physiology, for example, teaches that the immediate outcome of exercise in healthy people is a temporary general fatigue but that the long-term effect is lessened fatigue experienced later in the day. In studying nutrition, we learn that fatigue warns of the possibility that one has poor eating habits or eats poor-quality food.

Fatigue has a special relevance for nurses because of its frequency in both patients and clients. (Patients are people who are ill. Clients are people participating in health care programs.) Some students of fatigue believe it to be the most prevalent symptom of illness, physical or mental, and often the first indication of the occurrence of some abnormal process (MacBryde et al. 1970). Several others writing about fatigue attest that fatigue is an almost-universal complaint that occurs in association with almost any illness (Burkhardt 1956; Hargreaves 1977; Keliher 1959; Kuguelmas et al. 1965; and Spaulding 1964). Despite the universality of fatigue in illness, its nonspecificity gives it negligible importance in making a diagnosis. Lack of clarification of the concept of fatigue may have contributed to its elusiveness as a human phenomenon and to nurses' inability to operationalize it with any precision in the clinical setting.

Fatigue has been conceptualized in the past in simple energistic terms or as a loss of energy or a decrement in physical performance. Much of the research in fatigue has been conducted in industry and physical education. Nursing cannot use to any great extent concepts clarified for other purposes. For example, the goal of nursing is not to increase the patient's ability to work or to be productive of goods, nor is it to help the patient run or play faster and better. The role fatigue plays in health maintenance, illness, healing, and convalescence is ambiguous. As long as this ambiguity exists, nursing intervention and nursing research related to fatigue have little logic.

DEFINING FATIGUE

Just as the different conceptual frames of reference used in research on fatigue have compounded the vagueness of the concept, the countless definitions have accomplished the same effect. McFarland (1971) identified the problem by pointing out that there were as many different definitions of fatigue as there were studies of it. For example, Bartlett (1953) defined fatigue as "all those changes in expression of an activity which can be traced to the continuing exercise of that activity that leads to deterioration in expression of that activity or to results within that activity that are not wanted." Physiologists and industrial researchers defined fatigue as an impairment in work performance (Brown 1964; Davis 1943; DeLater, Lehman, and Gasconi 1976; Snook and Irvine 1969; and Yoshitake 1971). Others included subjective feelings of lassitude, producing the disinclination toward activity in their definition of fatigue (Cameron 1973). Bartley (1965, 1976) defined fatigue as a self-recognized state of an individual, a self-felt assessment of inadequacy and incapacitation, and an aversion to activity.

In an attempt to eliminate the confusion associated with the meaning of fatigue, Bartley (1965, 1976) offered other concepts to be used for areas that have been ascribed to fatigue. He used the term *impairment* to indicate a decline in the functional capacity of cells. *Disorganization* was used to refer to the decrease in the way that cells, tissues, or organs worked together or to a decrease of skill in performance. *Discomfort* was used to imply the unpleasant sensations in the muscles after prolonged work due to metabolic by-products such as lactic acid. Finally, Bartley (1965) used the term *work decrement* to indicate the decreased productivity or drop in muscular activity in energistic terms. At a more subjective level, he identified fatigue as "the individual's assessment of his condition with reference to his immediate task with his overall appraisal expressed in bodily feelings."

CLASSIFICATIONS OF FATIGUE

To compound and cloud the definition issue, fatigue has been classified and categorized according to its causative factors. Darling (1971) distinguished *effort fatigue* as that resultant from muscular work, *tropical fatigue* as due to heat intolerance, *altitude fatigue* as the result of decreased oxygen in high altitude, and *sensory fatigue* as the result of loud noises or poor lighting. Several authors categorized fatigue as mental, physical, physiological, nervous, pathological, or emotional (Coates 1964; Forbes 1943; Mason 1961; Putt 1975; and Rockwell and Burr 1974).

In addition to these specific classifications of fatigue, causation has also been depicted in broader categories such as natural or normal, acute, hyperacute, chronic, and morbid or persistent fatigue (Albeaux-Fernet, Bugard, and Roman 1958; Collier 1936; Grandjean 1970; Kuguelmas 1965; McFarland 1971; Rockwell and Burr 1974; and Schwab 1953). The numerous subdivisions of fatigue along with the lack of uniformity in terminology has added to the denotative confusion in use of the term.

ETIOLOGY OF FATIGUE

The causes of fatigue are as global as its definitions. In an attempt to be more specific, this chapter will emphasize the pathophysiological causes of fatigue as opposed to the commonly accepted causes. These fatigue-producing variables, which include pathophysiological causes, are

1. *Physical factors*. These included expenditure of energy due to intense or prolonged exercise or work, poor posture, infrequent position changes, and sedentary life-style.
2. *Mental factors*. These referred to prolonged mental work, monotony, or boredom.
3. *Emotional factors*. These included areas of anxiety, conflicts, frustrations, responsibilities, worries, depression, and personality type.
4. *Environmental factors*. These included illumination, altitude, noise, temperature, and climate.
5. *Physiological factors*. These referred to interference with normal body processes, which included areas of malnutrition, inadequate sleep and rest, and medications that drain energy supply.
6. *Pathological factors*. These factors included organic disease processes and pain.

PATHOPHYSIOLOGICAL FATIGUE

Cameron (1973) conceptualized fatigue as a general response to stress over a period of time, resulting in a subjective state of the individual with a measurable decrement in performance. The subjective state was seen as changes in feeling–

tone exhibited by lassitude, weariness, and a disinclination for exertion. These, he felt, represented biological warnings that the individual's resources were overtaxed.

According to Thetford and Schucman (1971), a stress situation was one in which the individual regarded his or her well-being as endangered. Stress is not inherent in a situation but is the individual reaction of an organism to the situation. Intensity of a stress situation is proportional to the threat seen in it. Donaldson (1975) stated that the duration of the stress response and not its intensity was responsible for the fatigue sensations. Coefer and Appley (1964) postulated that fatigue and the resultant metabolic disturbances were both causes of stress and by-products of it. According to Thetford and Schucman (1971), the individual stress tolerance was due to differences in individuals' physical and psychological constitution.

Seyle (1974, 1975, 1976a, 1976b) described the nonspecific reaction of the body to any demand, activity, or emotion that excited a stress response. He called this the "General Adaptation Syndrome." It is characterized first by a *stage of alarm* where there is activation of the hypothalamo-pituitary-adreno-cortical systems with subsequent discharge of the stress hormones, adrenocorticotropic hormone (ACTH), corticoids, and catecholamines. This is followed by a *homeostatic state* or stage of resistance to the stressor. If the stress state is prolonged, the *stage of exhaustion* sets in. Fatigue and the desire for inactivity manifest the attempt of homeostatic processes to replenish depleted reserves.

According to MacBryde and Blacklow (1970), human stress response involves the whole organism through the activation of two neurobiological emergency systems. These are the well-known *flight–fight system* and the less familiar *conservation–withdrawal system*. The flight–fight system prepares the individual for action to meet threats through activation of neuroendocrine and physiological mechanisms. The conservation–withdrawal system serves the function of protecting against exhaustion by giving signals of impending energy depletion. Responses to conserve energy are initiated by increasing the stimulus threshold causing a reduction of activity. With renewal of energy stores, this system becomes inactive.

These two systems are indirectly connected to the limbic system, the hypothalamus, and the reticular formation in the brain stem through the analyzer-integrator-effector circuits. These circuits process sensory information in the CNS. Past sensory input is categorized as to successes and failures. The behavioral response to internal and environmental changes is based on patterns that have been effective in the past. If an impulse is considered being inconsistent with the behavioral responses in memory, the flight–fight system is activated, followed by conservation–withdrawal activation (MacBryde and Blacklow 1970).

In the reticular formation of the midbrain is an activating system called the reticular activation system (RAS). Stimulation of this area will arouse an organism while destruction of this area results in a permanent comatose state. Neural pathways from the cerebral cortex lead impulses to the reticular formation and have a feedback effect that maintains the cortex in a state of arousal and alertness. Afferent pathways from the sensory organs have collateral fibers to the RAS so impulses from the environment can also maintain arousal (Grandjean 1970).

Hess (1957) described two areas in the diencephalon and mesencephalon that also act as emergency defense systems. The ergotropic system is sympathetically mediated and is known as the *dynamogenic zone*. With stress, the stimulation of this system causes dilation of the pupils, increased blood pressure and respirations, and increased motor excitability. Afferent fibers that originate in the exteroceptive sensory organs play an important role in activation of the ergotropic system so auditory, visual, and pain stimuli arouse the individual. Prolonged excitation of the proprioceptors results in inhibition of the ergotropic system. The endophylactic–trophotropic system is parasympathetically mediated, and stimulation of the supra- and preoptic areas of the anterior hypothalamus and inferior lateral thalamus causes decreased respiratory rate, decreased blood pressure, decreased salivation, and urination. This area is the antagonist of the dynamogenic zone and results in hypodynamia or adynamia of the skeletal musculature.

The reflexogenic zones of the mucous membranes in the walls of the visceral organs, heart, aorta, carotid sinus, lungs, bladder, and rectum, collectively known as the *intracentral reflexogenic zones,* play a part in adynamia when continued stress leads to inhibition of ergotropic activity. This protective mechanism against stress activates the endophylactic-trophotropic system and promotes restorative processes or vegetative proprioception (Hess 1957).

HIGH-RISK FATIGUE POPULATIONS

Metabolic State of the Surgical Client

The person who has had surgery is in a state of acute stress. As mentioned previously, in a state of stress cortisol is released from the adrenal cortex, and the catecholamines, epinephrine, and norepinephrine from the adrenal medulla.

Metabolic response to stress. The catecholamines stimulate the processes of lipolysis and glycogenolysis, while at the same time inhibiting insulin secretion, which is necessary for carbohydrates to be moved into the cell for glycolysis. Free fatty acids, which are liberated from lipolysis, go through a process of beta oxidation where two carbons are cleaved from the long-chain fatty acids to form acetyl CoA. Acetyl CoA usually combines with pyruvate, an end product of glycolysis, to continue the citric acid or Krebs cycle, the major source of energy production in the body. If insulin secretion is inhibited by epinephrine and increased production of free fatty acids blocks glycolytic breakdown of glucose as well as antagonizing insulin, glucose cannot enter the cell. Therefore, pyruvate from the breakdown of glucose is not available to bind with acetyl CoA. To maintain the Krebs cycle, acetyl CoA builds up, diffuses out of the cell, and goes to the liver. The liver, however, cannot metabolize all of it. Acetoacetic acid then forms and is released into the blood to produce a ketotic or acidotic state (Guthrie and Guthrie 1973; Tepperman 1973, pp. 183–186; and Williams 1974, pp. 530–538). The degree of acidosis that develops depends on the magnitude of the stress response to surgery and the person's physiological ability to compensate for these changes.

With acidosis, there is an efflux of potassium extracellularly. Insulin mediates the influx of potassium into the cell, but in a catabolic state insulin is antagonized by cortisol so will not be as effective in moving the potassium into the cell. With rising levels of serum potassium, hydrogen ion is exchanged for potassium ions for excretion. This can lead to an accumulation of hydrogen ion, which contributes to the acidemia.

Cortisol release stimulates gluconeogenesis by the liver primarily by increasing transport of amino acids from the extracellular fluid to the liver and by mobilizing amino acids from muscle tissue. Since cortisol antagonizes insulin, however, the glucose formed is unable to be transported into most body cells to be used for energy. Serum glucose levels rise (Guyton 1976, p. 1026). The body's decreased ability to use glucose for energy can contribute to fatigue sensations. Also, with mobilization of amino acids from muscle tissue for gluconeogenesis, there is decreased protein synthesis and increased catabolism of protein in body cells. This also can cause changes in available energy. A variety of agents have been identified that are capable of triggering the metabolic response to stress. They are anesthesia, pain and pain medication, sleep deprivation, boredom and disinterest, and age and sex.

Anesthesia. Anesthesia alone is capable of stimulating the stress response in surgical patients. There is depression of major body systems with general anesthesia. Until these systems return to presurgical levels of functioning, we can expect fatigue sensations in postanesthesia patients.

According to Norris and Campbell (1975), respiratory insufficiency occurred with anesthesia because individuals did not breathe deeply enough to permit adequate air exchange in the alveoli. This is caused by depression of the brain centers controlling respirations, depression of the cough reflex, and excessive secretions. Lowered levels of oxygen in the blood can cause lethargy and fatigue sensations.

Circulatory complications may occur with surgical procedures. There is an increased tendency for the blood to clot after surgery, especially following incisions of the lower abdominal cavity. While the exact mechanisms are not understood, there is definitely a slowing of the circulation with immobilization of patients throughout the surgery. Also, minor damage to vessel walls occurs because muscle tone, which normally protects the vessels, is decreased by anesthesia (Norris and Campbell 1975). Impaired circulation and perfusion of body tissues can potentiate fatigue responses.

With general anesthetics, the glomerular filtration rate of the kidneys decreases 19 percent; renal blood flow decreases 38 percent; and renal vascular resistance increases. The same effects have been observed with the balanced anesthetic technique and following the administration of narcotics and barbiturates. This can potentially inhibit the body's ability to finely regulate serum electrolytes and body wastes, causing abnormal variations in serum constituents (Lippman 1970). Electrolyte imbalances and accumulation of body waste products in the blood can lead to fatigue responses.

Pain and pain medication. Postoperative pain is most severe after thoracic or abdominal surgery, due to the proximity of the diaphragm (Sweeney 1977). According to Johnson (1977), the typical response to pain is sympathetic stimulation, which causes an increase in heart rate, elevated blood pressure, increased rate and depth of respirations, increased perspiration, and dilated pupils. The body cannot maintain continued sympathoadrenal activity so the autonomic nervous system activities become depressed and sensations of fatigue ensue. Fatigue brought about by the the body's reaction to the pain can decrease pain tolerance, setting off a vicious cycle (Johnson 1977).

Analgesics given for pain postoperatively can act in several ways. They can elevate the pain threshold altering pain perception. They can alter the mood or attitude of the person experiencing the pain. They can act on the nerve fibers and interfere with the transmission of noxious stimuli. Analgesics do produce a state of sedation and narcotics alter cerebral cognition, causing drowsiness and feelings of fatigue (Sweeney 1977).

Sleep deprivation. It is commonly recognized that symptoms of sleep deprivation are similar to fatigue. Early theorists saw sleep as a means of preventing, combating, or defending against fatigue. Hartmann (1973) distinguished two types of tiredness, physical and mental. Physical tiredness is relieved by slow wave sleep (SWS), which is stages three and four and is often called synchronized, nonrapid eye movement (NREM), or quiet sleep. He went on to describe this as the anabolic phase of sleep where protein and RNA synthesis takes place, especially in the central nervous system, and has a physically restorative function. People have increased requirements for SWS when they are in a state of general body tiredness or increased catabolism. This type of sleep is extremely pertinent to the postsurgical patient. Mental tiredness represents a need for desynchronized, dreaming, rapid eye movement (REM), or active sleep; this is also called *D*-

sleep. The restorative quality of REM sleep is needed after days of stress, worry, or intense new learning. Psychic processes are absent during dreaming. D-sleep has a renewing function for the enzymes involved in maintaining optimistic mood, energy, and self-confidence and systems involved in processes of emotional adaptation to the physical environment. The renewing aspect of D-sleep also is important to the person who has recently undergone surgery.

There appear to be several direct causal relationships between fatigue and sleep. Fatigue is relieved by sleep; lack of sleep causes fatigue; fatigue can stimulate sleep (Donaldson 1975; Grandjean 1970; Hobson 1968; and Mills 1976). Mills (1976) stated that at the end of the day a person's level of arousal is increased and, if sleep is of poor quality, the individual starts the next day above baseline arousal. The higher arousal level, in turn, causes sleep disturbances, and so on. Fatigue, Mills believed, can overcome the high arousal state and stimulate good sleep (1976).

Boredom and disinterest. Wilkinson (1961, 1962) stated that motivating influences can cancel effects of lack of sleep and resultant fatigue. According to Cameron (1973), the natural response to sleep deprivation is a low arousal level as a preliminary to sleep; this response can, however, be reversed by a demand for greater effort, by interest in work, by intense stimulation, or by a strong emotion. People behave in both adaptive and purposive ways and, if incentives are strong enough, individuals can work for long periods without fatigue. Interest and determination enhance the length of time at a task without fatigue responses. McClelland (1955) found high motivation led to more energy mobilization. MacBryde and Blacklow (1970) also found that motivation played an important role in fatigue. Pleasure and satisfaction raised the threshold for fatigue; disinterest and discomfort lowered it. The person in pain following surgery will have a lower threshold for fatigue. According to Luongo (1964), pleasure increases voluntary muscle tonicity and fosters inclination to act and thus has an inhibitory effect on fatigue. Boredom, grief, and pain decrease tonicity, amplitude, and power of muscles, thus stimulating fatigue sensations. Wendt and Palmerton (1976) proposed that suggestion is a powerful force; that is, what a person believes about his or her abilities greatly influences behavior. A person's perception and expectations about his or her prognosis can contribute to expressions of feelings of fatigue.

According to Coefer and Appley (1964), fatigue is a motivational phenomenon itself in that its accumulation leads to behavior change. The change in behavior is associated with the need for rest. The common factor in all classifications of fatigue states is the *motivational element directing the individual toward inactivity*.

Age and sex. Bafitis and Sargent (1977) found that human adaptive capacity, or the individual's ability to cope successfully with the stresses of life, is greatest between the ages of 3 and 20. After 30 years of age, adaptation gradually decreases but the variability in adaptation increases with age. Klumpp (1976) felt that fatigue in older persons in the absence of illness is due to lessening of cardiac reserve and circulatory status, decreased ability for mental and emotional effort, decreased glandular activity, atrophy due to disease, and loss of incentive, motivation, and interest. Variability in adaptation of elderly people depends on the extent to which these processes affect the individuals. Darling (1971) projected that total avoidance of fatigue leads to decreased adaptability. Klumpp (1976) supported this when he wrote that functional capacities are maintained and enhanced only through repeated stress.

One physician found fatigue more prevalent in patients over 40 years of age, but this group of patients also had a greater number of physical disorders. Two-thirds of the patients complaining of fatigue were women. Psychiatric disturbances were more common in fatigued women than in fatigued men (Spaulding 1964).

Although fatigue is not peculiar to women, they do have a unique kind of fatigue according to one theorist, who suggested that sex glands were a neuro-glandular system having as one function the production of energy. Women's glandular changes in the monthly menstrual cycle lead to fluctuating amounts of available energy (Hilliard 1960). Moos and colleagues (1969) found that there was a sharp rise in activation energy around midcycle that steadily decreased during the remainder of the cycle, reaching the lowest point in the menstrual and premenstrual phases.

MANIFESTATIONS OF FATIGUE

The physiological manifestations of fatigue are due to the decrease in the physiological and metabolic processes in the body required for interaction with the environment and the shift toward anabolic processes to replenish depleted energy stores. The changes seen are similar to those occurring during sleep, which are caused by the inhibition of all sympathetic activity and some parasympathetic activity. Inhibition of sympathetic and parasympathetic activity manifests itself as a decrease in motor activity and muscle tone and also in a reduction of cardiovascular activity leading to a lowered blood pressure, heart rate, and cardiac output. There is also a reduced sensitivity of the respiratory control center to CO_2, so respirations are decreased; a rise in blood CO_2 and a fall in blood pH are also seen (MacBryde and Blacklow 1970, p. 636). Nixon (1976) brought forth several biochemical changes associated with exhaustion and high levels of arousal: decreased serum iron, increased thyroid and sympathoadrenal activity, increased serum cholesterol, triglycerides, uric acid, glucose, blood coagulability, and increased fluid retention. Kuguelmas (1965) stated that when the blood of a fatigued individual was injected into a rested subject overt manifestations of fatigue were produced, causing tremulous muscular action, clumsy movements, increased respirations, pulse, pulse pressure, blood pressure, and metabolism, and decreased blood glucose.

According to Grandjean (1970), the manifestations of fatigue were seen as areas of cortical inhibition. They included decreased attention, slowed and impaired perception, impaired thinking, decreased motivation, and decreased performance in physical and mental activities. Davis (1943) stated that there is loss of fine coordination. According to Schwab (1953), a fatigued individual also made poor judgments, omitted details, and was indifferent to his or her surroundings.

Kashiwagi (1971) classified the varied manifestations of fatigue into three broad categories: weakened activation, weakened motivation, and physical disintegration. According to Yoshitake (1971), fatigue symptoms represented dull, sleepy factors, a decline of work motivation, and a projection of fatigue to the body or somatization of feelings of mental and sensory incongruity. Grandjean (1970) described these incongruity feelings as nonspecific physical complaints such as headache, rapid breathing, loss of appetite, indigestion, and insomnia. Gilbert (1971) maintained that the main outward sign of fatigue was a lack of a sense of well-being that was found in physically and mentally healthy persons. According to Schaefer (1976), fatigue dictated the results of one's pursuits: "success or failure," "achievement or resignation," and "alertness or sleepiness."

Beck categorized the symptoms of depression that represented the fatigue seen in these clients into five manifestations as follows: Affective manifestations were portrayed by apathy; cognitive manifestations were seen as defective concentration; motivational manifestations referred to "paralysis of the will"; the tiredness, drowsiness, and inability to initiate activity comprised the vegetative manifestations; finally, the changes in motor behavior were displayed by decreased activity and slowness in movement (Karno and Hoffman 1974).

PROGNOSIS OF FATIGUE

Levels

There are two basic levels of fatigue; protective and painful. Each level indicates a different prognosis. Protective fatigue forces the individual to avoid further fatigue by stimulating the desire for natural restoratives, thus allowing recovery. Kuguelmas (1965) called this *natural fatigue*. Grandjean (1970) stated that the sensation of this fatigue is not necessarily unpleasant if a person is able to rest, sleep, or have some leisure time for recuperation. Fatigue maintains the homeostatic processes of the organism by stimulating the desire for such restorative measures. It is a warning signal that signals the need for rest before complete exhaustion and collapse from the total depletion of the energy reserves occurs (Davis 1943; and Shands and Finesinger 1952). Protective fatigue not only guards the physical integrity of the individual, but also preserves personal self-esteem and ideal self-concept (Kuguelmas 1965; Shands and Finesinger 1952).

When recuperation is not allowed, fatigue becomes persistent, chronic, and painful. Collier (1936) called this *morbid fatigue*. Kuguelmas (1965) noted that persistent fatigue led to failure of recuperating powers resulting in exhaustion and activating a latent process of precipitating a pathological disorder.

Degrees of Intensity

In the literature and in clinical settings, tiredness and exhaustion are viewed as separate concepts from fatigue. According to Putt (1975), tiredness was seen as occurring normally after work or an activity of a physical nature. When tired, an individual can still function to capacity. Tiredness is a transient, temporary state that is relieved by rest or sleep; it is often a good feeling. Fatigue is a more extreme state. It has both mental and physical components and interferes with the optimal functional capacity. It is an unpleasant state and of longer duration than a tired state, but recovery follows recuperative measures. Putt (1975) stated that exhaustion is fatigue carried too far; it is the final state of fatigue where catabolic processes exceed anabolic processes. Exhaustion is a total decompensated state of illness. Spaulding (1964) confirmed this relationship by stating that there are different degrees of intensity of fatigue, tiredness being mild and exhaustion being overwhelming. These concepts can be viewed in the relationship shown in Figure 16-1.

Fatigue on a Continuum

Prognosis in fatigue can also be viewed on a health–illness continuum. *Energy,* as defined by *The Random House Dictionary of the English Language* (1966, p. 472) is "the capacity for vigorous activity, vigor, or the ability to act forcefully"; fatigue can be seen as the antonym of *exhaustion,* which is defined by *The Random House Dictionary of the English Language* (1966, p. 499) as "to use up or consume completely, to drain of strength or energy, wear out or fatigue

---

Figure 16-1 Intensity Progression of Fatigue

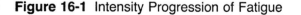

Exhaustion ⟶ Fatigue ⟶ Tiredness

greatly." Various descending levels of energy comprise the health side of the continuum. The illness side of the continuum is represented by tiredness, fatigue, and exhaustion (Figure 16-2).

Nixon (1976) arranged the aspects of fatigue in the natural order of their passage from health to health breakdown, using levels of arousal and performance. In healthy individuals, increasing arousal leads to increased performance. Gain in performance falls off in fatigue and exhaustion when persisting arousal leads to deterioration and ill health.

Recovery

The starting and stopping points of fatigue are undefined events. Further, the subject of recovery from fatigue is controversial. Several authors believe that sleep and rest are necessities (Davis 1943; Grandjean 1970; and Hargreaves 1977). Other authors state that rest is not the ultimate cure-all but that activity overcomes fatigue (Ford's Continuing Series of College Newspaper Supplements 1977; and Klumpp 1976).

ASSESSMENT OF FATIGUE

The conceptual clarification methodology developed by Carnevali (1977) was used to provide the framework and direction for a study of fatigue in nursing the surgical patient. According to Carnevali (1977), concepts are the organizers of knowledge/experience and are assigned meanings that refer to one or more sets of interrelated phenomena. She views conceptualization as a filing system in which the concept is organized into an idea package. This involves four steps: (1) determining the identifying properties, (2) organizing the ideas within the concept, (3) evaluating the concept in situations for usefulness, and (4) developing responses or appropriate management related to the concept.

Figure 16-2 Health–Illness Continuum of Fatigue

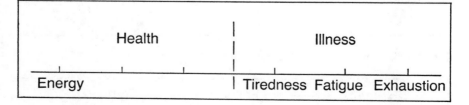

Three aspects of Carnevali's conceptual package were used to clarify fatigue in postoperative patients. Consistent with this package, data were collected in four ways: (1) by reviewing the patient's records, (2) by observation checklist, (3) by interview, and (4) by fatigue scale.

An observation checklist was developed. Content validity for the checklist was established by asking for a description of how patients looked and acted when fatigued. The information was categorized into major subdivisions, analyzed, and organized. Using the checklist, observations of subjects were made by two nurse graduate students to establish inter–rater reliability and to further establish both face and content validity (Figure 16-3).

Open-ended interviews were used to collect subjective data from patients. Interview items were aimed at gathering information from subjects who were considered expert informants, that is, people who were experiencing fatigue after

Figure 16-3 Observation Checklist

General Appearance

Physical appearance
1. Alert
2. Awake
3. Drowsy
4. Disheveled
5. Quiet

Coloring
1. Flushed
2. Pink
3. Pale
4. Ashen

Breathing
1. Normal rate (12–24 breaths/minute)
2. Fast rate (>24)
3. Slow rate (<12)
4. Regular
5. Irregular
6. Shallow
7. Deep
8. Sighs

Communication

Eyes
1. Opened wide
2. Closed
3. Eye contact present
4. Eyelids droopy
5. Fixed, staring
6. Look vacant

Facial expression
1. Grimacing
2. Eyes rolling
3. Brow wrinkling
4. Mouth open
5. Jaw tight
6. Smiling
7. Musculature relaxed
8. Yawning frequent

Speech
1. Complete sentences
2. Incomplete sentences
3. Short, abbreviated answers
4. Frequent pauses
5. Slow responses
6. Rapid responses
7. Clear tone
8. Soft tone
9. Loud tone
10. Slurred or mumbled
11. Specific statements of feeling tired

Figure 16-3 continued

Activity

Movements
1. Spontaneous changes
   in position
2. Minimal movements
   initiated
3. Sluggish movements
4. Restless movements

Posture
1. Upright posture
2. Lying on back
3. Lying on right side
4. Lying on left side
5. Shoulders slumped
   forward
6. Head hanging
7. Body not arranged in
   comfortable position

Ambulation
1. Slow pace with
   assistance
2. Slow pace alone
3. Fast pace
4. Shuffles feet

Food and fluid intake
1. NPO
2. Refuses meal
3. Eats at fast pace
4. Eats at slow pace
5. Verbalizes about hunger
6. Verbalizes about lack of
   hunger

Attitude

Attitude
1. Interested
2. Easily aroused
3. Cooperative
4. Apathetic
5. Hard to arouse
6. Irritable
7. Sleep-seeking
8. Emotional outbursts
9. Somatic complaints
10. Flat affect
11. Indecisive

---

surgery. Interviews usually started with the suggestion, "Tell me how you feel today," and built on patients' responses.

In the second phase of the interview, several standard questions were built into an interview schedule. These items reflected significant factors found in the literature as contributing to fatigue and asked for descriptions of several points on the Subjective Feeling Scale adapted from Yoshitake (1971) by Putt (1975). Points on the scale included (1) how patients felt in their heads, eyes, arms, and legs, (2) whether they were able to concentrate or think clearly, and (3) whether they were experiencing various aches and pains and how their voices felt.

Figure 16-4 Rhoten Fatigue Scale

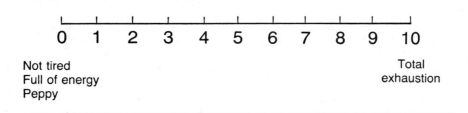

A fatigue scale (Figure 16-4), used by subjects to rate their fatigue, was developed. The scale consisted of 10 increments beginning at zero, which represented "not tired, feelings of energy, and peppy," to 10, which represented "total exhaustion." This scale was used in attempting to quantify patients' fatigue.

Fatigue Study

Selection of patients and procedure. A convenience sample of 5 patients who were 25 years of age or older admitted for abdominal surgery within 48 hours prior to interview was obtained. Patients who consented to participate in the study were observed simultaneously by 2 nurses using the observation checklist for 3 15-minute periods at 24, 48, and 72 hours postoperatively. Interviews of 20 to 30 minutes were conducted after each observation, using an open-ended item approach and a semistructured schedule. Interviews were taped. After each interview, patients were asked to assign their level or degree of fatigue on the Rhoten Fatigue Scale. The scale was held up and patients were asked to point to the description of how they felt on the 10-point scale. In addition to the observation checklist, interview and fatigue-scale data information about patients' illnesses, treatments, and socioeconomic levels were available along with demographic data.

Data analysis. Qualitative methods of data analysis were used for defining the concept and identifying the manifestations of fatigue and the characteristics of those at high risk for fatigue. (See Table 16-1.).

Sample characteristics. Sample characteristics were examined to explore the effects they might have on level of fatigue. Characteristics considered were as follows: (1) extent of surgery, (2) anesthesia length, (3) duration of IV fluids, (4) duration of nasogastric (NG) tube, (5) amount of pain medication and number of abnormal laboratory values. Extent of surgery, length of anesthesia, amount of pain medication, and number of abnormal laboratory values seemed significant and seemed to operate in a synergistic manner. The greater the number of these

Table 16-1 Characteristics of the Patients

Characteristic	A	B	Patient C	D	E
Sex	M	F	F	F	F
Age	71	39	63	61	35
Race	Caucasian	Caucasian	Caucasian	Caucasian	Caucasian
Type of surgery	Colectomy	Gastric stapling	Colectomy	Removal of colostomy scar, drainage of abdominal abscess	Cystectomy, splenectomy
Type of anesthesia	General	General	General	Spinal	General
Duration of anesthesia	2 hrs	1 hr, 50 min	2 hrs, 10 min	45 min	3 hrs, 15 min
Duration of IV fluids	3 days	3 days	3 days	none	3 days
Duration nasogastric tube	2 days	2 days	3 days	none	2 days
Pain medication	Morphine sulfate	Morphine sulfate	Morphine sulfate	Acetaminophen (Tylenol 3)	Morphine sulfate
Frequency of pain medication	Every 3–6 hrs for 3 days	twice a day	twice a day	2–3 times a day	Every 3 hrs for 3 days
Laboratory values					
Hematocrit (male: 40–54%)* female: 37–47%	low	normal	low	normal	low
Hemoglobin (male: 14–18 gm/100 ml) female: 12–16 gm/100 ml.	low	normal	low	normal	low
White blood count (5,000–10,000/cu mm)	normal	high	high	normal	high
Serum sodium (135–145 mEq/L)	normal	normal	normal	normal	normal
Serum potassium (3.5–5.5 mEq/L)	normal	normal	normal	normal	normal

*Normal ranges of laboratory values established by the hospital where data were collected.

variables present and the greater their magnitude, the higher the level of fatigue. See Table 16-1 for ranking of patients by sample characteristics.

Observation checklists. To identify characteristics that correlated with high and low fatigue, each item on the checklist (see Figure 16-3) was analyzed for frequency of occurrence in the 2 most-fatigued patients for the 3 days and in the 2 least-fatigued patients for 3 days. The patients were ranked from most to least fatigued by the investigators at 24, 48, and 72 hours.

Categories showing major differences between most-fatigued and least-fatigued patients were general appearance, eyes, facial expression, speech, movements, and attitude. Categories showing moderate differences between the two types of patients were coloring, breathing, and posture. Categories too infrequently observed to identify differences between the two types of patients were ambulation and food and fluid intake. Each major category contained items that more accurately separated most-fatigued from least-fatigued patients.

Interviews. Each criterion attribute of fatigue emerging from each patient's interviews was analyzed in terms of most fatigued to least fatigued. All 3 days were analyzed together and trends were identified.

Criterion attributes showing major differences between most-fatigued and least-fatigued patients were general sensation, pain, pain medication (frequency), concentration, attitude, and motivation. Those criterion attributes that showed very few differences between the two types of patients were sensation in eyes, head, extremities, and torso, and speech, movements, sleep, appetite, effect of pain medication, emotional state, and primary concerns.

Sensation. General sensations experienced by those most fatigued were pain, nausea, tiredness, discomfort, and general malaise. The least fatigued had fewer aches and pains, no nausea, and felt more energetic; they had a few discomforts, but overall felt more comfortable than the most fatigued.

Both the most and least fatigued felt that they wanted to close their eyes, although their eyes did not necessarily feel groggy or tired. Both types felt their eyes did not feel abnormal and that their vision was clear; both types of patients also felt that they were mentally clear.

The majority of both the most-fatigued and least-fatigued patients felt some tiredness or weakness in their extremities, particularly in the legs, which they described as heaviness, weakness, numbness, or slowness. One patient described heaviness in the torso.

Physical response. Both types of patients complained of vocal weakness, softness, and hoarseness. The most fatigued mentioned more frequently that they did not feel like talking.

Mostly, both the most fatigued and least fatigued felt their movements were slower. Both types felt good when they got up and both complained of restlessness. The most fatigued more frequently stated that they just wanted to sleep. Two patients felt more tired due to poor sleep, and one patient felt more energetic with less sleep and more tired with sound sleep.

Appetite varied from individual to individual and seemed unrelated to level of fatigue. One patient never mentioned hunger.

The most-fatigued patients experienced the greatest amount of pain. Pain was felt throughout most of their bodies, whereas the least fatigued had localized pain that they did not consider very uncomfortable. Most fatigued patients were medicated more frequently for pain. Both types of patients stated that the pain medication made them tired, groggy, or sleepy.

Mental response. The most-fatigued patients more frequently complained of not being able to concentrate or not wanting to concentrate on anything. The least fatigued felt their levels of concentration were normal.

The attitude of the patients who were most fatigued was one of not caring about things going on around them and trying to ignore them, but they had more complaints of being irritated by them. The least fatigued complained of feelings of boredom and lack of interest in things they had enjoyed before surgery.

The most-fatigued patients suffered a greater depletion of motivation than did the least-fatigued patients.

Three of the five patients had improved emotional outlooks following surgery. Two had cancerous tumors removed with good prognoses; the other had pain 3 years prior to surgery, which was eliminated by surgery. Improved emotional outlook did not have a significant bearing on how these subjects were ranked.

Primary concerns. Four of the five patients had IV catheters and nasogastric tubes, which they complained about. The sore throat and nausea associated with these interventions was a major preoccupation of these four patients.

Fatigue scales. The fatigue scale was used to determine whether the level of fatigue felt by the patients correlated with the level of fatigue assigned to the patient by the investigators according to the information gathered through the observations and interviews. Most patients ranked themselves at three to four on the fatigue scale. Generally, there was correlation between the rankings made by patients on the fatigue scale and rankings assigned by the investigators.

Findings. Several potentially useful findings emerged from the sample characteristics, observation checklist, interview, and fatigue scale tools used in this study. The rankings of the levels of fatigue made by the two observers based on their observations and interviews correlated with subjective rankings made by patients on the fatigue scale.

It is difficult to relate positively the findings to fatigue specifically, since fatigue does not exist as a pure phenomenon in the postsurgical client. Fatigue is confounded with the effects of pre- and/or postoperative illness, pain and discomfort, and the effects of pain medication.

BEGINNING OPERATIONAL DEFINITION

The overall definition of postoperative fatigue can be described as a general introverted sensation state following surgery that is usually accompanied by a large amount of widespread pain and discomfort and frequent administration of pain medication. The postoperative client lacks motivation to do anything but sleep and rest.

Nursing Concerns

Fatigue was not a primary concern for the postsurgical patient. Most patients admitted to some degree of tiredness, but their main perception of their state was not necessarily fatigue. Instead, they were bothered by things such as pain, IV catheters, and nasogastric tubes; these factors may contribute to fatigue in various degrees but they, not fatigue, were the main concerns.

Most of the patients said they felt less tired after they were up and around; however, most were content just to lie in bed. Perhaps the earlier and more frequently ambulation and activity is promoted the less patients will feel the tiredness and discomfort.

Overwhelming fatigue responses seemed to occur in patients who had had more extensive surgery and were experiencing a great deal of pain that required frequent medication. These patients need to be watched carefully, as they are less likely to do anything on their own initiative and would be more susceptible to postoperative complications. The usual nursing routines of turning, coughing, and deep breathing may not be frequent enough for these fatigued patients to prevent complications.

Findings about Fatigue Related to Additive Stress-Response Construct

The model presented in Figure 16-5 incorporates the findings of this study with its relationship to the stress response and the physiological dynamics of fatigue proposed in the literature.

According to the model, abnormal preoperative laboratory values are indicators that the organism is stressed prior to surgery. This preoperative stress state is compounded by the surgery and anesthesia and markedly compounded with extensive surgery associated with longer periods of anesthesia. Pain is a direct

Figure 16-5 Conceptual Model of Criterion Attributes Associated with Fatigue in the Surgical Client

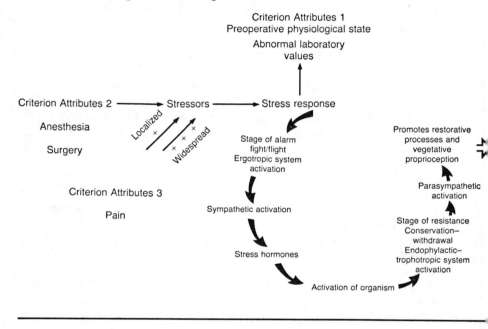

result of the surgery and also is capable of inducing a stress response, thus increasing its magnitude. According to Thetford and Schucman (1971), the stress situation is proportional to the threat seen in the situation. It seems reasonable that the greater the perceived pain, the greater the threat seen by the client and the more marked the stress response. Figure 16-5 shows the additive response to stress is more fatigue producing.

The first reaction to stress is a stage of alarm, which is also known as the fight–flight system or ergotropic system (Selye 1974, 1975, 1976a, 1976b; MacBryde and Blacklow 1970; and Hess 1957). This causes sympathetic system activation with the subsequent release of the stress hormones and activation of the organism. Over an extended period, this will lead to the depletion of body reserves. The body has a built-in protection mechanism against the ultimate depletion of its reserves. The stage of alarm is followed by a stage of resistance, also known as the conservation–withdrawal system or endophylactic–trophotropic system (Selye 1974, 1975, 1976a, 1976b; MacBryde and Blacklow 1970; and Hess 1957). This is caused by parasympathetic nervous system activation and promotes restorative processes and vegetative proprioception, thus stimulating feelings of fatigue.

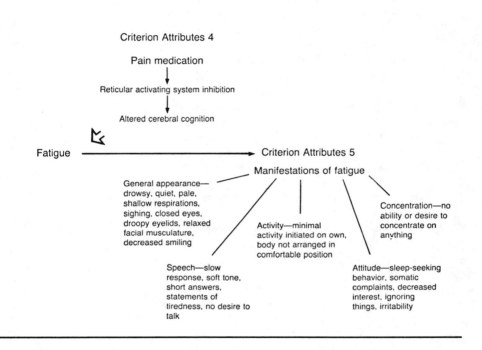

Criterion Attributes 4

Pain medication

Reticular activating system inhibition

Altered cerebral cognition

Fatigue

Criterion Attributes 5

Manifestations of fatigue

General appearance—
drowsy, quiet, pale,
shallow respirations,
sighing, closed eyes,
droopy eyelids, relaxed
facial musculature,
decreased smiling

Activity—minimal
activity initiated on own,
body not arranged in
comfortable position

Concentration—no
ability or desire to
concentrate on
anything

Speech—slow
response, soft tone,
short answers,
statements of
tiredness, no desire to
talk

Attitude—sleep-seeking
behavior, somatic
complaints, decreased
interest, ignoring
things, irritability

Pain medications, especially narcotics, given liberally to recent postoperative clients to alleviate the pain perception, contribute to fatigue sensations through a different mode of action. They inhibit the reticular activating system, which is an area in the reticular formation of the midbrain that maintains the cerebral cortex in a state of arousal and alertness (Grandjean 1970). Through CNS depression, medications also are capable of generating the manifestations associated with fatigue. At this point we cannot identify whether the fatigue response is due to the additive stress response or if it is a reflection of depressed cerebral cognition and the concomitant decreased motor activity.

Observable manifestations of the fatigue response in the postoperative client can be categorized into five major categories: general appearance, speech, activity, attitude, and concentration.

The following questions and hypotheses generated from the conceptual model are proposed for further study:

1. Is fatigue in the postoperative patient greater because of the stress response to surgery or because of the CNS depressive effects of the pain medication?
2. Do patients who complain of widespread pain experience more fatigue than those who complain of localized pain?

3. Do people who are undergoing stress responses accurately perceive the magnitude of fatigue that they are experiencing?
4. Can the magnitude of fatigue be predicted by the amount of fatigue manifestations?
5. Do the amount of fatigue manifestations correlate with the subjective ranking on the fatigue scale?
6. Can the fatigue manifestations be arranged in a hierarchical order in regard to the level of fatigue? Is one more significant than the other?
7. How does the quality of sleep affect fatigue responses? Does the quality of sleep in a hospitalized patient differ significantly from normal sleep, thus producing exaggerated fatigue responses?
8. Are the signs and symptoms of fatigue different from those of depression? If so, how?
9. What are the criteria for determining that a patient has recovered from fatigue?
10. Reduction of fatigue promotes more rapid healing than when fatigue is not treated.
11. Reduction of fatigue reduces the number of hospital days required for recovery from major surgery.
12. Reduction of fatigue reduces the time between when an individual identifies him- or herself as ill and when the person feels "well again."

REFERENCES

Albeaux-Fernet, M., Bugard, P., and Roman, J. The treatment of chronic fatigue with adenosine tri-phosphoric acid. *La Presse Med.* 66:1265, 1958.

Bafitis, H., and Sargent, F., II. Human physiological adaptability through the life sequence. *J. Gerontol.* 32(4):402–410, Jul. 1977.

Bartlett, F. Psychological Criteria of Fatigue. In W.F. Floyd and A.T. Welford (Eds.), *Fatigue*. London: H.K. Lewis and Co., 1953.

Bartley, S.H. *Fatigue: Mechanism and Management.* Springfield, Ill.: Thomas, 1965.

Bartley, S.H. What Do We Call Fatigue? In E. Simonson and P.C. Weiser (Eds.), *Psychological Aspects and Physiological Correlates of Work and Fatigue*. Springfield, Ill.: Thomas, 1976.

Brown, J.R. Environmental aspects of fatigue. *Appl. Therapeut.* 6:905–910, Nov. 1964.

Burkhardt, E.A. Fatigue: Diagnosis and treatment. *N.Y. State J. Med.* 56:62–67, 1956.

Cameron, C. A theory of fatigue. *Ergonomics* 16(5):633–648, 1973.

Carnevali, D. Conceptualizing, a Nursing Skill. In P.H. Mitchell (Ed.), *Concepts Basic to Nursing*. New York: McGraw-Hill, 1977.

Coates, D.B. The management of tiredness. *Appl. Therapeut.* 6:916–919, Nov. 1964.

Coefer, C.N., and Appley, M.H. *Motivation: Theory and Research*. New York: Wiley, 1964.

Collier, H.E. The recognition of fatigue with special reference to the clinical diagnosis of morbid fatigue in industry. *Br. Med. J.* 2:1322–1325, 1936.

Darling, R.C. Fatigue. In J.A. Downey and R.C. Darling (Eds.), *Physiological Basis of Rehabilitation Medicine*. Philadelphia: Saunders, 1971.

Davis, H. Symposium on fatigue: Introductory remarks. *Psychosom. Med.* 5:153–154, 1943.

DeLateur, B.J., Lehman, J.F., and Gasccni, R. Mechanical work and fatigue: Their roles in the development of muscle work capacity. *Arch. Phys. Med. Rehabil.* 57:319–324, Jul. 1976.

Donaldson, S. Critique: Effects of noise on fatigue in healthy middle-aged adults. *Commun. Nurs. Res.* 8:35–40, 1975.

Forbes, W.H. Symposium on fatigue: Problems arising in the study of fatigue. *Psychosom. Med.* 5:155–157, 1943.

Ford's Continuing Series of College Newspaper Supplements. More Power to You: Beat Fatigue with This High-Energy Rx. *Insider* Laura Eshbaugh (Ed.), 1977.

Gilbert, J.R. Highlights from a recent seminar on fatigue. *Can. Med. Assoc. J.* 105:309–310, Aug. 7, 1971.

Grandjean, E.P. Fatigue. *Am. Ind. Hyg. Assoc. J.* 31:401–411, Jul.–Aug. 1970.

Guyton, A.C. *Textbook of Medical Physiology*. Philadelphia: Saunders, 1976.

Hargreaves, M. The fatigue syndrome. *Practitioner* 218:841–843, June 1977.

Hartmann, E.L. *The Functions of Sleep*. New Haven: Yale University Press, 1973.

Hess, W.R. *The Functional Organization of the Diencephalon*. New York: Grune & Stratton, 1957.

Hilliard, M. *Women and Fatigue*. Garden City, N.Y.: Doubleday, 1960.

Hobson, J.A. Sleep after exercise. *Science* 162:1503–1505, Dec. 27, 1968.

Johnson, M. Assessment of Clinical Pain. In A. Jacox (Ed.), *Pain: A Source Book for Nurses and Other Health Professionals*. Boston: Little, Brown, 1977.

Karno, M., and Hoffman, R. The Pseudoanergic Syndrome. In A. Kiev (Ed.), *Somatic Manifestations of Depressive Disorders*. New York: American Elsevier, 1974.

Kashiwagi, S. Psychological rating of human fatigue. *Ergonomics* 14(1):17–21, 1971.

Keliher, T.F. Fatigue. *Gen. Prac.* 20(6):102–106, Dec. 1959.

Klumpp, T.G. Some thoughts on fatigue in the older patient. *Med. Times* 104(10):87–93, Oct. 1976.

Kuguelmas, I.N. Foreword. In S.H. Bartley (Ed.), *Fatigue: Mechanism and Management*. Springfield, Ill.: Thomas, 1965.

Lippmann, M. Renal blood flow and function under various anesthetics. *Am. Assoc. Nurse Anesth. J.* 38(5):393–396, Oct. 1970.

Luongo, E.P. Work physiology in health and disease. *J. A. M. A.* 188(1):27–32, Apr. 1964.

MacBryde, C., and Blacklow, R. *Signs and Symptoms*. Philadelphia: Lippincott, 1970.

Mason, R.E. *Internal Perception and Bodily Functioning*. New York: International Universities Press, 1961.

McClelland, D.C. *Studies in Motivation*. New York: Appleton-Century-Crofts, 1955.

McFarland, R.A. Fatigue in industry. Understanding fatigue in modern life. *Ergonomics* 14:1–10, Jan. 1971.

Mills, I. The disease of failure of coping. *Practitioner* 217:529–538, Oct. 1976.

Moos, R.H., Kopell, B.S., Melges, F.T., Yalom, I.D., Lunde, D.T., Clayton, R.B., and Hamburg, D.A. Fluctuations in symptoms and moods during the menstrual cycle. *J. Psychosom. Res.* 13:37–44, 1969.

Nixon, P.G.F. The human function curve. *Practitioner* 217:765–770, Nov. 1976.

Norris, W., and Campbell, D. *A Nurse's Guide to Anaesthetics, Resuscitation and Intensive Care*. New York: Churchill Livingstone, 1975.

Putt, A. Effects of noise on fatigue in healthy middle-aged adults. *Commun. Nurs. Res.* 8:24–34, 1975.

The Random House Dictionary of the English Language. New York: Random House, 1966.

Rockwell, D., and Burr, B. The tired patient. *J. Fam. Pract.* 1(2):62–65, Aug. 1974.

Schaefer, H. Epilogue. In E. Simonson and P.C. Weiser (Eds.), *Psychological Aspects and Physiological Correlates of Work and Fatigue.* Springfield, Ill.: Thomas, 1976.

Schwab, R. Motivation in Measurements of Fatigue. In W.F. Floyd and A.T. Welford, *Fatigue.* London: H.K. Lewis, 1953.

Selye, H. Stress without distress. *World Health* pp. 3–11, Dec. 1974.

Selye, H. Confusion and controversy in the stress field. *J. Human Stress* 1(2):37–44, June 1975.

Selye, H. *The Stress of Life.* New York: McGraw-Hill, 1976a.

Selye, H. Further thoughts on "stress without distress." *Med. Times* 104(11):124–144, Nov. 1976b.

Shands, H.C., and Finesinger, J.C. A note on the significance of fatigue. *Psychosom. Med.* 14:309–314, 1952.

Snook, S., and Irvine, C.H. Psychophysical studies of physiological fatigue criteria. *Hum. Factors* 11(3):291–300, June 1969.

Spaulding, W.B. The clinical analysis of fatigue. *Appl. Therapeut.* 6:911–915, Nov. 1964.

Sweeney, S. Pain Associated with Surgery. In A. Jacox (Ed.), *Pain: A Source Book for Nurses and Other Health Professionals.* Boston: Little, Brown, 1977.

Tepperman, J. *Metabolic and Endocrine Physiology.* Chicago: Year Book Medical Publishers, 1973.

Thetford, W.N., and Schucman, H. Motivational Factors and Adaptive Behavior. In J.A. Downey and R.C. Darling (Eds.), *Physiological Basis of Rehabilitation Medicine.* Philadelphia: Saunders, 1971.

Wendt, H., and Palmerton, P.R. Motivation, Values and Chronobehavioral Aspects of Fatigue. In E. Simonson and P. Weiser (Eds.), *Psychological Aspects and Physiological Correlates of Work and Fatigue.* Springfield, Ill.: Thomas, 1976.

Wilkinson, R. Interaction of lack of sleep with knowledge of results, repeated testing and individual differences. *J. Exp. Psychol.* 62(3):263–271, 1961.

Wilkinson, R. Muscle tension during mental work under sleep deprivation. *J. Exp. Psychol.* 64:565–571, 1962.

Williams, R.H. *Textbook of Endocrinology.* Philadelphia: Saunders, 1974.

Yoshitake, H. Relations between symptoms and feelings of fatigue. *Ergonomics* 14:175–186, 1971.

Chapter 17

Insomnia: From a Nursing Perspective

Mary Prokop

This chapter is based on observations in an adult nursing unit for eye-surgery patients. Cataract and retinal surgery are the most frequent procedures, and the majority of patients are over 50 years of age. The time is approximately 1 A.M. One of the patients' most often voiced concerns, "Nurse, I can't sleep," is heard. (It should be noted that eye surgery is associated with little pain.) A large number of eye-surgery patients are awake at night; some have difficulty falling asleep; others have problems with staying asleep; some wake up "too early." Older patients, especially males, seem to have the most frequent awakenings. Preoperative anxiety does not seem to explain the phenomenon adequately, as the behavior is observed commonly postoperatively as well. Patients often report having insomnia at home, although some state they only have trouble sleeping in the hospital. What accounts for so much insomnia? In charting that a patient had experienced insomnia during the night, the nurse might begin to wonder what the term really meant since it seems to include such a wide variety of sleep disturbances.

In an effort to clarify the problem of insomnia, a 3-month period of observation and literature review was instituted. This chapter presents the results of this initial work.

IDENTIFYING INSOMNIA

In addition to lack of clarity about what insomnia is, there seem to be additional problems. It has been observed that nursing assessment and response to patients having difficulty with sleep is almost reflex in nature. A typical sequence of events is, "If a patient can't sleep, give him a 'sleeper,' even though it is logical to assume that different problems require different solutions." The impediment to effective use of problem solving may stem from a "fuzzy" concept. We seem to be proceeding as if we are on common conceptual ground, that is, we all "know" what insomnia is and what to do about it. Such assumptions preclude further investigation and analysis of the phenomena. To formulate reality-based rationales for nursing action, concept clarification must be an ongoing process. After reviewing considerable literature on insomnia (Bradner 1976; Clift 1975; Dement 1975; Drucker-Colin 1977; Hartman 1973; Jouvet 1972; Jovanovic 1973; Kales 1969; and Williams 1971), I turned to observing insomnia in hospitalized patients.

Almost all patients observed also have some chronic health problem as a function of increased age that tends to interfere with sleep. Most of the patients interviewed reported that, although their sleep patterns have changed over the years, they have even more trouble in the hospital setting. Therefore, it seems that something in the hospital setting or the patients' response to it is particularly disruptive to sleep. No hypothesis reviewed is sufficiently comprehensive to explain what is observed in the clinical setting. It became necessary to return to the clinical area to gather more specific data in an effort to gain an understanding of the overall dynamics involved in this aspect of dyssomnia.

A typical patient reports

> At home when I wake up, I usually walk around the house for 20 minutes and then fall asleep; here I'd feel funny doing that so I can't go back to sleep now. . . . This pillow is impossible to sleep on, I should have brought my own. . . . What was that noise, it sounds like a cannon (addressograph), how can I sleep with that going on!?. . . . My arthritis is killing me and I can't sleep. . . . You know, when you get older you just don't sleep as well. . . . It's hard to sleep the night before you have surgery.

Initially, comments did not appear to point in any specific direction. What is the common denominator? What conceptual framework can be utilized in meeting the need of these patients for the most restful night's sleep possible under the circumstances?

Data collected from charts and through discussions with colleagues was not helpful in providing additional clues. Although the word *insomnia* is used in informal conversations, nurses rarely use it in charting a patient's problem list. This may be because only the bare minimum of problems is listed in attempts to reduce discharge paperwork. Another possible explanation is that nurses do not view most instances of sleep disturbance as serious. Sleep problems are accepted as a normal consequence or accompaniment of hospitalization. The one instance where insomnia was identified as a patient problem on a chart was when a physician had listed it. Nurses tend to look to a single solution, listing the relative effectiveness of pharmacological agents used in treatment. An analysis of a given patient's sleep problem by a nurse has yet to be reported. Sleep problems do not receive the attention given to other commonly recognized human disorders such as headaches or low back pain.

After a period of reflection, things started to coalesce in my endeavor. One common element in patients' comments about causes of insomnia is that all are types of stressors. Nocturnal awakenings seem to constitute a protective response to potential "danger" signals in the night (e.g., unfamiliar noises). Stress theory can be used as a basis for a conceptual framework in dealing with the sleep problems or dyssomnias of the patient population under observation.

It may be helpful to view the insomnia situation in terms of general systems theory in order to describe dynamics involved from the broadest possible perspective. The patient is the throughput on which the hospital and unit staff work as processor. The patient, as an open system, is ideally in a state of dynamic equilibrium with his or her environment. In this state, the patient maximizes use of personal energy reserves, thereby maintaining optimal-level wellness. It is beyond the scope of this chapter to deal with analysis of stressors on hospitalized patients except for those that decrease the Sleep Efficiency Index (i.e., time in bed ÷ total actual sleep time) (Williams, Karacan, and Hursch 1974). There are two major categories of stressors affecting this index: (1) characteristics of the environment (i.e., hospital) and (2) characteristics of the patient (Figure 17-1). The ultimate effects are increased or decreased levels of wellness–illness and of equilibrium–disequilibrium of patients' systems.

EFFECTS OF STRESS AND AGE ON SLEEP PATTERNS

The stressful nature of the physical and emotional concomitants of surgical procedures are well documented energy drains on the human system; heightened anxiety levels and physical discomfort involved often result in increased wakefulness.

> There is a tendency for stress and anxiety to be followed by increased sleep and D-time (dream sleep), but in some cases, this is masked or even reversed by the difficulty in falling and remaining asleep when anxious. And disturbed sleep is almost always associated with a decrease in percentage of rapid eye movement (REM) time, since REM time is more sensitive to noise or any physical disturbance than the remainder of sleep (Hartmann 1973, p. 90).

It has been found that stressful events such as surgery increase the need for sleep; although patients need more sleep, they often get less. Hartmann (1973) states that sleep serves two functions: (1) REM seems to help the person deal with emotional stressors and (2) stage 4 apparently enables a person to recover from

Figure 17-1 Preliminary Model for Dynamics of Nocturnal Awakenings in a Hospitalized Patient Population Aged 50 or More Years*

Stresses decreasing sleep efficiency	Intervening variables	Phases of stress intensification

Surgery
Anxiety, physical trauma

Unfamiliar environment
  Unrecognizable or loud noises at night
  Uncomfortable bed
  Significant others not present
  Decreased ability to tolerate change with increased age

Hospital routines ⟶
  Eye drops every 2 hours
  Awakening at 6 A.M.
  Use of sleep medication especially REM suppressants

Characteristics of patients
  Increased need for REM sleep to cope with emotional stress and assimilate new learning
  Increased need for stage-4 sleep as a function of physical demands on human system
  Decreased sleep efficiency past age 49
  Increased sleep latency (especially at 70–80 years)
  Increased number of night awakenings at 40 years for men and 60 years for women
  Increased frequency and percentage of stage-1 sleep (higher for men than for women) with increased age
  Decreased percentage of stage-4 sleep more marked in men than in women, greater as function of increased age

Intervening variables:
Kind of stressor

Number of stresses

Duration of stress

Perception of stress

Prehospitalization level of resistance ⟶

Increased health problems with increased age

Phases of stress intensification:
Upper limit of survival

Exhaustion

Resistance

Alarm

State of dynamic equilibrium

*Modeled after Byrne and Thompson, 1972.

physical trauma or exertion. In the hospital setting, we can expect to hear more complaints about obtaining insufficient sleep since people in a stressful environment require more sleep than usual.

The functions of sleep posited by Hartmann (1973) are complex. Some of the most salient features of his work refer to insomnia. For example, among aphasic patients, those whose aphasia was improving (i.e., relearning) had significantly higher REM time than those aphasic patients who were not improving. Also, total sleep time and REM time has been found to be decreased in children with mental deficiencies and old people with chronic brain syndrome when compared with age-matched controls. These studies suggest, according to Hartmann (1973), that mental functioning, or learning ability, is related to REM time. It is suggested that people have increased REM requirements during periods of learning as well as during periods of psychic stress.

Apart from events directly connected with surgery, such as preoperative teaching–learning and the anxiety involved, unfamiliarity of the hospital environment itself may be considered a stressor that decreases the efficiency of sleep. Patient complaints about loud night noises and uncomfortable pillows belong in this category. Another factor is that the ability to tolerate change decreases with increasing age; this further taxes coping mechanisms, increasing patient anxiety levels and decreasing the quality of sleep.

The largest category of factors decreasing a patient's Sleep Efficiency Index involves characteristics of patients themselves. Generally speaking, efficiency of sleep decreases as we grow older. Sleep efficiency remains at about the same level from 3 through 30 years of age, then it drops markedly for men. After 49 years of age, it drops for both men and women and continues to drop rapidly with increasing age. This means that after age 49, individuals spend less of the total time spent in bed asleep. It is important to reassure patients that their changing sleep patterns are normal. Abnormal signs of sleep disturbance should not be ignored, however.

With regard to sleep latency, there is little change between the ages of 3–70 for men and 3–80 for women. Men 70 to 80 years of age had the largest increase over all other subjects. *Sleep latency* is the time from lights out to the onset of first stage sleep. There is high variability in sleep latency at either end of the age spectrum; there is no easy explanation for this trend. We can expect some patients over 60 years of age in the clinical setting to take a long time to fall asleep.

The number of times an older person wakes up during the night is another factor interrupting sleep on the clinical unit as well as in the patient's home. After 40 years of age, the number of awakenings increases sharply for men and gradually for women until age 70–75 years, when it rises sharply for women as well. On the nursing unit, we can expect patients (especially after age 40) to awaken more frequently in the night as a natural occurrence. Women, however, should not evidence such frequent awakenings until their seventies and if it occurs earlier, the nurse can suspect a dyssomnia. In some cases, patients may need reassurance that their patterns are normal. Nurses need to be aware of normal versus abnormal awakening patterns related to age and sex.

Another interesting change in sleep patterns over the years involves the amount of stage 1 sleep during the course of the night. Stage 1 is the lightest stage and is associated with less restful sleep; its frequency is higher for men than for women throughout life, reaching a peak in old age. This is important because it tells us the patient over 55–60 years of age is more susceptible to awakening at night by stimuli that nurses typically regard as insufficient to disturb sleep. There is a concomitant decrease throughout adulthood in the percentage of stage 4, or delta, sleep. By the time they are 70–80 years old, males have no stage 4 at all. If Hartmann's (1973) hypothesis that stage 4 has an anabolic function for restoring the body after stress is correct, then decreased stage 4 sleep may be considered an additional stressor for the elderly surgical patient.

Comparing sleep characteristics of patients 50 years of age or older to that of young adults shows that it is more difficult for older patients to obtain efficient sleep before hospitalization. Older patients bring these difficulties as additional stressors into the clinical setting. Hospitalization, which may be seen as contributing to stress intensification, further disturbs dynamic equilibrium.

We need additional data derived from direct testing in the clinical area where sleep disturbances were first identified as a problem. For study purposes, it would be necessary to keep track of the exact number, age, and sex of patients along with admission sleep history including whether they have problems sleeping. Then the number of awakenings and, if possible, the stage of sleep, should be recorded; reasons given by patients for being awakened should be elicited. Once data about what percentage of awakenings are baseline for the particular unit and what, according to the patients, is the stimuli waking them are obtained, the environment could be altered to mitigate or eliminate aggravating factors. Subsequent studies could be undertaken to determine whether the patients' Sleep Efficiency Index was raised.

COPING WITH SLEEP DISTURBANCES IN THE CLINICAL SETTING

Based on observations of patients and a framework for looking at patient stress, I developed a model to depict the dynamics of nocturnal awakening in hospitalized patients aged 50 or more years (Figure 17-1). Even though the validity of the conceptual model derived thus far has not been ascertained, some implications for nursing action can be identified. As already mentioned, familiarity with normal changes in sleep patterns permits the nurse to detect dyssomnias and reassure patients who question the normality of their own sleep patterns.

Hospitals are designed and built to accommodate waking activities. Design alterations could be made to minimize noise, especially on units with older patients who, as a function of increased age, have decreased arousal thresholds. Carpeting in the halls and quiet addressographs might increase sleep efficiency markedly. Since we know now that older people do awaken more frequently during the night, the unit should be staffed sufficiently to accommodate this activity level and ensure safe trips to the bathroom, meet food and fluid needs, and provide interpersonal contact. More specific questions on patients' admissions as part of the data base would be helpful, for example, are patients long or short sleepers? What time do they go to bed and get up? Do they usually take sleeping medications and if so, what kind?

According to Hartmann (1973, pp. 53–70) long sleepers are people who tend to have personalities or life-styles characterized by worry, depression, and anxiety. Though they are more neurotic than short sleepers, they are more often creative and unconventional. Short sleepers tend to be nonworriers, somewhat conformist, energetic, ambitious, and extroverted. Long sleepers sleep 9 + hrs/ night; short sleepers sleep 6 hrs/night.

The question of whether or not to administer sleeping medication is a complex one. Fass (1971) points out that it is important to maintain REM suppressants if patients are used to taking them since sudden cessation causes "REM rebound," with accompanying nightmares and increased numbers of vivid dreams. Also, REM suppressants should be continued in persons with ulcers or angina, which may be exacerbated by REM sleep. Patients whose physician regularly prescribes a REM suppressant should be told of the REM rebound effect and surgeons involved should be asked to discuss their rationale for prescribing a REM suppressant when drugs such as Dalmane, a non-REM suppressant is available. One sleep-disturbing problem for eye patients is eye drops ordered for round-the-clock administration. Surgeons who routinely order antibiotic eye drops to be given every 2 hours despite the fact there is no proof of the practice being of value, should be asked to reconsider the desirability of this in view of recent sleep research.

Fass (1971) found nurses correct in evaluating a patient's sleep only 50 percent of the time; nursing needs to develop criteria for such evaluation. Clues such as rate and depth of breathing and eye movements could be considered as sleep indicators. The system of evaluation would have to be unobtrusive and undisturbing to the patient. Another variable for consideration could be number and frequency of movements in bed during a 60-second observation period, along with other variables mentioned, which would then be compared with patients' estimations of how well they slept.

Differential diagnosis is important too, since age is only one factor associated with dyssomnia. Depressed patients awake at 3 or 4 A.M. and cannot get back to sleep. If they do fall asleep again, it may be toward daylight. Fear has a well-known relationship to restless and fitful sleep; immobility or required change in sleeping position require years of adaptation. Meanwhile, various kinds of sleep disturbance occur in both young and old people. The menopause is a period of life when changes in sleep patterns typically occur. Night sweats and hot flashes occurring at night may interrupt sleep for considerable periods.

Another hospital routine that should be reevaluated on the unit observed involves the taking of vital signs at 6 A.M. instead of at 8 A.M.; many patients seem to dislike waking at the earlier hour. Formal study, as proposed earlier, would confirm or deny this assessment as well as the others outlined. If confirmed, this is the sort of patient-advocate role nursing can play. This chapter is only the first step in concept clarification of insomnia.

REFERENCES

Berthold, J.S. Theoretical and empirical clarification of concepts. *Nurs. Sci.* 2:406–422, Oct. 1964.

Bradner, J.A. (Ed.). Sleep disorders: Help for the patient who can't sleep. *Patient Care* pp. 98–133, Feb. 1, 1976.

Byrne, M.L., and Thompson, L.F. *Key Concepts for the Study and Practice of Nursing.* St. Louis: Mosby, 1972. P. 51.

Clift, A.D. (Ed.). *Sleep Disturbance and Hypnotic Drug Dependence.* Amsterdam: Excerpta Medica, 1975.

Dement, W.C. *Some Must Watch while Some Must Sleep.* San Francisco: Freeman, 1975.

Drucker-Colin, R.R., and McGaugh, J.L. (Eds.). *Neurobiology of Sleep and Memory.* New York: Academic, 1977.

Fass, G. Sleep, drugs, and dreams. *Am. J. Nurs.* 71:2316–2320, Dec. 1971.

Hartmann, E.L. *The Functions of Sleep.* New Haven: Yale University Press, 1973.

Jouvet, M. The States of Sleep. In T.J. Teyler (Ed.), *Altered States of Awareness.* San Francisco: Freeman, 1972. Pp. 51–59.

Jovanovic, U.J. *The Nature of Sleep.* Stuttgart: Gustav Fischer Verlag, 1973.

Kales, A. (Ed.). *Sleep: Physiology and Pathology.* Los Angeles: University of California, 1969.

Williams, D.L. Sleep and disease. *Am. J. Nurs.* 71:2321–2324, Dec. 1971.

Williams, R.L., Karacan, I., and Hursch, C.T. *Electroencephalography of Human Sleep: Clinical Applications.* New York: Wiley, 1974.

Chapter 18

Disorientation

Karma Castleberry and Frances Seither

"I NEVER FELT THAT WAY. IF YOU FEEL LIKE THAT, YOU MUST BE CRAZY!"

The word *disorientation* evokes strong emotions including frequent denial when individuals are asked to relate personal experiences with loss of orientation. Reluctance to share such experiences may be associated with negative connotations of disorientation. Belittlement and disrespect for this alteration in cognitive functioning is clearly evident, even though the common terms are tempered by humor. Phrases such as "out to lunch," "out of one's gourd," "out in left field," "spaced out," and "freaked out" suggest that the mind has separated from its conscious state. Other terms such as "mixed-up," "addled," "fuzzy-headed," "befuddled," "bemuddled," and "muzzy" suggest an internal kind of mental disorganization.

For many, the term *disorientation* connotes a psychotic disorder and words such as "cuckoo," "crazy," "loco," "nutty," "psycho," and "wacky" are used as synonyms. The tendency to equate disorientation and psychosis helps explain the pervasive denial of the phenomenon and the defensive behavior used to avoid detection. The response of a 75-year-old female interviewed at a bus stop illustrates the reluctance to discuss such experiences. In spite of assurances that disorientation is not uncommon and being given examples of the investigator's personal experience with disorientation, the woman emphatically denied that she had ever been disoriented about the time of day or her location. As the interview continued, the woman displayed increasing defensive behavior and agitation. Pointing a finger at the investigator, she shouted, "I never felt that way. If you feel like that, you must be crazy. You'd better have your head examined. I had a cousin who didn't know where she was and something was wrong with her head. She got put in the loony bin for 3 weeks!"

COMMON ATTITUDES AND EXPERIENCES

Willingness of people to admit or discuss experiences of disorientation has an inverse relationship with age. Interviews with a random sample of subjects in three age categories (adolescence, middle years, and old age) indicated that the younger group had less reluctance to describe personal disorientation even though they had found the experience frightening to some degree. Youths frequently described spatial disorientation while traveling in a car at night or when wakening from sleep during daytime travel. The predominant method of coping with the sensation was to mentally retrace the route or to study a map. An 18-year-old described feelings of panic while driving home on an interstate highway. As she passed signs signalling approaching towns, she suddenly realized that she did not know where she was or even the name of her home town. The questions, "What is wrong with me?" and "Am I getting senile?" flashed through her mind. Her anxiety continued to rise until she recognized a familiar landmark and was able to regain her orientation.

An 18-year-old male described the rationalization he used to overcome feelings of disorientation while searching for a fairgrounds in a nearby town. Failing to find the fair in the expected location, he concluded that the fairgrounds had been moved, thus reconciling the environment with his visual expectations. Students readily expressed feelings of spatial disorientation on entering a new school, particularly if their schedules were changed during the first week of class. Feeling "stupid" or "dumb" was a commonly shared reaction.

Middle-aged people's responses to the question, "Have you ever felt disoriented?" were often couched in humor. A frequent reply was, "You've come to the right person. I'm always disoriented." When they realized that the investigation was serious, interviewees quickly disqualified their responses by such statements as, "I'm almost never disoriented" or "I only get disoriented once or twice a year."

In the older age group (people over 65 years), there was marked resistance to sharing feelings of disorientation. Reactions to questions ranged from angry denial to repudiation of anxiety through humor. A 70-year-old male denied he had ever experienced such sensations but agreed that he had observed the behavior in others. When asked to describe what disorientation would be like, he replied, "Oh, just running along in neutral." For several elderly people, the question was so threatening that they refused to talk to the investigator after learning of the interview topic. In contrast, two sisters initially denied having ever been disoriented but later admitted they joked about the situation when such "stupid" behavior occurred. The relationship between age and denial of disorientation experience is not unexpected. Disorientation has long been associated with the mental deterioration believed to occur throughout aging. Thus, the older an individual becomes, the greater the anxiety about becoming disoriented. From a developmental perspective, individuals are permitted time to become oriented early in life. Once attained, orientation is expected to be continuous until the decline of cognitive functioning due to aging processes begins. Denial of cognitive deterioration may be a useful mechanism for maintaining a sense of stability and competence.

In spite of the connotation of mental illness or deterioration attributed to disorientation, there are numerous examples of the phenomenon in ordinary experiences of individuals who have no pathological disorder. People often report momentary disorientation of location when stepping off elevators and find themselves looking in both directions for a familiar landmark. Others indicate that, once disoriented in a new locale, they find it particularly difficult to feel oriented in that location again. For example, a college professor first approached a small campus on a rainy night and became disoriented, experiencing panic when he couldn't get his "bearings." For the next 5 years, he approached that area of the campus on a daily basis and continued to feel disoriented. The feelings of panic gradually lessened as he reminded himself that the disorientation was "usual." Another man told of visiting a small city on a regular basis. He, too, experienced feelings of disorientation during the initial contact. This recurred each time he entered the city, in spite of the fact that the streets were laid out in a systematic plan.

Automobile drivers often experience anxiety because the countryside looks suddenly strange while traveling over a seemingly familiar route. Habituation to redundant stimuli with the disappearance of the orienting response (alpha attenuation response) is a common adaptive mechanism of the CNS and explains the fleeting experiences of disorientation to highway driving. The momentary disorientation experienced by automobile drivers can also be explained by the automatic behavior syndrome, which is characterized by continuation of mechanical activity as orientation to the activity decreases.

While mild and episodic in most people's experiences, even fleeting disorientation can become hazardous in certain occupations. In an endeavor to investigate rumors of disorientation experienced by long-distance truck drivers, interviews were conducted at a truck stop on an interstate highway. Questions posed to truckers regarding such experiences were met with resistance and denial. One driver who had emphatically denied experiencing disorientation on the highway shouted as he pulled away from the truck stop, "You're wasting your time; they'll lie to you."

In certain occupations, such as fire fighting, sensory alteration may be the antecedent for loss of orientation. Firefighters frequently experience disorientation to both time and place while fighting fires in smoke-filled buildings in which they can no longer depend on sight or touch for orientation. Although firefighters are placed in simulated training sessions with blindfolds and heavy gloves during training, they require many months of actual experience in fires before they are able to rely on other orienting senses. This disorientation poses a particular hazard since firefighters must frequently depend on a limited supply of oxygen. It is not unusual for firefighters to complain that their oxygen tanks were not completely filled when in actuality, disorientation to time came during the frenzy of the fire-fighting activities. Scissor staircases cause momentary disorientation for many people who can quickly assess their error. For the fire-fighter, the failure to become oriented after climbing such a staircase can be life-threatening to both him- or herself and those in need of rescue.

Airline pilots may experience a sense of disorientation during take-off on dark nights. This phenomenon has been recognized for at least 25 years as a cause of night-time take-off accidents. There is an apparent displacement of the vertical that may occur when the sitting body undergoes longitudinal acceleration in the absence of visual pitch information. This sensation is attributed to failure to distinguish between the true vertical and the result of gravity and acceleration forces. Thus, the pilot may experience the illusion of excessive upward pitch and attempt corrective measures that direct the plane into a dive. The phenomenon has been reported more frequently over "textureless" terrain during an extremely dark but fogless night. These conditions may induce pilots to ignore their instruments in favor of using the terrain as a guide. Hours of experience in the air have not been a significant factor in protecting pilots from this form of disorientation (Buley and Spelina 1970).

NURSING AND THE CONCEPT OF DISORIENTATION

In spite of the numerous experiences with disorientation that occur in everyday life, the concept has received minimal attention. The term appears most frequently in medical literature as a symptom of certain physical conditions, a side effect of medications, or a result of the aging process. The common dictionary definition, "to cause to lose one's bearings; to displace from normal position; and loss of sense of time, place or identity" is the context in which disorientation is used most often in medical and nursing literature. Efforts to describe disorientation in any detail, however, are almost nonexistent. The concept has not been sufficiently developed to require a topic heading in *Index Medicus, Cumulative Index to Nursing, and Allied Health Literature* and *International Nursing Index. Psychological Abstracts* has listed a small number of references during recent years. Within the nursing literature, texts devoted to fundamentals of practice and medical–surgical nursing frequently fail to list the term in their indexes. In other textbooks, discussion of the concept is often restricted to one or two paragraphs. Within nursing periodicals, case studies are occasionally provided depicting nursing problems encountered in the care of the disoriented patient. Nursing techniques, which have been effectively used to facilitate return to orientation, are also described (Budd and Brown 1974; Hirschfeld 1976; Hogstel 1979; Morris and Rhodes 1972; Putnam 1976; Richard 1975; Schwab 1973; Twist 1976; and Voelkel 1978). A general indifference within the profession is suggested by the paucity of research and available information.

PREDISPOSING FACTORS

A number of conditions or factors seem to predispose or be etiologically implicated in the occurrence of disorientation. None of these factors occurs in all cases of disorientation nor does disorientation necessarily accompany the condition. Disorientation may be a side effect of certain medications such as L-dopa, amatadine, the tricyclines, antihypertensives, L-asparaginase, lithium, and some sedatives and tranquilizers (Davis 1976; Hodkinson 1975; and Holland, Fasanell, and Onuma 1974). Substance abuse can also produce disorientation. Some users of cannabis and LSD suggest that the production of disorientation is an event at least partially under the individual's own control and is related to the user's physical setting and mind set.

Cerebral involvement with systemic lupus erythematosis and scleroderma, Alzheimer's disease, metastatic brain lesions, arteriosclerotic disease, strokes, and brain tumors can be accompanied by disorientation (MacNeil, Grennan, Ward, and Dick 1976; Reichel 1976; Whitehead 1974; and Wise and Gingler 1976). Closely resembling the patient with actual organic brain damage is the patient whose disorientation develops after electric convulsive treatment (Arnot 1975). Metabolic conditions of hypoglycemia, diabetic precoma, hyperthyroidism, hyperparathyroidism, and uremia may cause temporary disorientation. Deficiencies of Vitamin B_{12} and magnesium, as well as generally poor nutrition, have also been implicated (Epstein 1976; Gatewood, Organ, and Mead 1975; and Hodkinson 1975). Severe electrolyte disturbances such as those occurring with peritoneal dialysis or in burn patients can cause disorientation (Richard 1975); correction of the deficiency or imbalance changes the disoriented state. Wahl (1976) noted that both MI and congestive heart failure patients may have disorientation as the presenting symptom prior to other clinical findings. Persons who experience excessive daytime sleepiness or narcolepsy, with episodes ranging from a few minutes to a few hours, have no orientation to time on awakening (Guilleminault, Billard, Montplaisir, and Dement 1975).

Disorientation can also result from sensory deprivation, sensory overload, or altered sensory acuity. This phenomenon has been described in normal volunteers under experimental conditions, in geriatric patients, and in patients in medical and surgical ICUs (Gimbell 1975; Kornfeld, Zimberg, and Malm 1965; and Wahl 1976). Windowless or heavily curtained rooms, the monotonous sound of air-conditioning, respirators, and monitors were explained by experienced ICU nurses as conducive to disorientation. Decreased sensory acuity, especially prominent in the elderly, limits the amount of auditory and visual orientation stimuli. Schwab (1973) and Jahraus (1974) noted a "distortion" of sensory input with failing hearing and eyesight. In a study of 60 disoriented postoperative patients, Morse (1969) concluded that sensory distortion was one of the multiple causes of disorientation of his population. Disoriented roommates, incomplete information, as well as nurses' agreement with patients' misconception can also be major sources of distortion for hospitalized patients.

Sensory overload from continuous monitoring, frequent awakening, bright lights, and extraneous noises contribute to disorientation. Patients' failure to anticipate these events also seems to be a factor. Many nurses have noted that careful preoperative preparation for such occurrences substantially decreases postoperative disorientation (Budd and Brown 1974).

Closely associated with sensory overload is sleep deprivation. Under experimental conditions, subjects experienced disorientation, memory loss, and visual disturbances as the number of hours awake increased (Freeman 1972). In a study of psychiatric complications of open-heart surgery, Kornfeld and colleagues (1965) failed to find a relationship between postoperative "delirium" and patient age, sex, marital status, or length of procedure. They found, however, that between the third and fifth postoperative day, 36 percent of patients experienced either perceptual distortions, hallucinations, or disorientation, which cleared when the patients received more sleep.

ASSOCIATED FACTORS

There is some evidence of a relationship between disorientation and depression. In a small sample of intensive care patients who developed disorientation after initially making good progress, depression was found to be closely associated with disorientation (Brock-Utne, Cheetham, and Goodwin 1976). Epstein (1976) reported that a small proportion of depressed elderly go through a phase of disorientation that usually subsides within a short period of time. It is at this point that the underlying depression becomes more apparent.

Disorientation frequently appears or increases at night. Kornfeld and co-workers (1965) identified paranoid behavior during day and nighttime disorientation in postoperative patients. Nurses report that certain patients become disoriented at night and then become oriented again in the morning, usually after breakfast. These patients, often elderly, become known as "sundowners." Butler and Lewis (1973) hypothesized that this phenomenon is due to loss of visual orientation when daylight ends and lights are turned off. Many nurses, however, note that patients in windowless rooms with constant lighting still exhibit sundown syndrome. This poses the question of the influence of the individual's biorhythms.

Other factors have been linked to the occurrence of disorientation. Based on a pilot study of patients admitted for medical problems who subsequently became disoriented, Nowakowski (1980) identified predisposing factors within the family system and within the health care system. Study patients were found to have abdicated decision-making responsibility regarding significant health care matters. Family and health care workers typically failed to discuss the patient's health or plan of care with them, and the patient did not ask for this information. Despite abdication of responsibility for such decisions, the patient felt dissatisfaction with decisions made by others. Nowakowski (1980) concluded that disorientation was a signal of anxiety occurring as a function of family and health care systems. She hypothesized that the "stress that contributes to loss of functioning in disorientation is stress of unresolved decisions."

Some authors consider disorientation a major problem in the elderly (Hodkinson 1975; Lowenthal and Berkman 1967; Twist 1976; and Wahl 1976). According to Hirschfeld (1976), an insufficient supply and/or utilization of oxygen and glucose may be causative factors. Symptoms of severe disorientation, however, are probably related to degenerative cerebral changes and are not symptoms of "normal" aging. Gustafson and Risberg (1974) reported normal blood flow and metabolism are not affected by age, at least not before age 70.

Wahl described progression toward disorientation as beginning with the older person's difficulty in screening out irrelevant stimuli coupled with poorer concentration ability. Pressure to act and hurry also impairs perception and confounds the difficulty. Hodkinson (1975) noted that disorientation may indicate physical illness in the elderly, especially if disorientation is of recent onset or exacerbation. A pneumococcal infection, for example, may be heralded by fever or increased pulse rate in a younger patient but by disorientation in the elderly.

Loss, whether of health, spouse, peers, employment, or familiar environment, is also a factor in disorientation (Hirschfeld 1976; and Twist 1976). Wahl views disorientation in the elderly as a phenomenon connected with a network of social relations; thus when family ties are broken, feelings of disorientation are universally experienced. Nursing home staff identify an initial disorientation, which seems to be a function of recent change and loss, in many of their newly admitted residents. It is not unusual for a resident to have moved from home to a hospital and then to a nursing home within a few week's time. Accompanying loss of a familiar environment is the necessity of adapting to a new environment. The resultant disorientation in elderly residents usually subsides within a week but may last as long as a month.

A synergistic effect seems to be produced when a combination of predisposing factors exists. Onset of disorientation was noted in an older man following the death of his wife. Alarmed, his daughter spoke to the family physician who suggested eliminating her father's tranquilizer prescribed to prevent a "grief" reaction. Discontinuing the tranquilizer and carefully monitoring other medications resulted in an abrupt end to disorientation. The synergistic effect is also exemplified by the case of a 60-year-old woman who climbed over her siderails each night. Stumbling into the hallway, she was completely disoriented to time and place. She had undergone bilateral cataract surgery several days before and had been lying flat in bed except for her brief nocturnal excursions into the hall. Episodes of "sundown" disorientation continued until eye bandages were removed and sensory deprivation as well as immobilization were alleviated.

MANIFESTATIONS

Manifestations of disorientation are dependent on the type and intensity of predisposing factors. Loss of orientation to time, including day, hour, and year is common and is the earliest form to appear. Loss of sense of place often follows, with the inability to recognize persons indicative of still further progression. Failure to know one's own identity is the most extreme form of disorientation. Behavior suggesting loss of orientation may range from increased questioning to physical combativeness. Early overt signs of disorientation include increased motor activity, often described as restlessness and a searching behavior involving both head and eye movements. Bed patients have a tendency to focus intently on objects hanging from above with a fascination that suggests unfamiliarity. Nurses often describe disoriented patients as having a "puzzled look" and seeming to worry a great deal. Touching or pursing the lips, making soft whistling sounds, or crying without apparent reason are all common behaviors of the disoriented. Picking at clothing or bedding, tearing paper into small pieces, and aimlessly moving hands and arms have also been reported. Increased hostility toward staff during administration of treatments and nursing care is often encountered. Both physical and verbal abuse may be exhibited as patients attempt to cope with feelings of fear and helplessness.

Numerous behaviors indicate a need to escape. It is not unusual to hear disoriented patients say, "Something is wrong. I've got to get out of here." Getting out or attempting to get out of bed at inappropriate times often reflects the need to flee an environment no longer comprehensible or to seek familiar surroundings. Older patients may dress themselves during the night and begin to pack their belongings. Escape behaviors seem to be more reflective of people with place disorientation. Restraints are often used to prevent escape; however, their effect upon disorientation is equivocal.

Loss of time orientation is often observed among individuals who have been severely injured or who are seriously ill. Older persons often place themselves in a framework of earlier events. A burn unit patient continued to worry that he would not get his load of produce delivered on time. In actuality, the man had not driven a truck for several years. An additional example is provided by the elderly woman who insisted on calling her sister by her maiden name and indicated no awareness that her sister had been married for many years. Similarly, a nursing home occupant described her relationship with her husband in such clear detail that new nursing personnel were amazed to find the woman had been a widow for 15 years. It is also commonplace to find an older individual who can recognize a neighbor he has not seen for several years but fails to identify a son or brother.

When individuals describe their state of disorientation, they state "I *am* disoriented" or "I *have been* disoriented." Unlike many physical conditions that can be described as an "attack," feelings of disorientation permeate the entire self. Failure to isolate experience to a particular organ system may help explain the pervasive feeling of helplessness and loss of control. Persons who have experienced disorientation can often share their fears and bewilderment as time, place, and person become increasingly vague. Adjectives used to describe the sensation include feeling "hazy," "foggy," "in a daze," or "in a muddle." Some disoriented persons describe the feelings as "fuzzy" or being in a dreamlike state. The disoriented person frequently has feelings of depreciation and describes him- or herself as "stupid" or "dumb." A young male accident victim related, "I felt mad because I couldn't get a handle on things. It made me feel ignorant, that something was wrong with my brain." Others stated feelings of tension and frustration. Many could share feelings of isolation from the world. One young man who became disoriented following severe personal stress was able to express that his wife seemed like a stranger. Pausing a few moments, he corrected himself with, "No, I was the stranger." Many patients reported feeling "scared" and indicated they had no idea what was happening to them. There was a universal feeling of helplessness and loss of control over themselves and their environment. A feeling of embarrassment was not uncommon and several were reluctant to have family or friends see them in their disoriented state. Others complained of feeling physically "drained" from increased tension.

PATIENT ADAPTATION

As individuals return to an oriented state, they often try to clarify feelings and perceptions. When the nurse suggested to an elderly woman that she might be disoriented, the woman replied, "No, I'm not as mixed up as I was. I just haven't been able to get everything straight in my mind." Other patients show recognition of nurses' efforts to reorient their thinking but find themselves unable to comply. One aging woman cautioned, "You're upsetting me with all your questions. I can't think right now, but I know you're trying to help." Patients also report, "Yesterday (or last week) everything was fuzzy, but today things are getting clear again."

Patients use a variety of devices to reorient themselves to person, place, or time. Questions such as, "What day is this?", "Where am I?" and "What's wrong with me?" are frequently posed to intensive care nurses. Patients find a need to trace events back in time prior to their accident, illness, or surgery; others have need to structure their environment in ways that limit the amount of unfamiliar stimuli experienced. Some patients find coping devices unique to their particular situation. One young accident victim frequently "got lost" when he left his bed and ventured out into the corridor. Reluctant to admit disorientation, he discovered that his name and room number were posted on the wall near the nurses' station. He quickly learned to seek this orienting cue when ready to return to his room. Another man reported that he looked for a newspaper each morning to find what day it was rather than admit his disorientation to time.

Some patients reported feelings of disorientation apparently undetected by staff. A badly burned firefighter reported having no knowledge of where he was or what had happened to him during his week of hospitalization, yet progress notes not only failed to indicate signs of disorientation but reported the patient. was talking coherently. Some patients display a facade of orientation to overcome feelings of chagrin. In response to the nurse's question, "Who is the President?" a smiling patient replied, "Honey, don't you know?" Others attempt to cope with lowered self-esteem by such remarks as, "I wish you knew me when I was well—the way I used to be." Individuals disoriented over long periods of time are reported to have occasional lucid moments. An elderly nursing-home occupant who was disoriented to person, time, and place was confined by a latch on the screen door of her room. One evening the nurse accidentally locked herself in the patient's room and was startled to hear a chuckle followed by a low voice saying, "Now you know how it feels." These vignettes provide evidence that individuals can experience disorientation that goes undetected by caretakers while others considered markedly disoriented may have periods of unexpected orientation. These examples suggest that problems posed by disorientation may be a function of the environment in which it occurs.

For some individuals, disorientation may have an adaptive function. For those experiencing sensory overload or sensory deprivation, disorientation can provide alterations in the sensory environment. In crisis situations that reach intolerable limits, disorientation may psychologically remove the person from the crisis environment. An example of this function is demonstrated by the widow who chose to live in a time preceding her husband's death. Disorientation also provides a signal for assistance from the external environment when other coping devices are inadequate. It is an expectation in many societies that individuals exhibiting severe disorientation will be placed in a dependent position concerning self-care needs.

A flow chart (Figure 18-1) provides a schematic description of the adaptive function of disorientation.

Figure 18-1 Flow Chart of Adaptive Function of Disorientation

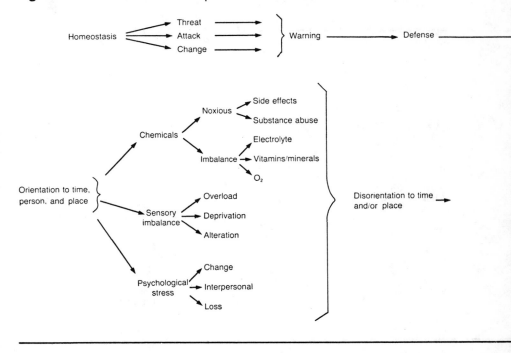

Nursing notes as well as published literature frequently have words such as "confusion" used synonymously with "disorientation." Thus, attempts to communicate various states of cognitive functioning as well as distinguish between them have been difficult (Dodd 1978; Lipowski 1967; Williams et al. 1979). For example, Dodd developed a tool to describe behavioral changes in mental status. Based on her operational definition, disorientation is viewed as a more severe impairment than confusion but less severe than delirium. In contrast, Davidhizar, Gunden, and Wehlage (1978) defined confusion as disorientation plus memory impairment. Williams and others differentiated between the two terms by stating that disorientation can be operationalized and tested in terms of loss of time, place, or one's identity. Confusion, on the other hand, tends to include "several disorders of consciousness, memory attention, comprehension, mood and interpretation of stimuli."

Certain commonalities can be identified regarding the concept disorientation that provide a framework for development of a typology (Table 18-1). This beginning typology describes five phases which, it is hoped, will further differentiate the concept. Most individuals experience Phase I at some time in their lives. For others, Phase I may begin the progression toward more severely

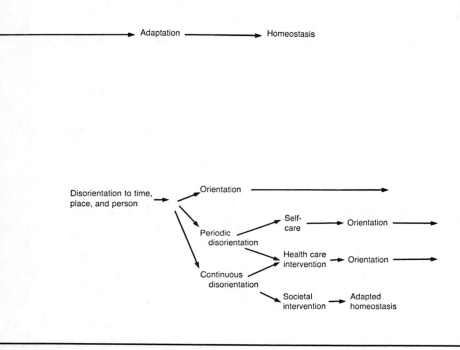

disoriented behavior. Because disorientation accompanies or results from a variety of biological and psychosocial conditions, the individual may progress through the phases at various rates of speed. For example, in severe injury, disorientation may not be recognized until Phase IV or V, while among the elderly the time in each phase may be distinct and prolonged. There are insufficient research data to determine if each phase occurs in an orderly progression.

Beginning efforts in clarifying the concept of disorientation have suggested numerous questions that warrant investigation. The following examples are provided to stimulate further research:

1. Does combativeness increase as disorientation progresses from Phase I through Phase V?
2. Do physical restraints increase the degree of disorientation?
3. Is there a relationship between age and degree of disorientation in restrained patients?
4. Is there a relationship between degree of physical activity in the elderly and the incidence of disorientation?
5. Do patients who wear their own clothing in health care facilities exhibit less disorientation than those who wear clothing provided by the institution?

Table 18-1 Beginning Typology of Disorientation

Phase	Symptoms
Phase I	Mild anxiety Feeling of something being "wrong" Questioning of perceptions "Fuzziness" or "fogginess" Mental "retracing" and searching for the familiar Momentary time or space disorientation
Phase II	Increased motor activity Aimless hand/arm movements "Searching" behavior involving head/eye position Feelings of bewilderment, helplessness Anger, inner-directed behavior Cognitive defect, labeled "dumb" or "stupid" Inability to identify time or place
Phase III	Attempts to "escape" Increased anxiety Picking at bedclothes Touching, pursing lips Whistling sounds, moaning, crying Hostility, verbal/physical abuse Inability to identify time and place
Phase IV	Combative/docile Inability to identify time, place, and other persons
Phase V	Combative/docile Inability to identify time, place, and self

6. Do patients in long-term facilities who are encouraged to meet their self-care needs exhibit less disorientation than those placed in a dependent position?
7. Is there a relationship between the incidence of disoriented behavior and the amount of environmental lighting?
8. Is there a relationship between the number of environmental changes and incidence of disorientation?
9. Is there a relationship between unresolved decisions concerning health care and the onset of disorientation?

REFERENCES

Arnot, R. Observations on the effects of electric convulsive treatment in man—Psychological. *Dis. Nerv. Sys.* 36:499–502, 1975.

Brock-Utne, J., Cheetham, R., and Goodwin, N. Psychiatric problems in intensive care. *Anaesthesia* 31:380–384, 1976.

Budd, S., and Brown, W. Effect of a reorientation technique on postcardiotomy delirium. *Nurs. Res.* 23:341–348, 1974.

Buley, L., and Spelina, J. Physiological and psychological factors in the dark night takeoff accident. *Aerospace Med.* 41:553–556, 1970.

Butler, R., and Lewis, M. *Aging and Mental Health.* St. Louis: Mosby, 1973.

Cohen, C. Nocturnal neurosis in the elderly: Failure of agencies to cope with the problem. *J. Am. Geriatr. Soc.* 246:86–88, 1976.

Copeland, J., Kelleher, M., Kellett, J., and Gourlay, A. A semi-structured clinical interview for the assessment and diagnosis of mental state in the elderly: The geriatric mental state schedule: I. Development and reliability. *Psychol. Med.* 6:439–449, 1976.

Copeland, J., Kelleher, M., Kellett, J., Gourlay, A., Cowan, D., Barron, G., and de Gruchy, J. Cross-national study of the diagnosis of the mental disorders. *Br. J. Psychiatry* 126:11–20, 1975.

Davidhizan, R., Gunden, E., and Wehlage, D. Recognizing and caring for the delirious patient. *J. Psychiatr. Nurs.* 16:38–41, 1978.

Davis, J. Overview: Maintenance therapy in psychiatry: II. Affective disorders. *Am. J. Psychiatry* 133:1–13, 1976.

Dodd, M. American mental status. *Am. J. Nurs.* 78:1501–1503, 1978.

Epstein, L. Depression in the elderly. *J. Gerontol.* 31:278–282, 1976.

Freeman, F. *Sleep Research.* Springfield, Ill.: Thomas, 1972.

Gatewood, J., Organ, C., and Mead, B. Mental changes associated with hyperparathyroidism. *Am. J. Psychiatry* 132:129–132, 1975.

Gimbell, L. The pathology of boredom and sensory deprivation. *Psychiatr. Nurs.* 16:12–13, 1975.

Guilleminault, C., Billiard, M., Montplasir, J., and Dement, W. Altered states of consciousness and disorders of daytime sleepiness. *J. Neurol. Sci.* 26:377–395, 1975.

Gustafson, L., and Riseberg, J. Regional cerebral blood flow related to psychiatric symptoms in dementia with onset in the presenile period. *Acta Psychiatr. Scand.* 50:516–538, 1974.

Hackett, T. The psychiatrist's view of the ICU: Vital signs stable but outlook guarded. *Psychiatr. Ann.* 6:14–27, 1976.

Henrichs, T., MacKenzie, J., and Almond, C. Psychological adjustment and psychiatric complications following open-heart surgery. *J. Nerv. Ment. Dis.* 152:332–345, 1971.

Hesse, K. Meeting the psychosocial needs of pacemaker patients. *Int. J. Psychiatry Med.* 6:359–372, 1975.

Hirschfeld, M. The cognitively impaired older adult. *Am. J. Nurs.* 76:1981–1984, 1976.

Hodkinson, H. The elderly mind. *Br. Med. J.* 2(5961):23–25, 1975.

Hogstel, M.O. Use of reality orientation with aging confused. *Nurs. Res.* 28:161–165, 1979.

Holland, J., Fasanell, S., and Onuma, T. Psychiatric symptoms associated with L-asparaginase administration. *J. Psychiatr. Res.* 10:105–113, 1974.

Jahraus, A. Who is confused? *Nurs. Homes* 23:6–7, 1974.

Kornfeld, D., Zimberg, S., and Malm, J. Psychiatric complications of open-heart surgery. *N. Engl. J. Med.* 273:287–292, 1965.

Lipowski, Z.J. Delirium, clouding of consciousness and confusion. *J. Nerv. Ment. Dis.* 145:227–255, 1967.

Lowenthal, M., and Berkman, P. *Aging and Mental Disorder in San Francisco.* San Francisco: Jossey-Bass, 1967.

MacNeill, A., Grennan, D., Ward, D., and Dick, W. Psychiatric problems in systemic lupus erythematosis. *Br. J. Psychiatry* 128:442–445, 1976.

Milstein, V., Stevens, J., and Sachdev, K. Habituation of the alpha attenuation response in children and adults with psychiatric disorders. *Electroencephalogr. Clin. Neurophysiol.* 26:12–18, 1969.

Moidel, H., Giblin, E., and Wagner, B. *Nursing Care of the Patient with Medical–Surgical Disorders.* New York: McGraw-Hill, 1976.

Morris, M., and Rhodes, M. Guidelines for the care of confused patients. *Am. J. Nurs.* 72:1630–1633, 1972.

Morse, R. Postoperation delirium: A study of etiologic factors. *Am. J. Psychiatry* 126:388–395, 1969.

Nowakowski, L. Disorientation—Signal or diagnosis. *J. Gerontolog. Nurs.* 6:197–202, 1980.

Putnam, M. Fiery and bewildered. *Nurs. Mirror* 142:67, 1976.

Reichel, W. Organic brain syndrome in the aged. *Hosp. Pract.* 11:119–125, 1976.

Richard, C. Nursing implications in the prevention of complications in peritoneal dialysis. *Heart Lung* 4:890–893, 1975.

Schwab, M. Caring for the aged. *Am. J. Nurs.* 73:2049–2053, 1973.

Twist, R. Psychogeriatric patients need encouragement and acceptance. *Psychiatr. Nurs.* 17:8–10, 1976.

Voelkel, D. A study of reality orientation and resocialization groups with confused elderly. *J. Gerontolog. Nurs.* 4:3–18, 1978.

Wahl, P. Psychosocial implications of disorientation in the elderly. *Nurs. Clin. North Am.* 11:145–155, 1976.

Webster, I. Aging and the relativity of time. *J. Am. Geriatr. Soc.* 24:314–316, 1976.

Whitehead, J. *Psychiatric Disorders in Old Age.* New York: Springer, 1974.

Williams, M., Holloway, J., Winn, M., Wolanin, M., Lawler, M., Westwick, C., and Chin, M. Nursing activities and acute confusional states in elderly hip-fractured patients. *Nurs. Res.* 28:25–35, 1979.

Wise, T., and Gingler, E. Scleroderma cerebritis: An unusual manifestation of progressive systematic sclerosis. *Dis. Nerv. Sys.* 36:60–62, 1975.

Wood, R. Psychological medicine: Organic illness. *Br. Med. J.* 1(5960):723–726, 1975.

Nipple Confusion in Neonates

June Kroh Kershner

One- to three-day-old neonates relay overt behavioral cues when they cannot properly grasp the nipple–areola junction in their attempts to suckle. Upon closer investigation, we could identify these cues as confusion. This confusion occurs when neonates cannot obtain a proper grasp of the maternal nipple–areola junction, either because the nipple is inverted or the breast is engorged. Some neonates demonstrate overt confusion over the mammary nipple after alternately being given the breast and the bottle.

The significance of dealing with nipple confusion in neonates is more than solving the physical problems of inverted nipples and engorged breasts. These are of vital importance, but the problem goes much deeper. While observing this phenomenon, we become aware of how American maternity–neonatal care practice encourages neonatal nipple confusion. Such practices as delaying the first breast feed, offering water and formula to the breast-fed newborn, restricting newborns to a four-hour schedule for feeding, ambivalent prenatal counseling, and separating mother and infant can enhance the problems underlying nipple confusion and thereby encourage bottlefeeding.

Nipple confusion is of utmost significance because, unrecognized and un treated, it may ultimately lead to maternal lactation failure.

DEFINING NIPPLE CONFUSION AND DESCRIBING ITS PROPERTIES

The confusion observed in the neonate is a lack of ability to distinguish, choose, or act purposefully to achieve a specific goal. One example of this purposeless behavior was observed while a neonate was attempting to breast-feed and was evidenced by the following behaviors.

The subtle cues that point toward neonate confusion included clinching eyes, rapidly blinking eyes, compressing lips, puckering face by a combination of lip compression and frown, slightly protruding tongue between lips, pouting by protruding lower lip, or making an ugly face by slightly raising upper lip as if in disgust and wrinkling nose.

More potent behavioral cues of confusion are increased activity of legs and arms, leg kicking, straightening and tensing legs and arms, and increased hand-to-mouth activity. The cry face, a combination of many subtle negative cues, was followed by such verbal cues as whining, fussing, or angry crying. The whining was prolonged, high-pitched, and not rhythmical; it was repeated only a few times in succession. Fussing tended to be short, low-pitched vocalizations without rhythm. The angry cry was forceful but low in volume and of short duration. It was rhythmical with vocalization and 1–2 second pauses.

Another characteristic of the newborn's confusion was that seemingly purposeless behavior related specifically to inability to properly grasp the nipple–areola junction. Increased confusion leads to greater frustration and the neonate's behavior becomes more restless and disorganized, often to the point of exhaustion (giving up).

SUGGESTED CAUSAL RELATIONSHIPS

Specific factors contribute to nipple confusion in the neonate. Nipple inversion, whether mildly flat or severely inverted, will contribute to neonatal confusion. If a woman with any degree of nipple inversion were correctly instructed during the prenatal period about specific nipple exercises for increasing nipple protractility, the newborn would subsequently be able to grasp the nipple properly. Even postnatally, the problem may not be recognized, and the mother has to bottle-feed because the infant nurses poorly and the poor nursing grasp makes her nipples increasingly sore. Improper grasp hinders good suckling, which ultimately inhibits milk production. Maternal anxiety increases both with nipple pain and the infant's poor nursing. Anxiety is one factor that hinders milk letdown so that an adequate supply is available to the infant.

Another condition contributing to nipple confusion is breast engorgement. When the breasts are engorged, the neonate has difficulty grasping the nipple–areola junction because the area is convex. The infant makes an effort to suck the inverted nipple and, in the process, causes soreness and injury to the nipple epithelium. In addition, normal breathing space is nonexistent, and the infant becomes frustrated in the attempt to nurse. The practice of waiting 3 to 5 hours or longer before the initial breast feed contributes to engorgement. A neonate's strongest sucking reflex often occurs within the first 30 minutes after birth. Putting the newborn right to the breast encourages milk production and stimulates the letdown reflex. Supplementary bottles encourage engorgement, whereas supplementary nursing enhances milk drainage. Rigidly scheduled feeding routines add to this problem. When a breast-fed infant is not permitted to feed on demand, crying with hunger between feedings may occur. Then the infant may be too exhausted to nurse when feeding time comes.

The practice of routinely supplementing healthy breast-fed newborns with bottled formula and water confuses the oral response. Applebaum (1970) graphically illustrates differences in sucking mechanisms at the breast and bottle (Figure 19-1).

Applebaum's (1970) diagram portrays how adapting to the breast may be more difficult and confusing to neonates who have become used to the easy flow of

Figure 19-1 Differences in Suck Mechanisms between the Breast and Bottle

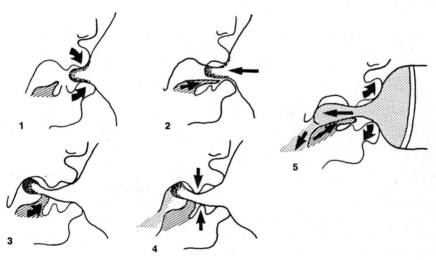

1. Lips of the infant clamp in a "C" shape at the concave junction of the nipple and areola, fitting "like a glove." Cheek muscles contract.
2. Tongue thrusts forward to grasp the nipple and areola.
3. Nipple is brought against the hard palate as the tongue pulls backward, bringing the areola into the mouth. Negative pressure is created by the action of the tongue and cheeks against the nipple, and the result is a true sucking action.
4. Gums compress the areola, squeezing milk into the back of the throat. Milk flows against the hard palate from the high-pressure system of the breast to the area of negative pressure at the back of the throat.
5. In contrast, the large rubber nipple of a bottle strikes the soft palate (causing gagging) and interferes with the action of the tongue. The tongue moves forward against the gum to control the overflow of milk into the esophagus. Lips are flanged into an "O" shape; compression does not occur because the cheek muscles are relaxed.

Source: Used by permission of R.M. Applebaum.

formula from the bottle nipple. Since less work is required for bottle feeding, desire for the breast may be lost. When complementary feedings have to be administered, the duration of breast-feeding is doubled when the extra feedings are given by teaspoon or dropper according to one study (Unger 1949).

PHYSIOLOGICAL, CULTURAL, AND BEHAVIORAL THEORIES RELATED TO NIPPLE CONFUSION

A search of the literature revealed little related specifically to nipple confusion in the neonate. Using this limited literature, I explored physiological, cultural, and behavioral theories indirectly related to nipple confusion in the neonate.

Some of the physiological theories or principles relating to neonatal nipple confusion have already been mentioned.

> One of the main difficulties with proper breastfeeding today is the so-called flat or inverted nipple. If this abnormality is not corrected . . . before breastfeeding begins, the procedure is usually not satisfactory or successful (Hoffman 1953).

As a clinician, he claims success with a method intended to loosen adhesions at the nipple's base. The nipple is made erect by stimulation using the opposing thumbs in a horizontal plane; the procedure is repeated with the thumbs in a vertical plane. As the nipple protracts, adhesions at the base are broken, and maximum nipple protractility is maintained for a proper nursing grasp (Hoffman 1953). Confusion results when the newborn cannot draw the nipple well into the mouth. It is important that the nipple's attachment to the breast be loose enough to permit it to be drawn to the back of the baby's mouth. In that way, the baby can keep the nipple in his or her mouth and the back of the hard palate is stimulated sufficiently to elicit the sucking reflex.

Applebaum's theory (1970) concerning the differences in oral mechanics of breast- and bottle-feeding and how this can contribute to the newborn's nipple confusion has already been cited.

Another theorist describes this confusion.

> The suckling reflex response to the breast can be interfered with and superseded by the "super-sign stimulus" of the larger, more easily flowing teat of the feeding bottle. The first type of intraoral stimulation introduced into the mouth of the infant creates a typical automated response to the stimulus (Gunther 1955).

Naish (1956) showed that infants who suck at the breast are stimulated by the maternal nipple to suck by a "compression" action of the lips, gums, and cheek muscles, thrusting the tongue first forward and then backward as the nipple and areola are pulled back into the posterior oral cavity. In contrast, Straub (1960) demonstrated that introduction of the rubber nipple creates a tugging response, with flanging of the lips, relaxation of the cheek muscles, and an anterior motion of the tongue thrusting forward between the gums and the rubber nipple. These authors support the concept that differences exist between orodynamics in bottle- and breast-feeding.

Cultural theories concerning nipple confusion in the newborn are unmentioned in the literature. Jeliffe (1962), in extensive studies in primitive cultures, made some interesting observations regarding breast-feeding. Breast-feeding problems are almost unknown of in cultures where bottle-feeding has not been introduced. He found that the unsophisticated tropical village mother is the world's expert in practical breast-feeding. He also found that bottle-feeding has had a deleterious impact on tropical infant nutrition—partly because of failure of breast-feeding (1978). The possibilities of confusion in breast-feeding greatly increase in areas where the bottle is becoming a symbol of progress and modern living, and breast-feeding is declining.

In the Mayan Indian culture of the Yucatan, essentially all babies are breast-fed. "Breastfeeding begins within minutes after birth and afterwards the baby is suckled whenever it shows signs of being hungry or upset" (Jordan 1978). A factor common to all Mayan women, as well as tropical peasant mothers, is the irregularity of breast feeds both during the day and night. Scheduled feeding is an American concept.

In the United States, the common practice of giving complementary feeds to newborns interferes with both sucking reflex and letdown reflex.

> By decreasing appetite, it can lead to diminished sucking at the breast by the infant; by suggesting the mother's inadequacy it can lead to anxiety and interference with her let-down reflex. It may also habituate to bottle-feeding because milk can be obtained with less effort. "Mixed milk feeding" can also confuse the baby, as the sucking mechanisms are different for breast and bottle (Jeliffe 1978).

In regard to behavioral theories, the newborn possesses two instinctive reflexes needed for successful breast-feeding: (1) *the rooting reflex,* in which the touch sensation on the cheek leads to turning the head and opening and closing the mouth as the baby seeks the nipple, and (2) *the sucking reflex,* in which the tactile "sign stimulus" of the nipple–areola area of the breast filling the mouth sufficiently and adequately leads to a milking action by the tongue against the hard palate (Barnett 1972). Rooting and sucking reflexes are often strongest immediately after birth, so vigorous nipple stimulation at that time can help in initiating a letdown reflex. The mother of a confused infant who cannot suckle properly will not experience this milk flow.

> The stimulus of suckling triggers nerve impulses from receptors in the nipple which ascend to the hypothalamus and evoke the release of oxytocin. The hormone is then carried in the blood stream to the mammary gland where it acts on a contractile effector tissue (the myoepithelial cells) and forcibly expels the milk from the alveoli and small ducts (Cowie and Tindal 1971).

Prolactin is the hormone that stimulates milk production by causing gland cells to synthesize fat, lactose, and protein necessary for milk. Prolactin levels are maintained by neurohormonal response to sucking and nipple stimulation (Larson 1978).

Nipple confusion in the neonate then may set up a complex chain of events. The confused neonate sucks improperly; maternal anxiety increases; milk letdown reflex diminishes; inadequate milk for infant results, nipple confusion increases.

Figure 19-2 Conceptual Model of Nipple Confusion

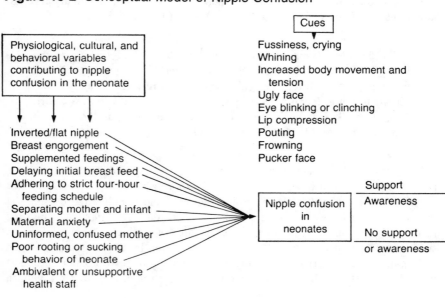

EXPLANATION OF BEGINNING CONCEPTUAL MODEL

A wide range of factors influence nipple confusion in the neonate, the behavioral cues given by the neonate, and the consequences of the neonatal confusion. Variables contributing to nipple confusion are of physiological, cultural, and behavioral origin.

Physiological variables include degree of maternal nipple inversion and whether there is breast engorgement. Cultural variables that are primarily Americanized maternity practices include supplemented feedings, delayed initial breast feed, adherence to a strict three- or four-hour schedule and separation of mother and infant. Behavioral variables include at least: degree of maternal anxiety, an uninformed mother ignorant about breast feeding; level of rooting and sucking behavior of the neonate. An ambivalent or unsupportive health care personnel may be another cultural variable.

The infant gives off a variety of negative behavioral cues, both verbal and nonverbal, when he or she is experiencing nipple confusion (Figure 19-2).

When these cues are observed, problems related to neonate nipple confusion can be confronted and, likely, eliminated. When nipple confusion is resolved,

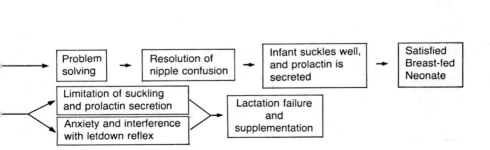

the infant can properly grasp the nipple–areola junction and suckle. This stimulates prolactin, which in turn stimulates milk production. This may permit the mother to be relaxed and experience an effective letdown reflex.

When neonate nipple confusion goes unnoticed, the infant never properly grasps the nipple–areola junction. Limited suckling limits prolactin secretion and milk production. Maternal anxiety may then increase because the infant is not breast-feeding well. Maternal anxiety response is inhibitory or antagonistic to the normal hormonal milk letdown reflex. Lactation failure ultimately leads to bottle supplementation.

In conclusion, two hypotheses about nipple confusion in the neonate can be stated.

1. The neonate who has a proper grasp of the nipple–areola junction appears less confused than the neonate who cannot properly grasp the nipple–areola junction.
2. The neonate who solely breast-feeds will show less nipple confusion than the neonate who breast-feeds and receives supplemental bottles.

REFERENCES

Applebaum, R.M. The modern management of successful breastfeeding. *Pediatr. Clin. North Am.* 17:217, 1970.

Barnet, H.L. (Ed.). *Pediatrics* (14th ed.). New York: Meredith, 1972. P. 87.

Cowie, A.T., and Tindal, J.S. *The Physiology of Lactation.* Baltimore: Williams & Wilkins, 1971. P. 186.

Gunther, M. Instinct and the nursing couple. *Lancet* 1:575, 1955.

Hoffman, J.B. A suggested treatment for inverted nipples. *Am. J. Obstet. Gynecol.* 66(2):346, Aug. 1953.

Jeliffe, D.B. Culture, social change and infant feeding. *Am. J. Clin. Nutr.* 10:34, Jan. 1962.

Jeliffe, D.B. *Human Milk in the Modern World.* Oxford: Oxford University Press, 1978. P. 24.

Jordan, B. *Birth in Four Cultures.* Quebec: Eden Press Women's Publications, 1978. P. 30.

Larson, B.L., and Smith, V.R. (Eds.). *Lactation: A Comprehensive Treatise. The Mammary Gland, Human Lactation, Milk Synthesis,* Vol. 4. New York: Academic, 1978. Pp. 195–196.

Naish, C.F. *Breast Feeding.* London: Lloyd-Luke, 1956. P. 38.

Otte, M.J. Correcting inverted nipples—An aid to breastfeeding. *Am. J. Nurs.* 75:3:454, Mar. 1975.

Straub, W.J. Malfunction of the tongue. *Int. Am. J. Orthod.* 46:404, 1960.

Ungar, R. Zwiemilchernahrung und stilldauer. *Kinderaerztl. Prax.* 17:289, 1949.

Chapter 20

Immobilization in Adolescents

Audrey J. Kalafatich

According to Bernabeu (1952) and Anna Freud (1952), the importance of movement and the use of motor discharge to handle stress poses a particular and unique problem when motor activity is impaired. In illness, two types of limitations on motor activity occur. In one type immobility is forced; in the second it is self-inflicted (i.e., voluntary). When the nature of the disease process is such that the individual is physically unable to move, as with paralytic polio-myelitis, or when mechanical devices such as a cast are used, the immobilization is forced. Self-inflicted immobilization occurs in illnesses, such as cardiac conditions or tuberculosis, that require bed rest. During illnesses requiring rest, the individual is compelled to impose or voluntarily imposes the immobility upon him- or herself. We would expect the effects of immobilization to be substantial in adolescents because of the need to discharge energies related to the stresses of this phase of development.

THE LITERATURE ON IMMOBILITY

The paucity of reports on studies of immobility required a literature survey of more than 30 years to describe how adolescents handle impaired motor activity. One small study found that reactions to immobility are similar regardless of whether restraint is forced or voluntary. Reactions of two patients with tuberculosis were compared with the reactions of children in plaster casts. Both sets of patients experienced inhibited emotions as well as inhibited activity. They feared death or consequences of movement so much that fear itself acted as a restraint on the children as strongly as mechanical restraint (Burlingham 1953).

Dubo (1950), in reporting a study of children with tuberculosis, seemed to disagree with Burlingham. She reported that her subjects asked for help; for example, they asked to be tied in bed to help them to maintain bed rest. Since one normal response to danger is increased physical activity, Dubo (1950) concluded that these children asked for protection against their instinctual impulse to action.

Bergmann (1945) studied patients from 2 to 16 years of age in the course of orthopedic treatment. These children showed "more movement and lively kinesthesia in their drawings and art work than productions of other children of the same age." This observation was supported by Bernabeu (1952), who found that in severely crippled children lack of mobility led to fixation on activity. Focus on activity by immobilized patients was also reported by Hetherington (1964) in a comparative study of the relationship between motor disabilities and cartoon references. Three groups with 20 10–12-year-old children in each group were compared. Group I included children with poliomyelitis; group II comprised children with cerebral palsy; and group III included children identified as normal. The children with poliomyelitis preferred activity cartoons and thought they were funnier than nonactivity cartoons. No preference between types of cartoons was shown by either children with cerebral palsy or those considered normal.

Denial of the occurrence or of the effects of the illness and the immobility led to a kind of "false" contentment in the children observed by Bergmann (1945), Robinson (1956), and Schechter (1961). Burlingham's (1953) observations of children led to the conclusion that physical restraint resulted in a "restraint of affect" as well. Prange (1957) reported his subjective reactions to a diagnosis of paralytic poliomyelitis and remembered his initial "It doesn't matter" attitude helped him to defend against anxiety by the use of denial.

A study of 30 children with limited mobility related to rheumatoid arthritis found that the life-styles of these children were structured around a drive for motor activity and the need to be "physical" (Cleveland, Reitman, and Brewer 1965).

Smith and Henry (1967, p. 460) identified psychological consequences of immobilization as including isolation from routines of peers, disruption of one's sense of time and space, as well as changes in the ways the future is anticipated.

A study of 12 children aged 6 to 17 who had limited mobility but who had never been fully mobile suggested that skills that have not been developed for use and that have not been part of a child's armamentarium for interacting with the environment are not missed. These 12 children with osteogenesis imperfecta, who had varying degrees of physical deformity and inadequate musculature, restricted their mobility to avoid spontaneous fractures and were little traumatized by lack of motor activity (Reite, Davis, Solomons, and Ott 1972).

Substitutes for movement are sought in many ways, and there is increased attention to various forms of activity. Wright (1955) saw clinging to the knowledge of past abilities and to what things used to be like before the illness as both a motivational factor in adjustment and as a depressive factor in terms of a hopelessness in the present and future.

The subjects of the studies by Bernabeu (1952) and Burlingham (1952) were found to have gained vicarious pleasure from activity of others in their attempts to handle their own immobilization. Not only were they preoccupied with the kinds of activity other people engaged in but they also used controlling behavior to get other people to do things that they could not do for themselves. In a sense, other people became the "legs" for the immobilized child; the immobilized child gained by substituting activity of others for his own activity. Prange (1957) stated that he resented the activity and agility of young nurses. He much preferred to have less agile, older nurses care for him.

Deprived of the ability to be active, tuberculosis patients observed by Wittkower were able to "seek and find a vicarious outlet in (increased) speech . . . and (increased) fantasy." Wittkower (1952) concluded that his subjects found "substitute gratification in pleasant thought. . . ."

A study of two groups of hospitalized children reports that children immobilized because of orthopedic problems had a four times greater incidence of elevated blood pressure. A group of 56 children with a mean age of 12 who were immobilized with orthopedic problems and a group of 48 with a mean age of 11 hospitalized for other reasons were compared. One hypothesis is that correction through stretching was the causal factor. But children who had casting without stretching had the same ratio of elevated blood pressure so immobilization was identified as an important factor. Whether this is related to increased vascular tone associated with hypercalcemia and/or whether there are emotional components or concomitants was not studied (Turner, Ruly, Buckley, and Strife 1979).

Houk (1980) discusses adolescent immobility within the larger framework of disability, including mental disability. She examines disability in terms of adolescent developmental tasks and supporting the accomplishment of these tasks rather than formulating the constellation of responses to the disabilities themselves. Mobility problems are not developed apart from the whole construct of disability.

In summary, individuals may be immobilized because of the nature of their illness; they may be "ordered" or requested to "bed rest" as with cardiac conditions, or they may impose immobilization on themselves.

A survey of the literature to determine how the subjects of mobility studies handled the impaired motor activity was done. Lack of mobility leads to a fixation on activity. Denial of the occurrence or of the effects of the illness and the immobility was seen in some patients as well as a "restraint of affect." Patients' sublimation of movement included increased attention to activity of others, controlling behavior to get other people to do the things they could not do for themselves, increased speech and fantasy, and a clinging to knowledge of past activity.

The next section reports some findings of a study I did and illustrates the concept of immobilization. This descriptive study was designed to use participant observation in order to examine and clarify in part, the responses of adolescent girls to prolonged immobilization produced by corrective treatment for scoliosis.

IMMOBILITY AND ADOLESCENCE

One characteristic change in moving from childhood to adolescence is an increase in physical activity. In addition to having excess physical energy, adolescents use action as a normal means of relief from tension and anxiety (Deutsch 1944). In some adolescents, action serves not to reduce anxiety to a manageable level, but rather to make it possible for them to avoid having to endure it at all (Deutsch 1944).

Adolescent subjects of this study were immobilized by a body cast. They faced treatment demands, especially demands of living in a body cast as well as having major surgery, which deprived them of the ability to be mobile. Gross body movement was limited by size and nature of the cast. Observational data were studied to permit description of the kinds of mobility behaviors or attempts at mobility that occurred in subjects during hospitalization.

For purpose of this study, mobility was defined as any kind of motor movement, substitutions for movement, and self-imposed nonmovement. Included in the category of motor movement behaviors was any kind of rhythmic motion such as rocking or stroking the self, excessive walking, tapping fingers and licking lips, and activities such as playing cards or playing games. The category of substitution for movement included increased verbalization, concern with the activity of others independent of the subjects, and use of others for self-stimulation, such as having others rub their bodies. Self-imposed nonmovement behaviors included subjects being nonmobile at times when motor movement was possible and generally expected. The nonmovement category included silence, withdrawal, pretended sleep, and the inability to do simple tasks or to follow simple directions.

The treatment regime the five subjects underwent included admission to the hospital for cast application and spinal fusion. Patients spent one week in the hospital prior to cast application. During this week, X rays were done, photographs taken, blood work done, and subjects became acclimated to the hospital. Following cast application (Risser Turnbuckle Jacket), one week after admission, each patient spent three weeks in bed in the cast during which time the cast was manipulated in order to straighten the patient's back. After this three-week interval, surgery for spinal fusion was done. Two days postoperatively, patients were discharged.

Patient Adaptation to Immobility

In analyzing the mobility behaviors, these 12 to 14 year olds displayed very little movement prior to cast application. This is the period when one would expect a great deal of gross body movement as they faced impending immobilization from the cast. Even though patients knew they were facing immobilization as a part of treatment, they imposed on themselves a certain immobilization. On admission and during the first few days of hospitalization, subjects remained in their beds or at their bedsides. Apparently, admission to the hospital was difficult enough for patients to cause them to restrict themselves to a circumscribed area in or around their beds. This phenomenon concurs with studies cited earlier in which admission to the hospital required patients to admit to the reality of illness and to their need for treatment. Another factor in maintenance of a circumscribed environment with limited mobility may be that of adjusting to the hospital environment as well. Patients were reluctant to become members of the ward group. In their little physical worlds, they did not appear to be a part of the hospital or its milieu and, therefore, could not engage in activities that would cause them to project themselves into the ward. Patients moved only if told to or if taken somewhere by either the investigator or by a member of the unit nursing staff. By the time they had spent 2 or 3 days in the hospital, patients were able to move about the ward a little more freely and began to actively interact with other patients. Other patients were usually in the same age group but were not in body casts; subjects were still able to deny to some extent their own impending cast applications.

Subjects fluctuated between nonmovement and motor movement as they waited to be called to the cast room for cast application and as they waited outside the cast room. They seemed to use nonmovement to withdraw from the external environment and also seemed during these periods of inactivity to be deep in thought. Motor movement displayed during this waiting period was a means for them to occupy the time. As they waited outside the cast room, they paced aimlessly. Motor movement, such as quivering lips, seemed to be in response to the anxiety patients felt as they waited.

Almost all mobility behaviors ceased as soon as patients were placed on the cast table, except for one subject who talked during the entire procedure. Increased verbalization is a common form of flight to get away, at least mentally, from a very difficult situation.

A marked decrease in mobility behaviors occurred immediately following cast application, followed by a noticeable increase on the day the cast was cut and the turnbuckles begun (3–4 days after application). By the time turnbuckles had been inserted, patients had mastered the skill of manipulating cast and body as one. More substitutions for movement occurred on this day than at any other time during hospitalization. Subjects increased verbalization in all areas, that is, they talked with no obvious purpose; they talked of self-activity and of the activity of others. Subjects were more free within the cast after the area had been cut out around the middle; more freedom within the cast seemed to be related to more freedom of speech. Also, patients at this time had recovered from the initial impact of the cast and seemed able to react directly to immobilization by seeking other outlets for activity.

The most outstanding mobility behavior during the 3-week period from the beginning of the turnbuckles until patients were prepared for surgery was the gross rocking motion seen in all of them. Each patient, while positioned on the side, would rhythmically rock body and cast back and forth. This rhythmic rocking was almost continuous and occurred independent of any other activity patients were engaged in. Leg movements in which they kicked the lower leg at the knee was also a means of physical motion and occurred independent of other activities. Both forms—gross body movement and leg kicking—were a means of self-stimulation. Since self-stimulation did not particularly occur during stress situations but rather almost constantly during the periods of observation, it is probably not a means of tension reduction. Patients were not questioned about movements and therefore it was not known how they interpreted these behaviors.

Several authors cited in the literature stated that immobilized patients received vicarious pleasure from activities of others. But Prange (1957) said that when he was immobilized with poliomyelitis he resented the agility of the young nurses. The behaviors of the subjects of this study seemed to be similar to both reactions; that is, they especially seemed to receive pleasure from the activities of the nurse–researcher; on the other hand, they resented her ability to come and go as she pleased. The subjects all showed interest in hearing about the nurse–researcher's activities when she was not at the hospital. They also needed to control the activities of the nurse–researcher while she cared for them. The subjects used the nurse–researcher as a substitute for their own leg movement by excessively having her run errands or get things for them.

Returning to the cast room for the preparation for surgery seemed to be stressful for patients as they increased mobility behaviors. Each patient resumed behavior similar to that demonstrated during the first visit when the jacket had been applied.

Mobility behaviors decreased on the day of surgery and during the postoperative period. Patients appeared to be too physically ill to display any mobility behaviors and, in addition, movement was painful.

Patients had a high frequency of occurrence of mobility behaviors the day they had their stitches removed. Return to the cast room to have stitches removed and the cast filled in found subjects repeating behaviors they had demonstrated on the two previous trips for casting and surgery preparation. They apparently found being in the cast room a difficult situation regardless of the reason for being there. Substitutions for movement, especially in the form of increased verbalizations, were most frequently displayed each time the subject returned to the cast room.

CONCLUSION

In summary, this study describes the reaction of early adolescent girls to a treatment regime that immobilizes the girls in body casts. The subjects of this study reacted with some motor movement, substitutions for movement, and with nonmovement when we would have expected them to be mobile.

Hypotheses and questions arising out of this study that need to be answered for further explication of the concept of immobility in adolescents include

1. Is there a sequence of processes young adolescents use in coping with long-term immobilization?
2. Threat to life is more important than extreme immobilization of early adolescents.
3. The degree of immobilization determines the health of coping strategies. (Almost total striated muscle paralysis will produce more flight-coping strategies than small circumscribed-area paralysis.)
4. Sudden immobilization produces greater numbers of flight-coping strategies than immobilization that is planned.
5. Immobilization with a long-term trajectory produces a greater number of flight-coping strategies than short-term immobilization.
6. Grief about loss was not evident in this study. Was it selectively inattended? Does the short-term nature of the immobilization or the anticipation of improved mobility or other factors ward off feelings of loss?
7. Does short-term immobility significantly delay or modify the accomplishment of adolescent developmental tasks?

REFERENCES

Bergmann, T. Observations of children's reactions to motor restraint. *Nerv. Child* 4:318–326, Jul. 1945.

Bernabeu, E. The effects of severe crippling on the development of a group of children. *Psychiatry* 21:169–194, 1952.

Burlingham, D. Notes on Problems of Motor Restraints during Illness. In R.M. Loewenstein (Ed.), *Drives, Affects, Behavior.* New York: International Universities Press, 1953.

Cleveland, S., Reitman, E., and Brewer, E. Psychological factors in juvenile rheumatoid arthritis. *Arthritis Rheum.* 8:1152–1158, Dec. 1965.

Deutsch, H. *Psychology of Women: Girlhood,* Vol. 1. New York: Grune & Stratton, 1944.

Dubo, S. Psychiatric study of children with pulmonary tuberculosis. *Am. J. Orthopsychiatry* 20:522, 1950.

Freud, A. The role of bodily illness in the mental life of the child. *Psychoanal. Study Child* 7:75, 1952.

Hetherington, M.E. Humor preferences in normal and physically handicapped children. *J. Abnorm. Soc. Psychol.* 69(6):694–696, 1964.

Houk, N.G. The Disabled Adolescent: Promoting a Positive Self-Concept by Achievement of Developmental Tasks. In P.L. Chinn and K.B. Leonard (Eds.), *Current Practice in Pediatric Nursing.* St. Louis: Mosby, 1980.

Prange, A.J., and Abse, D.W. Psychic events accompanying an attack of poliomyelitis. *Br. J. Med. Psychol.* 30(2):82, 1957.

Reite, M., Davis, K., Solomons, C., and Ott, J. Osteogenesis imperfecta: Psychological function. *Am. J. Psychiatry* 128:1540–1545, June 1972.

Robinson, H.A., Finesinger, J., and Bierman, J. Psychiatric considerations in the adjustment of patients with poliomyelitis. *N. Engl. J. Med.* 254(21):975–980, May 24, 1956.

Schechter, M. The orthopedically handicapped child: Emotional reactions. *Arch. Gen. Psychiatry* 4:247–253, Mar. 1961.

Smith, K.V., and Henry, J.P. Cybernetic foundations for rehabilitation. *Am. J. Phys. Med.* 46:379–467, Feb. 1967.

Turner, M.C., Ruly, E.J., Buckly, K.M., and Strife, C.F. Blood pressure elevation in children with orthopedic immobilization. *J. Pediatr.* 95:989–991, Dec. 1979.

Wittkower, E. Psychological aspects of physical illness. *Can. Med. Assoc. J.* 66:22, Mar. 1952.

Wright, M.E. The Period of Mourning in Chronic Illness. In M. Harrower (Ed.), *Medical and Psychological Teamwork in the Care of the Chronically Ill.* Springfield, Ill.: Thomas, 1955.

Chapter 21

Immobilization: Psychosocial Aspects

Becky Jane Christian

INTRODUCTION

Immobility is inconsistent with human life. It poses a threat to the nature and survival of the individual. Inherent in the human condition is the ability and drive to be mobile. Through mobility people are able to exert control over their environment. If mobility is restricted, the ability of the individual to retain control is threatened. Without control, we are at the mercy of our environment. Immobilization threatens survival.

Speed, mobility, flexibility, and versatility are the essences of our active lives. Activity is the power to start something; the power to move ahead, progress, or advance; the power to play and compete; the power for many kinds of work; the power to excite and arouse; the power to respond and change; and the power to maintain and present oneself using a design of one's choosing. Airplanes, hydroplanes, automobiles, dune buggies, motorcycles, speed boats, bicycles, and skateboards are all incorporated into our self-images and become part of our own identities. With so many expectations and options for an active life, even a short period of immobility may have serious overtones for one's life-style. More than ever immobility is of concern in nursing care.

WHAT THE WORDS TELL US

Webster's Dictionary (1971, p. 1130) defines immobilization as "the rendering of a part incapable of being moved." The scope of immobilization is substantial, going from minor decrease in range of motion of a small area (e.g., a sprained digit) to a more complete loss of mobility such as that incurred with a spinal cord injury (e.g., quadriplegia) in which the body is capable of little or no purposive movement. Existence of the broad spectrum of immobility is the basis for definitional problems inherent in concept clarification.

341

Immobilization is referred to in the common vernacular by descriptions of a person being "laid up," "flat-on-one's-back," "a shut in," "bedridden," "zoned," and "out-of-it," as well as "favoring" or "splinting" the movement of a body part. Each of these expressions describe types and degrees of immobilization indicating the broad range of the phenomenon.

Words typically used to denote immobilization are "motionless," "restrained," "restricted," "limited," "confined," "rigid," "fixed," and "immovable." These terms have a negative connotation in representing loss of inflexible state that is unchanging and characterized as disabling. Negative values are further explicated in the designations of "cripples," "wheelies," "burdens," and "vegetables." Nicknames such as "crip," "quad," "pegleg," "gimpy," or "rubber legs" are not uncommon. Immobilization is often used as if the person were a "quad" instead of identifying a person who has a limitation. The language of immobilization evokes derision in others and stigmatizes the victim. This compounds the problems of people who are immobilized. Another source of disapproval is when a person is thought to be able to be mobile or does not become mobile as fast as others think he or she should. In these cases, a person may be treated like a faker.

Negative connotations of immobilization are compounded by cultural ideals of youthfulness, wholeness, and beauty. Individuals who are immobilized are often unable to approach societal ideals because of distortion, destruction, or harm to a body part. People who are unable to approximate societal ideals may develop problems in somatic identity and body image. People who perceive themselves as different, inferior, or deviant when devalued by others have identity changes. This change in social identity is called *stigmatization* (Goffman 1963). There is little question about the significance of immobilization to people's self-perception or to the perception of society as a whole (Blackwell 1978). Stigmatization applies more to people immobilized permanently or over a long period of time. Stigmatization occurs to a lesser extent when immobilization is temporary. Permanence and pervasiveness of immobilization determine the body image and life-style associated with immobilization and are viewed by the person as a loss. It is awareness of this loss that precipitates a crisis (Shontz 1975). It is this loss of one's previous mobility and the subsequent changes in life-style that threaten the survival of the immobilized person. Denial, rage, and apathy are typical temporary (and useful) defenses against full awareness of loss.

IMMOBILIZATION: POINTS OF VIEW

Immobilization is one common method used in medical management. It is one outcome of many illnesses, physical disabilities, and trauma. It is an eventual concomitant of aging. Most students of immobilization have explored some physiological aspect of immobilization. There are also psychological and social concomitants and sequelae of immobilization, which have been studied less frequently. This chapter is concerned with these less frequently studied components of immobility.

Limitations imposed by immobilization influence the speed with which the individual is capable of interacting with the environment. Society places a high value on efficiency and productivity, both of which are reduced when immobilization decreases the rate of operation and interaction. Hampered by the rate of physical activity, the immobilized individual fails to function successfully in one or more spheres of activity. The relationship between immobilization and reduction in the rate of interaction with the environment can be illustrated on several levels. Primarily, there is concern with survival. The dependence associated with immobilization focuses attention on basic needs. The main question explicit in fact, is, "Who will take care of me when I cannot take care of myself?" This was exemplified by Debbi, an 18-year-old girl with quadriplegia. She feared what would happen to her when her parents died, feared for her survival of inclement weather, and feared for falling while transferring from bed to wheelchair. A second aspect of immobilization affecting interaction in the environment involves efficiency of the immobilized individual. Even getting dressed becomes a major task requiring much planning and, often, assistance. Debbi was essentially independent in dressing activities; after many position changes and repeated attempts to pull up her jeans, however, it still cost almost an hour of time and much frustration. A third way that immobilization interferes with normal activities relates to individual productivity. The person who is immobilized is limited in ability to perform motor activities. For Debbi, even motor skills such as writing, typing, and dialing a telephone number are major undertakings requiring a significant amount of time to perform as well as correct use of adaptive devices.

RELATIONSHIP BETWEEN AGE AND ONSET OF IMMOBILITY

The relationship between the age when immobility occurs and the developmental tasks an individual is trying to complete at that time may be significant in that requirements for coping may compound tasks necessary for normal growth and development. For example, activity and independence are characteristic of the adolescent. When immobilization is interposed on an adolescent, developmental needs can no longer be met. Debbi had established her independence from her parents by moving into an apartment on graduation from high school. When she was rendered quadriplegic, she was not only paralyzed in the use of her body but also immobilized in her efforts to remain independent.

ONSET, DURATION, INTENSITY, AND SEVERITY OF IMMOBILIZATION

Temporal aspects of duration, onset, and occurrence alter immobilization in terms of the severity of the conditions and the limitation imposed on the life-style of the individual. Duration of immobilization involves the permanence of the condition; the more permanent the condition, the greater the demands on the individual. Onset refers to the time frame in which the immobilization occurs, ranging from a sudden, traumatic immobilization to a chronic, progressive state; both types influence the manner in which the individual adjusts to the condition. The immobilization of an individual also varies according to the intensity and severity of the condition; these factors are related to the duration of the immobilization. Intensity and severity are contingent on the condition causing the immobilization as well as the permanence and pervasiveness of the restricted mobility.

Debbi's immobilization was a devastating experience for her. Her quadriplegia is permanent and pervasive, resulting from trauma sustained in a motor-vehicle accident. Changes in body structure and functions resulting from quadriplegia affect every body system encompassing physiological as well as psychosocial functions. This represents a crisis situation in that Debbi required a complete change in her life-style, relationships, progress in growth, as well as some degree of dependence.

SPATIAL RELATIONSHIPS AND IMMOBILITY

There is distortion of spatial relationships with immobilization. Because of changes in speed of movement, distances may seem much greater and tasks to be performed much more complicated, both in terms of time and space. The body's use of space changes with alteration in body image, loss of mobility, and loss of function. For the immobilized person, life is usually lived in a smaller space than other people live in. Much planning has to go into moving in space or utilization of greater amounts of space. Extending personal space to include a work life may be very stressful to an immobilized person.

LIFE-STYLE AND IMMOBILITY

Changes in spatial relationships create, in fact demand, changes in life-style. Debbi's life-style will be used to illustrate the magnitude of life-style changes associated with immobilization. Debbi's quadriplegia severely restricted her activity level. Her previous life-style involved the use of automobiles, frequent dates, dances, and parties, and shopping and sports activities as a means of socialization with her peer group. She was employed on an assembly line in a factory and shared an apartment with a friend. Her sexual activity involved experimental behavior in confirming her identity as a woman. She enjoyed playing with and caring for her sister's children. With her immobilization from quadriplegia, Debbi can no longer participate in these activities. She cannot drive a car at this time. She cannot dance. She cannot actively participate in sports. She cannot work at the factory. She cannot be independent. Her confinement to a wheelchair severely limits her accessibility to the environment. Her parents' home had to be modified to accommodate a wheelchair. Many stores are inaccessible to her and stairways and curbs are major obstacles. She worries about her appearance and desirability. She worries about her sexuality, her ability to bear children, and her ability to care for children. She is a different person because she is immobilized.

EMOTIONAL LIFE AND IMMOBILITY

Affective components of immobilization are related to loss, grief, change, stigma, and body-image trauma. Immobilization results in loss of mobility and function. This prompts grief about the loss and, ultimately, the individual must acknowledge the change and develop coping strategies for dealing with the loss. Confronting one's own feelings of shame and self-pity as well as confronting the feelings of others are other emotional components of immobility. The immobilized person faces the stigma of failing to achieve social values important in our culture. This is the essence of the psychosocial crisis that occurs when an immobilized person becomes fully aware and apprised of his or her situation and required adjustments. In describing herself, Debbi initially verbalized feelings regarding threats to her body integrity by describing herself prior to the immobilization. Changes in her self-perception were noted in a later description of herself as "the same inside, regardless of the disability." This perception of there being no essential difference in her body integrity served to decrease the magnitude of the threat. Debbi verbalized feelings of loss and the stigmatization of being different from her peers by pondering her ability to bear children, her desirability, and her inability to dance. She exhibited concern about friends "not knowing what to say" to her, sending her "get well" cards when she "really isn't sick" and hopefully promising her that everything will be better when she can walk again. Debbi's inability to walk and participate in other activities important to adolescents such as sports, dancing, and driving must be recognized as loss before she can successfully cope with her immobilization.

Sensory Deprivation

Sensory deprivation is a phenomenon that often occurs with immobilization. Restrictions on movement limit seeking sensory stimulation for the victim. But the stress of the stigmatization on family and friends causes them to create emotional distance that isolates the victim even more. The victim may also at times experience sensory overload such as when he or she is unable to withdraw physically from an environment that is too stressful, too taxing, or too noisy.

OTHER CONSIDERATIONS

Population

Immobilization is not selective in terms of population affected. It can occur congenitally, as a single occurrence in life, periodically throughout a person's lifetime, and as a chronic, progressive condition. Functional capabilities of immobilized people vary from total inability to care for self to independent self-care.

Economics

Immobility carries with it certain economic consequences. Immobilized people are often viewed as poor employment risks, expensive, and requiring continual assistance from others. Productivity of immobilized people may be viewed as low and they are not considered cost-effective. The amount of time required for immobilized people to perform their jobs may make their level of productivity prohibitive in terms of time and money. This generalization fosters the dependence and unemployment associated with people who are immobilized. For immobilized individuals to be gainfully employed, many adjustments and special arrangements must be made. Accessibility to buildings and facilities, transportation, specialized equipment, and assistance from other employees are just a few of these requirements. Generally, it is easier to make people dependent than to make special considerations that allow opportunities to be independent.

Families of Victims

Families of immobilized people experience a psychological crisis just as the victims do (Rapoport 1965; and Shontz 1975). They require anticipatory guidance and support in understanding both behavior and capabilities of their immobilized members (Carlson and Blackwell 1978; and Crate 1965). Debbi's parents and siblings acknowledge her immobilization and are willing to change their lives to a degree and provide support.

WHAT THE LITERATURE REVEALS

Burlingham (1953, p. 171) identified two types of immobilization that occur with illness: (1) forced immobility and (2) "self-inflicted" immobility or bed rest. *Forced immobility* is a condition in which an individual is physically unable to move or in which a mechanical restraining device such as traction or cast prevent movement. *Self-inflicted immobility* occurs when an individual is required to impose the immobility on him- or herself due to the nature of the illness, such as a cardiac condition or tuberculosis.

A study comparing forced and self-inflicted immobilization used two children with tuberculosis and an unreported number of children in plaster casts. Burlingham reported that neither group of patients experienced any inhibition of actions and concluded that reactions of both groups were similar regardless of the type of restraint (Burlingham 1953).

In a study of 25 children with tuberculosis, Dubo used nursing observations as well as individual and group sessions to study children's reactions to illness. Dubo found these children sought assistance to help them maintain bed rest. She concluded that the children were asking for protection against their instinctual impulse to action (Dubo 1950).

In a longitudinal descriptive study of 8 children with poliomyelitis, Bernabeu (1958) found that lack of mobility leads to fixation on activity. A study of psychological factors evident in 30 children with juvenile rheumatoid arthritis indicated they had an unusually strong need for physical expression and a life-style characterized by motor expression (Cleveland, Reitman, and Brewer 1965).

Sibinga and colleagues (1968) studied the effects of immobilization and sensory restriction on affected children, who manifested significantly more severe and frequent emotional disturbances than the control group of 14 children who had not experienced immobilization and sensory restriction.

A study of psychological functioning of 12 children aged 6 to 17 with osteogenesis imperfecta indicated that physical deformities or poorly developed musculature forced children to impose voluntary restriction on their own motor activity to reduce possibility of fractures. Little psychic trauma related to physical restriction was evidenced. It was concluded that "from a psychic standpoint, what has not developed or has not been experienced is not missed, nor is it experienced as a loss" (Reite, Davis, Solomons, and Ott 1922).

Sublimation of the drive to move after becoming immobilized was demonstrated by Wright (1955). Victims were observed clinging to knowledge of past abilities, focusing on pre-illness behaviors, and giving increased attention to various forms of activity. Two investigators found that immobilized children gained vicarious pleasure from the activity of others as a way of handling their own immobilization. In addition to their own preoccupation with activity, children used controlling techniques to get others to do things they could not do for themselves (Bernabeu 1958; and Burlingham 1953).

Orthopedic patients 2 to 16 years old found "more movement and lively kinesthesia in their drawings and art work than the productions of other children of the same ages." It was also found in one study that restraint of one limb may have inhibited other nonaffected body parts. Increased speech was suggested as compensating for restricted mobility (Bergmann 1945, p. 326). In describing an unreported number of children with tuberculosis, Wittkower (1952) found they evidenced increased speech, language, and fantasy activity.

Denial of the occurrence or the effects of illness and immobility led to "false contentment" in children with orthopedic injuries (Bergmann 1945; and Schechter 1961) and children with poliomyelitis (Robinson, Finesinger, and Bierman 1956; and Schechter 1961). Sample sizes were not reported for these studies. Burlingham (1953) concluded from observations of two children with tuberculosis and children in plaster casts that physical restraint resulted in a "restraint of affect." Immobilization of children with dermatologic conditions caused an increase in anger and aggression followed by increases in symptom formation (Musaph 1968).

Several descriptive case studies identify various coping behaviors used by immobilized children. An 11-year-old girl, immobilized for correction of scoliosis, used self-control and control of others to cope with her anxiety resulting from immobilization and hospitalization. In another study, self-control was demonstrated by cognitive mastery, withdrawal, compulsivity, and verbalization of fears and fantasies (Dadich 1972).

Coping behaviors of three physically handicapped children showed each child coped by attempting to control the situation; however, their coping behaviors varied from being good-humored and willing to accept ideas and help from others to demanding behavior that prompted frustration and punitive behavior. Researchers concluded that, although children with physical handicaps received attention to correct the handicaps, little was done in the clinical setting to prevent attendant psychosocial disturbances (Rose 1975).

Wessell (1975) described the use of humor by an immobilized adolescent girl as an outlet for anxiety and aggression. This girl also used withdrawal, silence, pretended sleep, and inability to do simple tasks or follow directions as a means to withdraw from the environment.

In a case study of the reactions of a school-aged girl to hospitalization and immobilization, one investigator reported that the situation represented a crisis. The child experienced overwhelming anxiety, loss of behavioral control, and regressive mobility (Al Ageel 1978). Another case study of a 5-year-old boy immobilized with osteomyelitis found coping mechanisms included aggressive behaviors and compensatory ways of achieving mobility and control over environment (Terry 1979).

In summary, studies of immobilized individuals indicate that in order to cope with lack of mobility, affected people use various behaviors to substitute for movement. Some typical substitutions included increased attention to activity, gaining vicarious pleasure from activities of others, controlling the behavior of others' activity, increased speech and language, use of humor and fantasy, and nonmovement as a means of withdrawal from the environment. Most of the studies cited are descriptive and are based on few subjects. Only one study reports emotional crises. No studies were found that report on psychosocial crises as defined in this chapter.

ADOLESCENT DEVELOPMENT THEORY AND IMMOBILIZATION

Adolescence is characterized by the culmination of developmental tasks inherent in each preceding stage of development (Erikson 1959). The nature of adolescence is such that the tasks of each previous developmental stage are reexamined by the adolescent as part of the task of developing identity. The developmental requirements of adolescence involve the acquisition of an appropriate body image, a sense of identity including sexual identity, the formation of peer relationships, a redefinition of roles, and concern with physical activity.

Immobilization is antithetical to the nature of adolescents. Characteristically, adolescents evidence an increase in physical activity. Adolescents use action as a normal method of avoiding stress or relieving tension and anxiety. Adolescence, then, is a dynamic period in which individuals seek independence and develop self-identity. In contrast, immobilization represents forced dependence, a state that is fixed, unchanging, and restrictive. The combination of adolescence and immobilization can be a devastating experience. The immobilized adolescent is confronted with the following tasks associated with adolescent development: increased independence, mobility, establishment of self-identity and body image, change in activity level, and change in abilities. A crisis exists because of vital concern about increased dependence, estrangement from peers, physical vulnerability, and altered body interest and body image. Adolescents need to be mobile to effectively manage stress.

Case Study

To collect data on the phenomenon of immobilization in an adolescent, I cared for 18-year-old Debbi, who had sustained a spinal-cord injury (a lesion involving cervical vertebrae 6 and 7) in a motor-vehicle accident, which resulted in quadriplegia. Debbi was from a small, rural community, the youngest of five children with three brothers and one sister. All of her siblings were married and no longer lived with their parents. Debbi graduated from high school and began working at a local factory. Several weeks prior to her accident in September, she had moved into an apartment with her friend who also worked at the factory. Debbi was admitted to the spinal-cord unit at the rehabilitation center after 3 months of acute care; she had been a patient at the center for 2 months when these observations began. She was observed for approximately 1 month for 2 to 3 hours per day, 4 to 5 days per week. Observations terminated with Debbi's discharge to her parents' home.

In response to her immobilization, Debbi primarily used humor as a coping mechanism. She joked about her appearance and stated that she was afraid to go swimming, then laughed and said she had always been afraid to swim. Her aggression was directed at various members of the health care team and stemmed from her frustration at inabilities and limitations in function. Withdrawal and passivity were used to avoid verbalizing about her accident and her future as an immobilized person. Debbi sought to control my behavior by changing the times of the sessions as well as seeking assistance in her activities of daily living. She showed much concern with my outside activities related to mobility.

SYNTHESIS

The data from the 60 hours of observation of Debbi were examined. Data were organized according to critical variables observed in the phenomenon of immobilization as observed in Debbi. These variables and the relationships among them represent a move toward clarifying the concept of immobilization. The literature on immobilization was used to expand the concept and to put data about Debbi in perspective of the larger concept.

Classification isolates aspects of a phenomenon, thus increasing the precision with which people can identify and communicate about a concept. Precision provides uniformity of definition while decreasing ambiguity. Identification and classification of categories of functional limitations also provide a standard to use in determining the level of client immobilizations.

Eight classes of immobilization were identified, using two aspects of activity. The first aspect relates to control. Voluntary or self-selected immobilization is when a person chooses to restrict activity to promote and preserve his or her own health state. This suggests that the person assists him- or herself in maintaining the level of energy for sustained mobility. Forced and self-inflicted immobilization is when the person is unable to provide personal care due to immobilization. This condition requires the individual to be assisted by another person. The second aspect relates to cause of immobilization (Table 21-1).

Further examination of both Debbi's data and the literature permitted another type of categorization based on the critical variables involved (Figure 21-1).

Debbi's data alone permitted a third type of classification using psychosocial behavior as the organizing variable (Figure 21-2). These psychosocial reactions are significant to the individual's adjustment to immobilization as well as assumption of self-care.

A model for sequential assessment of immobilization was developed for use in assessing immobilization as well as capabilities for self-care.

Table 21-1 Classification of Immobilization According to Type of
Limitation

	Type of Immobilization	
Class	Limitation of Movement	Description
1	Voluntary/self-selected	Immobilization of self to promote or preserve health (e.g., observing a daily schedule that includes time for rest and meditation)
2	Forced/self-inflicted	Medical management of a condition requiring restraint from moving (e.g., cardiac conditions, tuberculosis, acute illness, postoperative conditions)
3	Forced/mechanical	Medical management of a condition, using a mechanical restraining device (e.g., cast or traction)
4	Forced/pharmacologic	Medical management of a condition using drugs to immobilize mentally or physically
5	Self-inflicted/painful	Immobilization to relieve pain of an affected part (e.g., sprained muscle, rheumatoid arthritic joint)
6	Forced/functional weakness	Muscular weakness limiting movement (e.g., progressive muscular diseases)
7	Forced/incomplete functional loss	Physical inability to move part (e.g., caused by poliomyelitis, cerebral vascular accident, head injury)
8	Forced/complete functional loss	Physical inability to feel sensation or move body part (e.g., caused by paralysis, amputation)

A theoretical model was developed to specify relationships between the concept of immobilization, the major theory of mobility, and the concepts of survival, loss, grief, body image, stigma, coping, crisis, and change.

Questions for further study include

1. How does perception of psychosocial threat influence reaction to immobilization?
2. What are the relationships between physiological changes and psychosocial integrity of immobilized individuals?
3. Are there differences between psychosocial reactions to congenital and acquired immobilization?
4. How does the developmental stage at age of immobilization influence psychosocial reactions?
5. What is the nature of perceptual differences between immobilized individuals?

6. Do perceptual differences influence the length of immobilization?
7. What are the critical variables in the immobilized individual's ability to do self-care?
8. Is there a difference in stress level if the model for sequential assessment of immobilization is used by both nurse and client?

Figure 21-1 Classification of Critical Variables in Immobilization

1. *Change in function:* Forced/complete functional loss, quadriplegia, cervical 6–7 lesion
2. *Time/duration:* Permanent
   a) *Onset/acquisition:* Sudden, traumatic
   b) *Occurrence:* Developmental stage of adolescence
3. *Intensity/severity:* Devastating, crisis situation
4. *Associations/loss:* Paralysis of legs, trunk, partial upper extremities
   a) *Body image:* Change related to loss of movement and sensation, inability to ambulate, confinement to wheelchair, appearance
   b) *Self-identity:* Loss of independence and high-activity, question of sexuality
   c) *Stigma:* Appearance not "normal" for adolescent, "sick role"
   d) *Lifestyle:* Dependence, decreased activity, job loss, reordering of priorities
   e) *Productivity:* Job loss, dependence on parents, question of future employment
5. *Affective elements:*
   a) *Individual:* Acknowledges condition and motivates change
   b) *Family/support system:* Parents and siblings acknowledge condition, are willing to provide acceptance and support, peers supportive but expectations unrealistic
   c) *Society:* Community supports
6. *Psychosocial Reactions:* Uses anger, aggression, humor, withdrawal, denial, manipulation, control; substitutes movement to cope with immobilization

---

Figure 21-2 Classification of Psychosocial Reactions

1. *Anger/Aggression/Anxiety:* Behaviors the individual uses to cope with feelings of anger and anxiety regarding the threat to psychosocial integrity (e.g., humor, sarcasm, criticism, profanity, verbal abuse, argument, physical abuse)
2. *Withdrawal/Denial:* Behaviors the individual uses as protection from having to deal with threats to psychosocial integrity (e.g., ambivalence, passivity, regression, false contentment, clinging to past behaviors, nonmovement)
3. *Manipulation/Control:* Controlling behaviors the individual uses over other people's activities and environment
4. *Substitution for Movement:* Behaviors that individual uses to compensate for restricted mobility (e.g., increased attention to activity; vicarious pleasure from the activities of others; increased use of speech, language, and fantasy)
5. *Acknowledgment:* Behaviors the individual uses to achieve independence in activities of daily living and to maximize existing potential.

Figure 21-3 Model for Sequential Assessment of Immobilization

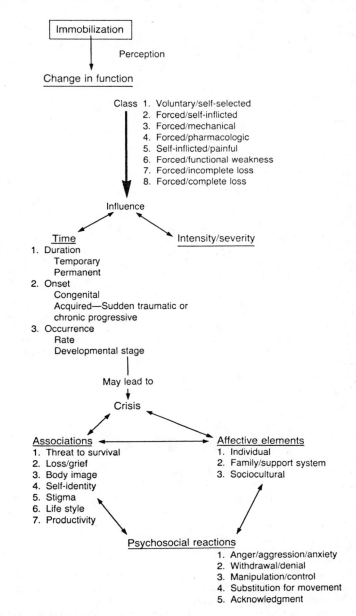

Figure 21-4 Model for Conceptual Clarification of Immobilization

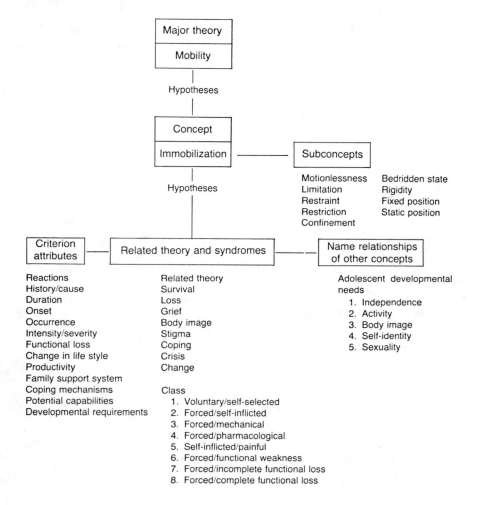

CONCLUSION

The intent of this study* was to clarify the concept of immobilization in terms of psychosocial variables by observing one subject who had a great degree of immobilization, by examining observation records for tendencies and regularities, and by searching for factors that comprise psychosocial aspects of immobilization. A classification system of immobilization as a whole using volition and cause as parameters was devised. Another classification system uses the critical variables that determine degree of trauma. A model illustrating relationships among a theory of mobility, immobility, and concepts related to psychosocial crisis in immobilization was created. Out of the data collected and the model that was constructed, questions for further study were identified.

REFERENCES

Al Ageel, M. Reactions of a hospitalized school-age child to separation and restricted mobility. *Matern. Child Nurs. J.* 7:163–173, Fall 1978.

Bergmann, T. Observations of children's reactions to motor restraint. *Nerv. Child* 4:318–326, July 1945.

Bernabeu, E. The effects of severe crippling on the development of a group of children. *Psychiatry* 21:169–194, 1952.

Blackwell, B. Stigma. In C. Carlson, and B. Blackwell (Eds.), *Behavorial Concepts and Nursing Intervention* (2nd ed.). Philadelphia: Lippincott, 1978.

Burlingham, D. Notes on Problems of Motor Restraint during Illness. In R. Lowenstein (Ed.), *Drives, Affects, Behavior.* New York: International University Press, 1953. Pp. 169–175.

Carlson, C. Grief. In C. Carlson, and B. Blackwell (Eds.), *Behavioral Concepts and Nursing Intervention* (2nd ed.). Philadelphia: Lippincott, 1978. Pp. 87–112.

Carlson, C. Loss. In C. Carlson and B. Blackwell (Eds.), *Behavioral Concepts and Nursing Intervention* (2nd ed.). Philadelphia: Lippincott, 1978. Pp. 72–86.

Cleveland, S., Reitman, E., and Brewer, E. Psychological factors in juvenile rheumatoid arthritis. *Arthritis Rheum.* 8:1152–1158, Dec. 1965.

Crate, M. Nursing functions in adaptation to chronic illness. *Am. J. Nurs.* 65:72–76, Oct. 1965.

Dadich, K. An eleven-year-old girl's use of control while immobilized in halo-femoral traction. *Matern. Child Nurs. J.* 1:67–74, Spring 1972.

Dubo, S. Psychiatric study of children with pulmonary tuberculosis. *Am. J. Orthopsychiatry* 20:520–527, Jul. 1950.

Erikson, E. Identity and the life cycle: Selected papers. *Psychol. Issues* 1:118–146, 1959.

Coffman, E. *Stigma: Notes on the Management of Spoiled Identity.* Englewood Cliffs, N.J.: Prentice-Hall, 1963.

---

*Patients with some type of emotional immobilization, such as psychiatric clients with catatonia, were not included in this examination.

Musaph, H. Aggression and symptom formation in dermatology. *J. Psychosom. Res.* 13:257–264, 1968.

Rapoport, L. The State of Crisis: Some Theoretical Considerations. In H. Parad (Ed.), *Crisis Intervention: Selected Readings*. New York: Family Service Association, 1965. Pp. 22–31.

Reite, M., Davis, K., Solomons, C., and Ott, J. Osteogenesis imperfecta: Psychological function. *Am. J. Psychiatry* 128:1540–1545, June 1972.

Robinson, H., Finesinger, J., and Bierman, J. Psychiatric considerations in the adjustment of patients with poliomyelitis. *N. Engl. J. Med.* 254:975–980, May 24, 1956.

Rose, M. Coping behavior of physically handicapped children. *Nurs. Clin. North Am.* 10:329–339, June 1975.

Schechter, M. The orthopedically handicapped child: Emotional reactions. *Arch. Gen. Psychiatry* 4:247–253, Mar. 1961.

Shontz, F. *The Psychological Aspects of Physical Illness and Disability*. New York: Macmillan. 1975.

Sibinga, M., Friedman, C., Steisel, I., and Sinnamon, H. The effect of immobilization and sensory restriction on children with phenylketonuria. *Pediatr. Res.* 2:371–377, 1968.

Terry, G. A 5-year-old boy's aggressive and compensatory behavior in response to immobilization. *Matern. Child Nurs. J.* 8:29–38, Spring 1979.

Wessell, M., Sr. Use of humor by an immobilized adolescent girl during hospitalization. *Matern. Child Nurs. J.* 4:35–48, Spring 1975.

Wittkower, E. Psychological aspects of physical illness. *Can. Med. Assoc. J.* 66:220–224, Mar. 1952.

Wright, M. The Period of Mourning in Chronic Illness. In M. Harrower (Ed.), *Medical & Psychological Teamwork in the Care of the Chronically Ill*. Springfield, Ill.: Thomas, 1955.

Chapter 22

Pressure Sores

Mary L. Shanon

Pressure sores, or *decubitus ulcers,* constitute an endemic problem among institutionalized and debilitated patients. Extrapolations from available data indicate that five to ten percent of the approximately 1,000,000 Americans hospitalized per year develop pressure sores—50,000 to 100,000 persons. By any definition, pressure sores are a major nursing problem. Though etiology and pathology of this condition have been extensively studied and basic causation explained, the nursing profession has been virtually unable to make a real impact on its prevention and control. Numerous treatment regimens—some with merit and some without—have been proposed for pressure sores. Yet in the final analysis, solution to the problem in the majority of cases is relief of soft-tissue pressure, reduction of friction, prevention of shearing force damage, and maintenance of normal nitrogen balance. None of these interventions is impossible to accomplish, but all require consistent attention of nursing personnel.

Additional causes of pressure sore development are unique to certain types of patients. A congenital or acquired bony deformity may cause internal pressure that results in a pressure sore. Pressure from an internal fixation device used in the treatment of fractures can do the same. Paraplegic patients also may suffer internal abrasions of fascia and subcutaneous tissue as a result of uncontrolled spastic, repetitive muscle movements (Tepperman, DeZwirek, Chiarcossi, and Jimenez 1976; and Roaf 1976).

Any person confined to the bed or to a chair for prolonged periods of time without ability to alter position becomes a candidate for the development of pressure sores. While most pressure sores can be prevented by aggressive nursing care, some cannot. Certain cachectic patients in extreme negative nitrogen balance will ultimately develop skin breakdown in spite of good nursing care. Pressure sores are also inevitable in patients who are admitted to the hospital after having been discovered too ill to move themselves or found unconscious and lying in one position for a prolonged period of time.

In this chapter, discussion will center on the definition of pressure sores, the scope of the problem, identification of the patient at risk, the pathophysiology, the objective of treatment, a proposed model for predicting and preventing pressure sore formation, and questions that are relevant for future nursing research.

DEFINITION AND CLASSIFICATION

Pressure sores are areas of soft-tissue necrosis that may be superficial or may involve all tissue planes. The necrotic areas occur as a result of tissue ischemia from prolonged pressure between the body and the surface on which it rests (Husain 1953).

Guttmann (1955) identified the stages of pressure sore development as follows:

1. *Stage of transient circulatory disturbance.* Pressure has been of sufficient duration and compressive force to cause reddening of the skin, which disappears with relief of pressure.
2. *Stage of definite superficial circulatory and tissue damage.* Pressure has been of sufficient duration and compressive force to cause reddening and congestion of the affected area, which do not disappear with relief of pressure. The epidermis and dermis may be excoriated or blistered, and the deeper layers of skin may also be involved.
3. *Stage of deep, penetrating necrosis.* Destruction from pressure involves all tissue layers—skin, subcutaneous tissue, fascia, muscle, and even bone. It frequently involves wide areas and is characterized by necrosis and sinus tracts.

A more definitive description of pressure sore development is provided by Shea (1975), using a classification system based on objectively measurable histologic variables. He identifies the following four grades of pressure sores:

Grade I. An acute, inflammatory response involving all soft-tissue layers. The extreme of Grade I involvement is a moist, superficial, irregular ulceration limited to the epidermis exposing the underlying dermis and resembling an abrasion. Clinically, it presents as a painful, irregular, ill-defined area of soft-tissue swelling and induration with associated heat and erythema overlying a bony prominence.

Grade II. Histologically this type of pressure sore reveals a mixed acute and chronic inflammatory process involving the full thickness of the dermis down to the subcutaneous fat. Clinically, a Grade II lesion presents as a shallow full-thickness skin ulcer whose edges are more distinct than those of Grade I due to early fibrotic and pigmentation changes that blend into a broader indistinct area of heat, erythema, and induration.

Grade III. Histologically characterized by extensive soft-tissue necrosis that is limited by the deep fascia. There is an intense reactive fibrosis, inflammation, and retraction in both dermis and the subcutaneous fat that distorts any previous tissue distinctions. Clinically, Grade III presents as an irregular full-thickness skin defect that extends into the subcutaneous fat and exposes a draining, foul-smelling, infected necrotic base. The skin edge is rolled with an altered dark and light pigmentation that sharply outlines the ulcer. The joints adjacent to the ulcer are flexed and have a limited range of motion.

Grade IV. Histologically there is extensive necrosis of soft tissues and osteomyelitis of the underlying bone because the deep fascia has been penetrated. Joint involvement causes the development of septic, subluxed, or dislocated joints in contiguous areas. Clinically, Grade IV resembles Grade III except that it is a much more extensive lesion with more profuse amounts of both drainage and necrosis. Bone is identified in the base of the ulcer and X rays reveal extensive bone involvement with both osteomyelitis and loss of bone substance.

In the discussion of classification of pressure sores later in this chapter, only two types of pressure sores are identified. There are more definitive typologies as is illustrated by the Shea (1975) classification. From a clinical standpoint, however, recognition and treatment of Shea's Types I and II are not remarkably different from the "superficial benign" type identified by Groth (1975). Shea's Types III and IV correspond clinically to Groth's "deep malignant" type. It seems that the simpler two-category typology based on treatment will be less likely to cause confusion.

SCOPE OF THE PROBLEM

The enormity and variability of the pressure sore problem is apparent when data on its incidence is studied. Two nursing audits of large general-hospital populations and one comprehensive community study done in the early 1970s showed the incidence of this complication to be less than three percent. Several later studies of total populations at risk, however, showed the occurrence to be significantly higher.

Rubin, Dietz, and Abruzzese (1974) audited 18,000 admissions at St. Luke's Hospital Center in New York City and found 262 patients with pressure sores, an incidence of 1.5 percent. Sixty-seven patients in this study were admitted with pressure sores of undetermined origin. Gerson (1975), reporting on a nursing inventory of 5,648 patients in three active treatment hospitals, identified 152 patients with pressure sores, an incidence of 2.69 percent.

One of the most comprehensive studies on incidence of pressure sores (Petersen and Bittman 1971) was a survey done in the County of Arhus, Denmark (population 517,000). The report encompassed 98 percent of all hospital departments and nursing homes. Data were also collected by questionnaires from 98 percent of all general practitioners and visiting nurses. The investigation showed that 43.1 patients per 100,000 population had pressure sores. A number of patients had multiple pressure sores that raised the number of pressure sores to 61.5 per 100,000 population. These findings of pressure sores in 3 percent of hospitalized patients was similar to Gerson's (1975).

Manley (1976) surveyed 772 patients at Groote Schuur Hospital in Capetown, South Africa and found a 4.5 percent incidence of pressure sores. An additional 5.2 percent showed beginning pressure signs, that is, reddened skin.

Jordan and Clark (1978) reported 7.4 percent (interpolated) of hospitalized patients at risk in the Glasgow Study. The study was an attempt to reach all patients "in care" on a given day in the 15,000-bed area served by the Glasgow Health Board. "In care" was interpreted as all hospital inpatients and all persons receiving a home visit from a district nurse on the day of survey, January 21, 1976. Hospitalized patients deemed to be low-risk for pressure sore development were not considered in the study—maternity cases, ambulatory psychiatric, and physically mobile mentally retarded patients. The hospitalized at-risk patient population was 8,685 or 57.0 percent of the potential 15,000 bed occupants and the home-care patients numbered 2,030. A total of 10,751 patients (10.2 percent of Glasgow's 1,105,645 population) were studied. Overall incidence of pressure sores was 8.8 percent. Incidence in all study patients over 70 years of age was 11.6 percent; this group accounted for 50 percent of the study population.

Two smaller studies done as a result of interest generated in Great Britain by the Glasgow Study also showed high incidences of pressure sores. Woodbine (1977) surveyed all wards in the district of Macclesfield and found that 48 of the 51 (94.1 percent) patients had pressure sores. In a second study, she surveyed orthopedic ward admissions during June–August, 1977. Data showed that 12 of the 49 patients admitted developed pressure sores (24 percent). Nine of these were over 78 years of age. Lowthian (1979) studied the entire hospital population of 168 patients on April 26, 1978, at the Royal National Orthopedic Hospital, Stanmore. He found 6.5 percent to have pressure sores as defined in the Glasgow Study (the study excluded all patients with no break in skin integrity). Of Lowthian's population, only 11 percent (29) of the subjects were 70 years of age or older versus 50 percent of the Glasgow Study population. His findings parallel the Glasgow Study in increased incidence of pressure sores (13.8 percent) in the aged.

While general hospital populations reflect risks of less than 10 percent, risk in other groups is as high as 85 percent. Spinal-cord injury patients are a striking example of a population at risk. The incidence of pressure sores in World War

II paraplegics ranges from 57 to 85 percent (Kosiak 1959). One study reveals pressure sores occurred in approximately 80 percent of spinal-cord injury patients (Spence, Burk, and Rae 1967). Incidence of pressure sores in geriatric patients is not as high as spinal-cord patients but is significantly higher than that of the general patient population. Norton, McLaren, and Exton-Smith (1962) reported an incidence of 24 percent in 250 patients admitted to a hospital geriatric unit. Williams (1972), in a sample of 26 nonambulatory patients with a mean age of 61.88 years, found that 26.92 percent developed pressure sores. The elderly and spinal-cord injury patients are two groups proven to be at greater risk of pressure sores.

Numbers of pressure sore problems are significant to health care providers, but the cost of care is important to the national economy. Schell and Wolcott (1966) estimated that pressure sores increased each patient's medical care costs by $5,000. Spence and colleagues (1967) estimated costs per patient ranging from $2,000 to $10,000. Fernie (1973) estimated that treating 25,000 pressure sore patients in the United Kingdom cost £60 million. Inflation makes these costs considerably higher. Scales (1977) estimated the cost to the National Health Service to be £100 million per year, while Dyson (1978) estimated the per patient cost to the British National Health Service for curing "a simple bed sore taking three weeks to heal" to be £777. An account of actual costs for treating four paraplegic patients for in-hospital decubitus care in British Columbia was $218,649; projected actual costs at 1977 prices to the Provincial Health Care System were $349,379 (Robinson, Coghlan, and Jackson 1978). Cost in the United States in 1977 was estimated to be $15,000 or more per patient (Sather, Weber, and George 1977). Assuming that 5 percent of the approximately 1,000,000 Americans hospitalized will develop pressure sores and using Sather and co-workers' (1977) $15,000 estimate for care cost per patient, the price tag is a staggering $750,000,000 without accounting for inflation.

Pressure sores increase costs of health care for everyone as insurance premiums increase. Insurance companies estimate that 25 percent of the cost for spinal-cord injury care is for pressure sores (Houle 1969). Hospitals raise rates for long-term nonsurgical patients occupying beds that might be more profitably used for short-term patients. But personal costs are highest for patients who must endure financial hardship, pain, disability, and loss of work time directly attributable to pressure lesions.

WHO IS AT RISK?

Experienced nurse practitioners can often empirically identify patients at risk for pressure sore development. They usually make their judgment from assessing the patient's diagnosis, age, ability to move, level of consciousness, nutrition, presence or absence of infection, adequacy of circulation, and/or incontinence.

A summary of the factors that increase patients' risk shows

1. Patients at greatest risk are those suffering from paralytic conditions resulting in paraplegia, quadriplegia, or hemiplegia. These persons do not feel discomfort from prolonged pressure with its attendant tissue ischemia so they have no motivation to change position. Additionally, loss of motor nerve function causes atrophy of musculature and subcutaneous tissue in the affected parts. This atrophy deprives the paralyzed area of the body of a significant portion of its padding. Bony prominences become even more prominent while the skin over them becomes more traumatized from pressure, and breakdown occurs.

2. The second greatest risk is probably in patients with decreased sensorium. Anything that decreases patients' levels of consciousness to a degree that renders them incapable or unwilling to alter body position makes them prime candidates for development of pressure sores. Patients who are unconscious or heavily sedated by analgesics, tranquilizers, or soporifics become unresponsive to normal stimuli for changing body position. Patients who are surgically unconscious are at significant risk. When placed on an operating-table surface for more than 4 hours, patients become candidates for iatrogenically induced pressure sores (Oates 1978; and Nightingale 1978). Petersen (1976) states that "only one place is more dangerous to patients than the operating table, and that is the traction table for the treatment of fractures of the femoral neck." The reason given is that the body's reactive force against the traction being exerted on the leg is centered from the sacrum down to the perineum. The subsequent incidence of pressure sores in patients treated in this manner for a femoral neck fracture is 11 percent.

3. Deficiencies of patients who are undernourished and anemic, suffering from hypoproteinemia, vitamin deficiencies, and possibly dehydration render cells susceptible to breakdown and necrosis.

4. Elderly patients, particularly those 85 years of age or older, are likely to develop skin breakdown if confined to bed or chair rest. People in advanced years often have circulatory changes, loss of muscle mass, loss of subcutaneous tissue, locomotion problems, incontinence, and visual impairment. Most of these alterations discourage frequent position changes. If, in addition, elderly persons are restrained because of disorientation, pressure sore formation becomes a virtual certainty.

5. Patients' medical diagnoses may be relevant. Diseases associated with circulatory impairment, cachexia, disturbed sensorium, disability, severe anemia, increased bodily temperature of sustained duration, and severe infections predispose to pressure sores. Conditions in which one or a combination of these factors may be present are cancer, arteriosclerotic disease,

paralysis, malnutrition, diabetes mellitus, congestive heart failure, and cerebrovascular accidents.

REPORT ON THE LITERATURE

Rubin and associates (1974), as the result of their survey of 18,000 patients, named the precipitating factors in 262 pressure sores studied.

Major surgery	16
Orthopedic problems	21
Malignancy	18
Diabetes	8
Incontinence	22
Debilitation other than malignancy	81
Unrecorded	96
	262

Petersen and Bittman's (1971) report of pressure sore incidence in Arhus County, Denmark named precipitating factors as

Cerebral or generalized arteriosclerosis	56
Cancer	28
Cerebral hemorrhage	26
Fracture of femoral neck	24
Paraplegia or quadriplegia	22
Disseminated sclerosis	19
Other neurological disease	17
Rheumatic disease	13
Cardiac failure	11
Sequelae of amputation	9
Diabetes mellitus	9
Other limb fractures	8
Renal disease	4
	246

The study also identified sites of pressure sore formation in the body. It shows over 60 percent of them developing in three locations: sacrum, heel, and ischium. These findings essentially agree with the Glasgow Study (Jordan et al. 1978) and Manley's Capetown study (1978).

Other factors have been identified as being significant in production of pressure sores. Diastolic blood pressure levels may be a predictor of risk. " . . . only four of 26 subjects whose skin remained intact had a diastolic blood pressure of less than 60 mm Hg, while all four persons who developed pressure sores had readings of less than 60 mm Hg (Gosnell 1973).'' A study of 26 patients indicated that those receiving corticosteroids were more likely to develop decubiti and that men were more predisposed than women to pressure sores (Williams 1972)—a finding not consistent in other studies.

Gerson (1975) found that male and female patients developed pressure sores with equal frequency in a report of 5,648 patients studied. In the Jordan study (1978), there were almost twice as many women as men in the population. Incidence of pressure sores was 9.2 percent and 8.0 percent respectively, a not statistically significant difference. Manley (1978) found no difference in pressure sore incidence among hospitalized males and females. Woodbine (1979), however, noted in both phases of her study that more females than males had pressure sores. In Survey A, which included all wards in the district (51 patients), incidence was 69 percent in females versus 31 percent in males. In Survey B of all orthopedic admissions (49) during a 3-month period, 32 percent of the females developed pressure sores compared to 14 percent of the males. Gerber and Van Ort (1979), in a study of 29 patients, found that females with pressure sores healed significantly more slowly than males. These conflicting findings among studies need further investigation.

Another potentially significant factor identified by Manley (1978) is that of race. On the survey day, 25 percent of all white patients had pressure sores while only 3.2 percent of colored and 1.8 percent of black patients had them. He raised a question of possible physiological tissue differences among races.

Patients of at least one type appear to be at decreased risk for the development of pressure sores—patients with amyotrophic lateral sclerosis (A.L.S.). Furukawa and Toyokura (1976) report a survey of 202 of these patients done between 1965 to 1975. No patient developed a pressure sore at any stage of the illness; the reason is unknown. The possibility of skin and blood vessel changes was raised by the investigators. Forrester (1976) hypothesized that increased sympathetic cutaneous vasoconstrictor activity in the lower part of A.L.S. patients' bodies might be responsible. Constricted blood vessels are harder to completely occlude than are large dilated blood vessels. One published report appears to refute Furukawa and Toyokura's results. Parish, Smith, and Collins (1978) state that two of five A.L.S. patients treated at a chronic disease facility in Philadelphia, suffered from large sacral bedsores. It should be useful to investigate why debilitated, bed-ridden A.L.S. patients develop pressure sores so infrequently. Certainly patients with this diagnosis would be considered to be at increased risk for their development. They suffer from muscular weakness, atrophy, and spasticity as well as motor neuron degeneration. Yet they rarely develop pressure sores. Is it coincidental that in Furukawa and Toyokura's (1976) survey of 202 A.L.S. patients, none had pressure sores? If not, then is the absence of pressure sores in these patients related to A.L.S. pathology? Or is it related to soft tissue and/or innervation changes resulting from the disease?

Furukawa and Toyokura's (1976, 1978) findings, coupled with Forrester's (1976) hypothesis and the research of Gosnell (1973) and Trumble (1930), suggest that increased resistance to compressibility of blood vessels is responsible for the scarcity of pressure sores. If so, the following hypothesis might be tested:

> Increased and sustained resistance to the compressibility of blood vessels as measured by a diastolic blood pressure greater than 60 mm Hg prevents the development of pressure sores in the patient normally responsive to pain.

This assumes that patients must alter their positions when discomfort from sustained pressure occurs. Sensory innervation is not impaired in A.L.S., so these patients shift their positions in response to discomfort. This, together with increased resistance to compressibility of blood vessels, might be sufficient to prevent pressure sores in almost all cases.

PREVENTION OF PRESSURE SORES IN THE NORMAL INDIVIDUAL

Since the human body is subject to the effects of gravity and a pressure of 15 pounds psi is present on all body surfaces (Husain 1953), why is it that healthy persons do not develop pressure sores? It is because of the enormous amount of body surface available to dissipate the pressure? According to Trumble (1930), a man weighing 150 pounds who is 5 feet 8 inches tall has a skin surface of 2,790 square inches. In recumbent position, the weight psi would be less than one-third pound or 17 mm Hg if he were supported by only one-fifth of his total body surface. If the body were supported by 20 percent of its total body surface, pressure sores would be unlikely to develop because pressure interface between the body's points of contact with its supporting surface would be less than capillary closing pressure. On an ordinary hospital mattress, less than 20 percent of the body surface is in effective contact (Bell et al. 1974).

One study of capillary pressures revealed that average pressure in the arteriolar limb of the capillary bed was 32 mm Hg, in the midcapillary region 20 mm Hg, and at the venous end 12 mm Hg. Venous congestion from pressure produced a rapid rise of capillary pressure as did hyperemia of the skin. In hyperemia, capillary pressure rose to 60 mm Hg in the arteriolar limb and 45 mm Hg in the venous limb of the capillary (Landis 1930). Other studies have shown that in the reclining position, capillary closing pressures are exceeded by pressure of the supporting surface against the body (Lindan 1961; Kosiak, Kubicek, Olson, and Day 1958; and Kosiak 1961). Lindan (1961) assumed that mean capillary pressure was 25 mm Hg, and any pressure in excess of 30 mm Hg was potentially damaging to soft tissues. Normal, healthy male subjects of average size registered the following pressure readings (using a surface whose compressibility was equivalent to 1³/₄ inches of foam rubber):

Supine position

Buttocks	40–70 mm Hg
Heels	30–50 mm Hg
Posterior chest wall	30–40 mm Hg

Side-lying position

Hip	70–95 mm Hg

Prone position

Knees	30–60 mm Hg
Costal Margins	30–50 mm Hg

Although the compressibility of the surfaces on which the studies were made was varied, he concluded that "even with subjects lying on a sprung surface which is more compressible than the ordinary hospital bed, an impairment of blood microcirculation may easily occur (Lindan 1961)."

In a study of seated subjects, pressures over the ischial tuberosities and the area 10–12 cm around them ranged from 100 to 40 mm Hg. These findings led to the conclusion that "the highest pressure to which a patient's skin is subjected in ordinary hospital circumstances is in the vicinity of 100 mm Hg (Lindan 1961)."

Kosiak (1958, 1961) concluded that pressures over the ischial tuberosities were considerably higher than 100 mm Hg. He found the weight-bearing area available to seated persons to be considerably less than the area available in a reclining position. Approximately 75 percent of body weight is supported by the buttocks and upper thighs, with most of the weight being under the ischial tuberosities. In experiments with various sitting surfaces ranging from unyielding to a 2-inch foam-rubber cushion, pressures over the ischial tuberosities varied from 300 mm Hg to 150 mm Hg. He concluded that if only one-half of the 150 mm Hg pressure were transmitted to the ischial tuberosities, pressure sores would develop in every case in time.

In the same series of experiments, a type of chair that dramatically lowered pressures over the entire sitting surface of the buttocks and thighs was tested. The chair, an alternating-pressure contoured device, was padded and had movable slats with an excursion range of ⁷/₈ inch. Maximum pressure recorded in the "down" phase was 48 mm Hg, which closely approximates normal capillary pressure. Kosiak was able to reduce pressure on all weight-bearing surfaces to zero by increasing excursion in the "down" phase of each movable slat. Such a contoured chair would minimize pressure sore development in chair-fast patients (Kosiak et al. 1958).

In patients whose upper-extremity strength was sufficient to lift their body weight, a simple pressure switch device imbedded in the seat cushion was developed to train patients to relieve pressure for 5–10 seconds every 10–20 minutes (Fordyce et al. 1968). The need for relieving this pressure is graphically described in relation to late chronic pressure sores

These ulcers result from recurrent, intermittent periods of low pressure (50–150 mm Hg) and appear most frequently over the ischial tuberosities of paraplegic patients who sit for prolonged periods of time in wheelchairs. This recurrent, intermittent, relatively low force, just above capillary pressure, produces chronic ischemic changes in the subcutaneous tissue between the ischial tuberosity and the skin. This chronic ischemia leads to development of a dense fibrotic avascular scar, which presents as a firm, palpable subcutaneous mass directly over the bone. Continued intermittent pressure causes liquefaction necrosis of this fibrotic nodular area and a bursa gradually forms over the ischial tuberosity. With continued pressure, the skin completely loses its nutrition and a small opening appears, followed by discharge of the contents of the bursa. Although this opening in the skin is quite small, there is a large fibrous walled sac that usually leads to the ischial tuberosity deep beneath the skin. This direct connection from the ischial tuberosity to the outside environment allows secondary infection to occur with osteomyelitis of the ischium (Stauffer 1978).

Findings of Lindan (1961) and Kosiak (1958) concerning amount of pressure exerted on supporting soft tissues of the body help to explain why healthy individuals do not remain in one position long enough to suffer pressure damage. Discomfort and actual pain from tissue ischemia causes release of algogenic polypeptides which produce pain. These polypeptides activate nociceptive afferent nerve fibers, which relay to the brain the need for a volitional or reflex change of position (Daniel, Terzis, and Cunningham 1976). Thus, continual alteration of body position takes place in order to prevent prolonged pressure on any body surface.

Recently, biomedical engineers have begun work relating to pressure-loading characteristics, mechanical properties of human skin for deformations, interface pressures, and equipment to prevent pressure sores. Significant new information about pressure sore prevention will soon be available as a result of this research.

PATHOPHYSIOLOGY OF PRESSURE SORES

Pressure sores have been extensively studied by clinical investigators; study findings have implicated numerous factors. It is generally accepted by most clinicians that ischemia caused by supracapillary pressure is one of the primary factors in the production of pressure sores (Kosiak 1961). Laboratory experiments have shown that application of 130 mm Hg pressure to the tails of rats for 18 hours produced massive necrosis in every animal. Results were the same with the application of 100 mm Hg pressure for 48 hours (Brooks and Duncan 1940). Their findings led these investigators to conclude that

> (1) With the application of pressures sufficient to produce pathologic changes, the duration of the pressure is of more importance than its amount and (2) Pressure only slightly below that necessary to render a part totally anemic may result in massive necrosis if the time of application is prolonged (Brooks and Duncan 1940).

Tissue changes, researchers observed, involved epithelial hyperplasia and muscle degeneration with myositis and fibrous replacement of muscle.

Another study found complete arterial ischemia of a rat's extremity for 4 to 4 1/2 hours was followed by dilation of arteries in the ischemic limb and patency of veins following removal of constriction. This led to the hypothesis that "degenerative muscular changes were probably due to severe capillary damage." Because of stasis and alteration of normal capillary permeability, there was a decrease in inflow of blood to cellular units and a considerable depression in rate of exchange of cellular metabolites (Harman 1948).

Husain (1953) found microscopic changes in rat muscle with pressures of 100 mm Hg applied for 2 hours. Cellular degeneration was apparent microscopically. The same pressure applied for 6 hours produced similar but more severe changes. Cellular infiltration, extravasation, and hyaline degeneration was found in tissue examined microscopically 24 hours after the application of only 60 mm Hg for 1 hour (Kosiak 1961).

It appears that primary effects of pressure on human tissue occur in the capillary bed. Burton and Yamada (1951) demonstrated that rate of flow through minute vessels was related to the perfusing pressure. They found a rapidly progressive decrease in blood flow when transmural pressure was reduced; that flow stopped completely in the capillaries, even though transmural pressure was maintained between 20 to 40 mm Hg. This level was designated as the "critical closing pressure" and could be produced by increasing externally applied pressure or by decreasing intravascular hydrostatic pressure. One study demonstrated capillary flow to be unstable at low perfusion pressures and that either cessation or temporary reversal of flow could occur at low levels of positive pressure (Nichol et al. 1951).

A 1961 study reported marked susceptibility of tissue in rats to relatively low constant pressures for short periods of time (e.g. 70 mm Hg for 2 hours). There was somewhat greater resistance to tissue change following the application of equal amounts of intermittent pressure. This was true even at pressures as high as 240 mm Hg for 3 hours. Reactive hyperemia, which is seen in tissue following release of pressure, is generally believed to be a normal protective response. Hyperemic response is generally proportional to temporal length of occlusion and to temperature of the affected part. Duration of the reaction increases with time of occlusion up to 1 hour and usually lasts one-half to three-fourths as long as the occlusion. Anoxemia is believed to be the primary reason for reactive hyperemia (Kosiak 1961).

Intense pressures of short duration are responsible not only for interference and perhaps complete cessation of capillary circulation but also for changes in larger vessels with possible venous thrombi formation. Presence of venous thrombosis interferes with normal reactive hyperemic vasodilatation after pressure is removed, with the result that tissues continue to remain ischemic and breakdown ultimately occurs (Kosiak 1961). Fernie (1973) believes that "the simplistic view of external pressure in excess of mean capillary pressure causing closure of the capillary bed neglects any supportive role of the nonfluid elements of the tissues."

Not all tissue subject to supracapillary pressure necroses. One investigator hypothesized

> Where tissue is subjected to pressures for only short periods of time, the normal reactive hyperemic response partially compensates for the temporary ischemia with the result that the tissue does not undergo morphologic degeneration. Even when excessive pressures are applied for a sufficient period of time to result in early degenerative changes, it would appear that complete relief of pressure may often permit restoration of circulation and cellular metabolism without ulceration (Kosiak 1961).

Although supracapillary pressure is the major factor in producing pressure sores, at least three other factors are of great importance—shearing force, friction, and severe negative nitrogen balance. *Shearing force* is that phenomenon initiated by friction between the patient's skin and the bed. An example with which every nurse is familiar is that of elevating the head of the bed to allow the patient to eat or converse with visitors. With change in bed position, the patient's body predictably slides toward the foot of the bed. Both pressure, which acts perpendicular to skin surfaces, and shear forces, which act parallel to skin surfaces, tend to concentrate over the sacrum. Sacral skin, rather than sliding freely when the patient's position is changed, is held in its original bed location by the effect of friction. The deeper segment of superficial fascia, which is loose and mobile in the sacral region, slides between fixed skin surface and the deep fascial layer. This action places the primary effect of shearing force on the deeper portions of the superficial fascia.

> The blood supply to the posterior sacral tissues arises principally from the posterior branches of the lateral sacral arteries and the superficial branches of the superior gluteal arteries. The former pass through the posterior sacral foramens to supply the local muscles and then pierce the deep fascia to reach the superficial fascia and skin. A shearing force concentrated in the deeper portion of the superficial fascia places the blood vessels in the involved area under stretch, and perhaps angulation, since the vessels are more or less anchored at their points of perforation through the deep fascia. Multiple thromboses of small vessels with subsequent necrosis are constant pathological findings in ducubitus ulcers. In time, the shearing force produces extensive tissue dissection or cleavage in the plane of greatest concentration of force. This is observed clinically as a large area of undermining which extends circumferentially about the base of the ulcer and lies at the level of the deeper portion of the superficial fascia (Reichel 1958).

Another major factor in the production of skin breakdown is *friction*. Movement of the patient against the resting surface is impeded by the friction coefficient of the skin itself and resting surface material. Friction interface between the two surfaces is variable but always present. In its simplest form, friction causes abrading of superficial skin surfaces similar to that of a mild burn. Continuous movement against a surface with a high friction coefficient will almost always impede skin movement sufficiently to cause shearing with its subsequent damaging effects. It is possible to have friction without significant shearing force (e.g., in moving the palmar surface of the hand repeatedly against a bed sheet). It is not possible, conversely, to have shearing force without significant friction.

Both shearing force and friction are increased in the presence of moisture. Adams and Hunter (1969) report that friction of cat's footpads increased by 51 percent with mild- to moderate-sweating and dropped to 6 percent less than the friction of dry pads with profuse sweating. While these two factors are as important as pressure in producing pressure sores, they have not been studied extensively. Satisfactory measurement methods are still elusive.

The last major factor in the production of pressure sores is that of *severe* negative nitrogen balance. Mulholland believes that a severe protein deficiency renders soft tissue more susceptible to breakdown when it is exposed to local pressure (Mulholland et al. 1943). He found in a study of 35 patients with bed sores that all had plasma protein levels below normal. With aging, body protein needs become greater, 0.6 grams per kilogram of body weight versus 0.35 grams per kilogram in the young adult (Munro 1972), yet protein consumption usually declines because of lessening physical activity, which leads to a lack of appetite. Cost of quality protein to the person with a decreased income also becomes a factor. The normal aging changes that result in loss of lean body mass and a decrease in serum albumin levels (Forbes and Reina 1970; Exton-Smith 1978) become further accentuated with lack of protein ingestion. Whenever elderly patients or any other patients with minimal protein ingestion are confined to bed or chair rest, they run significantly increased risks for the development of pressure sores. A patient who actually develops a pressure lesion may have a severely negative nitrogen balance because of protein loss through the lesion. It is estimated that up to 30 grams of protein per day can be lost through a single large draining pressure sore (Hubay, Kiehn, and Drucker 1957).

Closely related to protein levels in the body is the level of ascorbic acid necessary for the synthesis and maintenance of collagen, the chief protein component of connective tissue. Husain, as a result of laboratory research on scorbutic guinea pigs, feels that repair of tissue injury is related to the supply of Vitamin C in the body (Husain 1953). He therefore recommends an adequate supply in order to prevent or minimize severe pressure lesions.

The research of Taylor, Dymock, and Torrance (1974) shows that the administration of 500 mg of ascorbic acid per day to a group of ten surgical patients suffering from pressure sores resulted in a mean reduction of the surface area of the ulcers of 84 per cent after one month. The control group had a surface area reduction of only 42.7 percent at the end of the same period.

TYPES OF PRESSURE SORES

To the clinician, there are two distinct types of so-called pressure sores. One is a pressure-initiated necrosis caused by either pressure or shearing force, while the other is frequently a superficial lesion initiated by friction between the skin and its supporting surface. Groth (1975) called the first the "deep, malignant" type and the latter the "superficial benign" form. Actually, the superficial benign form does not remain long in that state; it heals or becomes worse. All skin breakdown—whether from pressure, shearing force and/or friction—has the potential for becoming a "deep, malignant" lesion.

One explanation of the pressure necrosis mechanism relates to differences in tissue properties that allow the deep, malignant type to develop (Shea 1975). Skin, the most superficial body tissue, is composed of an avascular epidermal layer and a second fibro-elastic dermal layer. Immediately beneath the dermis is a loose connective tissue layer composed primarily of fat cells with small amounts of intercellular substance and little vascularity. Its principal functions are to act as a shock absorber and to permit movement of skin over deeper layers of tissue. This subcutaneous fat layer has little tensile strength. Shearing force easily compromises its blood supply by causing angular stretching of vessels. Under the subcutaneous fat layer is the deep fascia. This tissue layer is dense, firm, and relatively avascular. Its composition is primarily collagenous, which makes it resistant to usual day-to-day mechanical forces assailing the body and less susceptible to vascular compromise. Its function is protective, but it also gives the body contour and shape. Beneath the fascia are muscles; muscle tissue is resistant to tension but sensitive to compression. This sensitivity makes muscle tissue vulnerable to pressure damage. Not only are muscle fibers themselves vulnerable to pressure but nerve fibers and blood vessels supplying muscles with metabolic and nervous conduction needs are vulnerable as well.

Deep pressure sores develop within muscles close to a bony surface or projection initially (Husain 1953; and Shea 1975). Pathological studies demonstrate muscular lesions before superficial skin lesions appear and show the presence of muscle lesions of varying stages accompanying frank bedsores (Husain 1953). Muscle tissue is more susceptible to disturbances from pressure than is skin or adipose tissue (Groth 1975).

Muscle tissue under pressure demonstrates histologic changes in muscle including loss of striation, conversion of sarcoplasm into homogeneous material, fragmentation, granularity, and eventual necrosis of the muscle fibers. Absorption of the necrosed part of the muscle fibers leads to the production of empty sarcolemmal husks. Experiments on compressed muscle tissue show that it is the site of diminished blood flow, which favors thrombosis and the localization of bacterial infection in its substance if bacteremia is present before or during compression (Husain 1953).

Kosiak's (1959) studies do not support the contention that pressure effects are greatest over the bone and are subsequently dissipated. His tissue-pressure experiments indicate that all layers are compressed sufficiently to produce degenerative changes simultaneously at every level. He cites as evidence that ulceration almost always involves all tissue layers down to the bony prominences. This finding raises the question of whether necrosis develops at different rates within various tissues.

Objectives of Treatment

While there is disagreement as to the order of tissue changes in deep, malignant pressure sores, there is basic agreement that necrosis is what ultimately happens. Since it is an irreversible tissue change, prevention of its occurrence is the most effective management. The relief of soft-tissue pressure, the prevention of shearing force, the minimization of friction, and the maintenance of a normal nitrogen balance will ensure prevention of pressure sores in almost all clinical situations.

In those cases where aggressive preventive measures are not consistently practiced or in those patients where skin breakdown is inevitable, the objective of treatment obviously changes. In every possible case where pressure sores exist, the aim of treatment is cure with minimal damage and scarring at the injury site. Attaining this objective is possible by conservative measures with the superficial, benign pressure sore because there is not extensive soft-tissue necrosis. With the deep malignant type of pressure sore, however, the degree of soft-tissue destruction usually negates fully attaining the objective by conservative measures, and surgical repair becomes necessary.

Types of Treatment

The number and variability of treatment regimens used in the management of pressure sores suggests that there is no one clinically superior method of treatment. This supposition may be fallacious, however, because no large scale studies using a well-controlled and valid research design have yet been done on this problem.

It is beyond the scope and purpose of this chapter to explore in depth the variety of regimens recounted in the literature. These methods can, however, be categorized in tabular form as shown in Table 22-1. The table reveals that all methods currently use physical methods, chemical methods, mechanical devices, diet, and/or surgery as the basis for their efficacy. The treatment methods listed are not intended to be exhaustive, nor does the table show that many times treatments are combined in the management of patients with pressure sores.

Creating a Model for Future Nursing Research

A causal model based on biochemical-physical cellular dynamics, gross physiological changes, economics of pressure-sore treatment or a variety of other possibilities can be created. The etiologic causal model might be the most useful for nursing because of its application to patient assessment, prevention, and intervention. Such a model could pinpoint critical areas for research such as determining the pressure-sore risk score for patients. In order to use such a model effectively, however, certain generalizations about pressure sores would need to be taken into consideration by the researcher. These include

1. Certain types of patients have a high risk of pressure-sore development. Patients who are more likely to develop them are those who are paralyzed, those who have a decreased sensorium, those who are debilitated and malnourished, those who are elderly, and/or those who have certain medical conditions such as circulatory impairment, cachexia, disturbed sensorium, physical disability interfering with movement, severe anemia, fever, or infections.

Table 22-1 Treatment Methods for Pressure Sores

Nutritional Methods	Mechanical Methods	Physical Methods	Chemical Methods	Surgical Methods
High-calorie, high-protein diet	Polyurethane foam (egg-crate mattress, reston)	Turning bedfast patient every 1 to 2 hours	Enzymes for topical administration (e.g., tryspin, fibrinolysin, collagenase, insulin)	Debridement
Intravenous fluids containing vitamins and electrolytes	Gel pads	Changing position of the chairfast patient every 30 minutes	Povidone-iodine solution (e.g.. Betadine)	Primary closure
	Polyether foam pads (e.g., Dupic)	Use of whirlpool bath every 1 to 2 days	Vitamin C	Incision and drainage
	Sheepskin	Use of wet to dry dressings	Antibiotics for secondary infection	Rotation of pedicle grafts
	Op-site	Heat lamp to pressure area	Vegetable gum typically (e.g., karaya)	Removal of bony prominences
	Substitute skin coverings—lyophilized porcine and bovine skin	Ultraviolet irradiatic ٦ to pressure area	Absorbable gelatin sponge and/or powder (e.g., Gelfoam) topically	Split thickness graft
	Net suspension bed	Ultrasonic treatment to pressure area	Sugar	Muscle transposition
	Turning frames (e.g., Circ Olectric, Stryker, Foster)	Carbon dioxide laser for debridement	Zinc cream	Sensory skin flaps in paraplegics
	Constant turnbeds (e.g., Co-Ro)		Insulin topically	Delayed pedicle grafts
	Alternating pressure mattresses		ACTH	Amputation
	Low-air-loss beds		Dextran polymer beads (e.g., Debrisan)	
	High-air-loss beds		Antacids topically	
	Air-fluid bed		Merthiolate	
	Water-immersion bed		Oxidizing agents (e.g., hydrogen peroxide)	
	High-density fluid bed (e.g., MUD)		Antiseptics (e.g., tincture of benzoin pHisoHex)	
	Sawdust bed		Anabolizing hormones (e.g., nilevar)	
	Mattresses—air, water, feather		Hyperbaric oxygen	
	Pillows		Silicone cream	
	Molding devices			
	Plaster casts			

2. Patients who are high risks for the development of pressure sores can be identified by the nurse through assessment of the following variables: medical diagnosis, age, ability to move, level of consciousness, nutritional status, presence of infection and/or fever, adequacy of circulation, and bladder and bowel control.

3. There are four basic causes of pressure sores: sustained soft-tissue pressure, friction, shearing force, and negative nitrogen balance.

4. The four basic causes of pressure sores are preventable or controllable by effective nursing management.

5. Some pressure sores are not preventable, such as in the patient who has suffered soft-tissue pressure injury as a result of accidental trauma.

6. Laboratory research indicates that ischemia from soft-tissue pressure is the major cause of most pressure sores.

7. The lowest limit of pressure capable of producing soft-tissue necrosis in humans has not been conclusively established. It is known that if capillary closing pressure is exceeded for sustained periods of time, skin breakdown will occur.

8. Mean capillary closing pressure is 25 mm Hg. Any pressure greater than 30 mm Hg is assumed to be potentially damaging to tissue.

9. Soft tissue is markedly susceptible to change with relatively low constant pressures for short periods of time (e.g., 70 mm Hg for two hours).

10. There is greater tissue resistance to change and/or damage if the soft tissue pressure is intermittent than if it is constant.

11. Intense pressure of short duration causes interference and perhaps complete cessation of capillary circulation as well as changes in the larger vessels with the result that venous thrombi may occur.

12. Not all tissue subjected to supracapillary closing results in pressure necroses.

13. The duration of soft-tissue pressure is more important than the amount of pressure in determining whether breakdown occurs.

14. Primary pressure effects occur in the capillary bed and interfere with the exchange of cellular metabolites.

15. Prevention of tissue ischemia from supracapillary pressure may be accomplished by achieving greater body surface contact with its supporting surface.*

16. Shearing force is a significant factor in the causation of pressure sores, particularly in the sacral area.

---

*On a regular hospital mattress only 10–20 percent of the body surface is in effective contact. For a patient weighing 175 pounds the pressure exerted on this 10–20 percent support surface would vary between 30–60 mm Hg, all pressures in excess of capillary closing pressure.

17. Friction, another significant factor in the production of pressure sores, may produce superficial lesions similar to burns.

18. Shearing force is never present without significant friction; friction may be present without significant shearing force.

19. Negative nitrogen balance, the fourth major factor in the causation of pressure sores, renders soft tissues more susceptible to breakdown.

20. Healing of pressure sores cannot take place if the patient is in severe negative nitrogen balance.

21. Limited laboratory research indicates that ascorbic acid accelerates soft-tissue healing of pressure lesions.

22. Multiple factors indirectly influence the development of pressure sores in the patient who is bed-ridden or chair-ridden. These include the patient's medical diagnosis, medications, activity status, temperature, neurological status, elimination control, and therapy.

23. There are at least two different major types of pressure sores: the superficial, benign type and the deep, malignant type.

24. The superficial, benign pressure sore is usually caused by friction and resembles a burn.

25. The deep, malignant pressure sore is truly a pressure initiated necrosis.

26. Deep, malignant pressure sores may involve all tissue planes down to the underlying bone. It is unclear whether the soft tissues involved necrose at different rates.

27. The most effective treatment for either type of pressure sore is prevention of the lesion.

28. Prevention of pressure lesions is accomplished by preventing the occurrence of or by interrupting the progression of prolonged soft-tissue pressure, shearing force, significant friction, and/or negative nitrogen balance.

With these generalizations in mind, plus a knowledge of the "direct" and "indirect" factors involved in the formation of pressure sores, nurse-researchers could generate a variety of models for pursuing needed knowledge about prevention and/or treatment. An appreciation of the importance of the direct factors (i.e., sustained soft-tissue pressure, shearing force, significant friction, and negative nitrogen balance) is essential in the construction of a model for research purposes. Of equal importance is an appreciation of the role of various "indirect" factors. The list of these indirect variables is extensive. Some of the ones identified by various writers include incontinence, skin maceration due to incontinence or diaphoresis, anemia, edema, obesity, dehydration, altered mental status resulting from medications, surgery, or personality disorder, nature of underlying disease process, reduced general resistance, decreased mobility, restraints, paralysis, loss of vascular tone, devitalization of deep tissue, presence of anesthetic areas, steroids, radiation therapy, type of mattress, and high-friction coefficient of bed coverings.

Following is one possible model that takes into account the major direct and indirect factors in the production of pressure sores (Figure 22-1). The need for others is readily apparent. Nurse-researchers must concentrate their efforts on defining and evaluating measures that contribute to prevention of pressure sores, on devising and evaluating tools for identifying patients likely to develop pressure sores, and on developing and refining valid instruments for use in assessing and evaluating the effect of nursing care on prevention and/or treatment of the patient with pressure sores.

FUTURE DIRECTIONS FOR RESEARCH

Among the research questions that remain to be answered or need to be replicated about pressure sores are:

1. Is there a variation in susceptibility among patients to the effect of localized pressure?
2. Is there a variation in the response of healthy tissue to the effect of localized pressure?
3. Do different types of healthy tissue (e.g., muscle, fat) show variations in their response to localized pressure?
4. Can we define in humans a minimal degree and amount of pressure that will consistently result in the initiation of a pressure sore?
5. What is the effect of small postural changes (i.e., movements not involving a large amount of rotation of the trunk) on the distribution of pressure on the tissues of the bedfast or chair-ridden patient?
6. Does a person's body type and weight influence the risk for pressure-sore development?
7. Does a patient's sex play a part in susceptibility to pressure-sore development?
8. Does a patient's race play a part in susceptibility to the development of pressure sores?
9. What is the role of aging in pressure-sore susceptibility?
10. Do changes in mental state influence the predisposition to pressure sores?
11. Does skin hydration, elasticity, and padding play a part in susceptibility to pressure sores?
12. What is the effect of low serum protein levels on the production of pressure sores?
13. Is the state of urinary and fecal continence a significant factor in a patient's likelihood to develop pressure sores?
14. Is there a significant relationship between an individual's diastolic blood pressure and his tendency to develop pressure sores?
15. Is there a significant relationship between the amount and type of medication that an individual receives and the subsequent development of pressure sores?

Figure 22-1 Etiologic Causal Model of Pressure Sore Production

Patient variables

1. Immobility
   a) Denervation
      Quadriplegia
      Paraplegia
      Hemiplegia
   b) Trauma
      Neurological injury
      Orthopedic injury

2. Decreased mobility
   a) Debilitation
   b) Aging
   c) Diagnosis
   d) Medication

3. Decreased or altered
   sensorium
   a) Unconsciousness
   b) Semiconsciousness
   c) Lethargy
   d) Depression
   e) Disorientation

4. Chronological age
   a) 85 and Over
   b) 75 to 85
   c) 65 to 75
   d) 55 to 65

5. Nutritional status
   a) Cachexia/debilitation
   b) Dehydration
   c) Hypoproteinemia
   d) Anemia
   e) Vitamin deficiency

6. Diagnosis
   a) Combination of following
      diagnoses
   b) Paralysis/spinal-cord
      injury
   c) Cancer
   d) Orthopedic injuries
   e) Vascular disease
   f) Neurological disease or
      injury
   g) Diabetes mellitus

Environmental variables

1. Unrelieved external pressure
   a) Confinement to bed
   b) Confinement to chair

2. Increased interface pressure
   a) Unyielding support surface
   b) Unyielding support-surface
      covering
   c) Decreased effective
      support surface for body
      weight

3. Inadequate supervision of
   patient mobility
   a) Infrequent alteration of
      position by patient
   b) Infrequent alteration of
      patient's position by
      personnel

4. Restriction of movement
   a) Restraints
   b) Certain treatments and
      orthopedic appliances

5. Traumatic injury resulting in
   prolonged immobility
   a) Pressure damage
   b) Circulatory damage
   c) Friction damage
   d) Shearing damage

6. Increased friction
   a) Nature of support surface
   b) Moisture
   c) Increased patient
      movement

7. Musculoskeletal alterations
   a) Loss of subcutaneous tissue
   b) Loss of muscle mass
   c) Increasing prominence of bony support surfaces

8. Soft-tissue changes
   a) Medication-induced changes, as with steroids
   b) Disease-associated changes, as with amyotrophic lateral sclerosis
   c) Race-related changes

9. Incontinence
   a) Bladder
   b) Bowel

10. Major surgery
    a) Any procedure lasting 4 or more hours
    b) Orthopedic procedures of hip and femur

11. Medications
    a) Narcotics
    b) Sedatives
    c) Analgesics
    d) Soporifics
    e) Steroids

12. Infection
    a) Severe generalized infection
    b) Localized infection in pressure-supporting areas
    c) Sustained elevated body temperature

7. Shearing force
   a) Pulling patients up in bed without lifting them clear of mattress
   b) Elevating head of bed

8. Lack of adequate nutritional management
   a) IV fluids only
   b) Formula feedings
   c) Inadequate oral intake

9. Failure to maintain dry environment
   a) Wet or soiled bed linens
   b) Skin maceration due to wetness and chemical irritation

The greater number of patient and environmental variables present and interacting, the greater the risk of pressure sore formation.

Pressure sore formation

16. Does the presence of clinically demonstrated infection predispose the patient to the development of pressure sores?
17. Is the patient whose body temperature is greater than 99°F significantly more likely to develop pressure sores?
18. How frequently should patients be turned to prevent pressure-sore development?
19. What chemical agents are effective in the prevention and/or treatment of pressure sores?
20. Which mechanical devices are effective in the prevention and/or treatment of pressure sores?
21. What physical methods are effective in the prevention and/or treatment of pressure sores?
22. How do different types of support surfaces prevent or promote pressure-sore development?
23. Are different types of support surfaces needed for different types of patients in order to minimize the danger of pressure-sore development?

Until we as nurses begin to clarify the concepts upon which our practice is based, we are doomed to perpetuate nursing care largely based in empiricism. Such a nonscientific basis in the practice of a profession is indefensible. The increasing number of prepared clinicians and scholars in nursing should be able to evolve objective, tested models on which optimal care can be based. This must be our goal, and the clarification of concepts must be one of our first steps in attaining it.

REFERENCES

Adams, T., and Hunter, W.S. Modification of skin mechanical properties by eccrine sweat gland activity. *J. Appl. Physiol.* 26(4):417–419, 1969.

Bell, F., Fernie, G.R., and Barbenel, J.C. Pressure sores: Their cause and prevention. *Nurs. Times* 70:740–745, May 16, 1974.

Brooks, B., and Duncan, W. Effects of pressure on tissues. *Arch. Surg.* 40:696–709, 1940.

Burton, A.C., and Yamada, S. Relation between blood pressure and flow in the human forearm. *J. Appl. Physiol.* 4:329, Nov. 1951.

Daniel, R.K., Terzis, J.K., and Cunningham, D.M. Sensory skin flaps for coverage of pressure sores in paraplegic patients. *Plast. Reconst. Surg.* 58(3):317–328, Sept. 1976.

Dyson, R. Bed sores—The injuries hospital staff inflict on patients. *Nurs. Mirror* 146(24):30–32, June 15, 1978.

Exton-Smith, N.A. Nutritional problems of elderly populations. In *Nutrition of the Aged.* (Quebec: The Nutrition Society of Canada) 1978.

Fernie, G.R. Biomechanical aspects of the aetiology of decubitus ulcers on human patients. University of Strathclyde, Glasgow, Scotland, Ph.D. Thesis, 1973.

Forbes, G.B. and J.C. Reina. Adult lean body mass declines with age: Some longitudinal observations. *Metabolism: Clinical and Experimental* 19:653–663, 1970.

Fordyce, W.C., and Simons, B.C. Automated training system for wheelchair pushups. *Public Health Rep.* 83:527–528, June 1968.

Forrester, J.M. Amyotrophic lateral sclerosis and bedsores. *Lancet* 1(7966):970, May 1, 1976.

Furukawa, T., and Toyokura, Y. Amyotrophic lateral sclerosis and bedsores. *Lancet* 1(7964):862, Apr. 17, 1976.

Furukawa, T., and Toyokura, Y. Amyotrophic lateral sclerosis and bedsores: Plethysmographic analysis (editorial). *Lancet* 1:159, Jan. 21, 1978.

Gerber, R.M., and Van Ort, S.R. Topical application of insulin in decubitus ulcer. *Nurs. Res.* 28(1):16–19, Jan.–Feb. 1979.

Gerson, L.W. The incidence of pressure sores in active treatment hospitals. *Int. J. Nurs. Stud.* 12: 201–204, 1975.

Gosnell, D.J. An assessment tool to identify pressure sores. *Nurs. Res.* 22(1):55–59, Jan.–Feb. 1973.

Groth, K.E. Klinische beobachtungen and experimentelle Studien uber die Entstchung des Dekubitus, *Acta Chir. Scand.* [Suppl.] 87:76, 1942. Cited in K.H. Berecek, Etiology of decubitus ulcers. *Nurs. Clin. North Am.* 10(1):157–170, Mar. 1975.

Guttman, L. The problem of treatment of pressure sores in patients with spinal paraplegia. *Br. J. Plast. Surg.* 8:196, 1955.

Harman, J.W. Significance of local vascular phenomena in production of ischemic necrosis in skeletal muscle. *Am. J. Pathol.* 24:625, May 1948.

Houle, R.J. Evaluation of seat devices designed to prevent ischemic ulcers in paraplegic patients. *Arch. Phys. Med. Rehab.* 50:587–594, 1969.

Hubay, C.A., Diehn, C.C., and Drucker, W.R. Decubitus ulcers in the post traumatic patient. *Am. J. Surg.* 93:705–713, 1957.

Husain, T. An experimental study of some pressure effects on tissues, with reference to the bedsore problem. *J. Pathol. Bacteriol.* 66:347–358, Oct. 1953.

Jordan, M.A., and Clark, M.O. Report on the incidence of pressure sores in the patient community of the greater Glasgow health board area on 21st January, 1976. The Bioengineering Unit, University of Strathclyde, and the Greater Glasgow Health Board, Glasgow, 1977. Reported in M.O. Clark, et al. Pressure sores. *Nurs. Times* 74(9):363–366, Mar. 2, 1978.

Kosiak, M., Kubicek, W., Olson, M., Danz, J., and Kottka, F. Evaluation of pressure as a factor in the production of ischial ulcers. *Arch. Phys. Med. Rehab.* 39(10):623–629, Oct. 1958.

Kosiak, M. Etiology and pathology of ischemic ulcers. *Arch. Phys. Med. Rehab.* 40(2):62–69, Feb. 1959.

Kosiak, M. Etiology of decubitus ulcers. *Arch. Phys. Med. Rehab.* 42(1):19–29, Jan. 1961.

Landis, E.M. Micro-injection studies of capillary blood pressure in human skin. *Heart* 15:209–228, May 1930.

Lindan, O. Etiology of decubitus ulcers: An experimental study. *Arch. Phys. Med. Rehab.* 42:774–783, Nov. 1961.

Lowthian, P. Pressure sore prevalence. *Nurs. Times* 75(9):358–360, Mar. 1, 1979.

Manley, M.T. Incidence, contributory factors and costs of pressure sores. *S. Afr. Med. J.* 53(6):217–222, Feb. 11, 1978.

Mulholland, J., et al. Protein metabolism and bed sores. *Ann. Surg.* 118(6):1015–1023, Dec. 1943.

Munro, H.N. Protein Requirements and Metabolism in Aging. In L.A. Carlson (Ed.), *Nutrition in Old Age*. Uppsala, Sweden: Almquist and Wiksoll, 1972.

Nichol, J., Girling, F., Jerrard, W., Claxton, E.G., and Burton, A.C. Fundamental instability of small blood vessels and critical closing pressures in vascular beds. *Am. J. Physiol.* 64:330, Feb. 1951.

Nightingale, K.M. Out of sight: Out of mind. *Natnews.* 15(9):15–18, Sept. 1978.

Norton, D., McLaren, R., and Exton-Smith, A.N. *An Investigation of Geriatric Nursing Problems in Hospital.* London: National Corp. for the Care of Old People, 1962.

Oates, G.D. Prevention of perioperative pressure sores during pelvic surgery. *Lancet* 1(7900):202, Jan. 25, 1975.

Parish, L., Smith, G., and Collins, E. Decubitus ulcers and amyotrophic lateral sclerosis (editorial). *Lancet* 1(8065):658–659, Mar. 25, 1978.

Petersen, N.C., and Bittman, S. The epidemiology of pressure sores. *Scand. J. Plast. Reconstr. Surg.* 5:62–66, 1971.

Petersen, N.C. The Development of Pressure Sores during Hospitalization. In R.M. Kenedi, J.M. Cowden, and J.T. Scales (Eds.), *Bedsore Biomechanics.* Baltimore: University Park Press, 1976. P. 222.

Reichel, S.M. Shearing force as a factor in decubitus ulcers in paraplegics. *J. A. M. A.* 166(7):762–763, Feb. 15, 1958.

Roaf, R. The Causation and Prevention of Bedsores. In R.M. Kenedi, J.M. Cowden, and J.T. Scales (Eds.), *Bedsore Biomechanics.* Baltimore: University Park Press, 1976. P. 6.

Robinson, C.E., Coghlan, J.K., and Jackson, G. Decubitus ulcers in paraplegics: Financial implications. *Can. J. Public Health* 69(3):199, May–June 1978.

Rubin, C.F., Dietz, R.R., and Abruzzese, R.S. Auditing the decubitus ulcer problem. *Am. J. Nurs.* 74(10):1820–1821, Oct. 1974.

Sather, M.R., Weber, C.E., and George, J. Pressure sores and the spinal cord injury patient. *Drug Intell. Clin. Pharm.* 11:154–168, Mar. 1977.

Scales, J.T. Beware of the hospital bed. *Nurs. Mirror* 144(9):39–41, Mar. 3, 1977.

Schell, V., and Wolcott, L. The etiology, prevention and management of decubitus ulcers. *Mo. Med.* 63:100–110, 1966.

Shea, J.D. Pressure sores: Classification and management. *Clin. Orthop.* 112:89–100, Oct. 1975.

Spence, W.R., Burk, R.D., and Rae, J.W. Gel support for prevention of decubitus ulcers. *Arch. Phys. Med. Rehab.* 48:283–288, June 1967.

Stauffer, E.S. Pressure trauma to soft tissue and bone. *Orthop. Clin. North Am.* 9(2):283–289, Apr. 1978.

Taylor, T.V., Dymock, I.W., Torrance, B. The role of Vitamin C in the treatment of pressure sores in surgical patients. *British Journal of Surgery* 61(11):921, Nov. 1974.

Tepperman, P.S., DeZwirek, C.S., Chiarcossi, A.L., and Jimenez, J. Pressure sores: Prevention and step-up management. *Postgrad. Med.* 62(3):83–89, Sept. 1977.

Trumble, H.C. The skin tolerance for pressure and pressure sores. *Med. J. Aust.* 2:724, 1930.

Williams, A. A study of factors contributing to skin breakdown. *Nurs. Res.* 21(3):238–243, May–June 1972.

Woodbine, A. Pressure sores—2: A survey in Macclesfield. *Nurs. Times* 75(26):1129–1132, Jul. 5, 1979.

Part III

Analysis and Synthesis: Developing the Construct of Basic Human Protective Mechanisms for Nursing

The major thrust of this section is moving all concepts dealt with specifically in the preceding section to an abstraction that includes them all. A further intent is to relate them to the discipline of nursing. Newman (1979, p. 2) specifies this relationship in her first two criteria.

1. The focus is on the life process in people
2. The purpose is to understand the patterns of the life process that relate to health.

All were concepts synthesized under a large umbrella concept named "basic human physiological protective mechanisms." Analysis of the protective function of each phenomenon permitted defining each concept in view of its protective aspects, identifying attributes held in common by concepts, identifying associational relationships among concepts, and organizing concepts in set–subset relationships.

The results of study of the umbrella concept, basic human physiological protective mechanisms, are presented as beginning theory for nursing.

In Chapter 24, a number of subjects about concept clarification for nursing are addressed including the significance of naming for the discipline of nursing, evaluation of concept work in nursing, possibilities for using concepts to guide further study and nursing practice, and the need for feedback about concept clarification work from within the profession.

REFERENCE

Newman, M. *Theory Development in Nursing*. Philadelphia: Davis, 1979.

Chapter 23

Synthesis of Concepts: Evolving an Umbrella Concept—Protection

Catherine M. Norris

Synthesis of the work of examining the ten concepts clarified in this volume and preliminary study of five concepts identified in the Preface allows conceptual systematization and the discovery of relationships among these diverse phenomena. Using the term *umbrella concept* to mean a complex concept, all of the concepts studied appear to share enough elements to permit their organization under an umbrella named *basic physiological protection mechanisms*. This chapter summarizes the work of evolving this umbrella concept of protection using a theory construction format.

ELEMENTS OF PROTECTION

In looking at this synthesis, readers may require some definition in order to understand the perspective of this text. In this work, the term *basic physiological protection mechanisms* refers to functional behavioral responses that attempt to remove threat to bodily organs or systems. These functional behavioral responses are perceived intellectually as needs, drives, or discomforts. Functional behavioral responses are, in this sense, warnings. Protective mechanisms have at least seven elements or components, which can be stated as postulates relating concepts to the larger umbrella concept. These seven elements have seven aspects in common:

1. They warn.
2. They are time-limited for action (i.e., protection).
3. They require action.
4. When acted upon, they give relief.
5. Accompanying or following relief, pleasure and relaxation are often experienced.
6. People continually make decisions about protective mechanisms.

7. Some of the protective mechanisms share common attributes (i.e., particular ways of protecting).

Warning as Protection

Functional behavioral responses that attempt to remove threat represent an
alert or alarm about potential loss of some aspect of dynamic homeostasis. The
alert or alarm can be responded to before actual homeostatic disequilibrium
occurs. The following phenomena are listed with the protective function they
hold in common described in the second column.

Concept	*Explication of Protective Warning Function*
Nausea	Nausea is a warning to the organism that the stomach is preparing to eject its liquid and solid contents. It is a protective warning that the stomach contents are not acceptable at this level of the organism.
Vomiting	(1) Ejection of the liquid and solid contents of the stomach prevents noxious agents from entering the circulatory fluids of the body. It protects the body by eliminating materials experienced as "dangerous." (2) Vomiting is orgasmic discharge in situations of great rage, disgust, or other emotions, followed by feelings of relief. It protects the organism from emotional shock and overwhelming emotional experience.
Morning sickness nausea with or without vomiting	The most accepted theory of morning sickness is that human chorionic gonadotropin-B (HGB) secretion increases rapidly after fertilization of the ovum. Either HGB is an irritant to the gastric mucosa or irritation occurs because of the quantity secreted. The nausea and vomiting represent the body's attempt to protect by eliminating the irritant.
Thirst	Thirst is triggered by the hypothalamus when there is an inadequate amount of body water available for intra- and extracellular metabolic work of the body. It represents a warning that the body needs water and protects against dehydration.

Concept	*Explication of Protective Warning Function*
Hunger	Signals to the satiety center in the hypothalamus convey messages that nutritional reserves have been depleted and the organism perceives a sense of hunger drive. Hunger, in contrast to appetite, expresses the need for nutrients necessary to ongoing metabolic processes (e.g., growth and repair). Hunger protects in that it warns against malnutrition and its extreme form, starvation.
Insomnia	Insomnia occurs in terms of interaction between the cerebrum and the sleep center in the hypothalamus when messages perceived by the organism indicate the need to be alert. The messages relate to some threat—real, imagined, or symbolic—and the insomnia protects through keeping the body ready to respond to perceived danger. It is often the first warning of impending illness.
Fatigue	Fatigue is perceived by the organism as a lack of energy or a tired feeling. It warns that energy production is not keeping pace with energy demands. Further, it warns that the organism needs rest to protect against exhaustion that cannot be relieved by routine resting. Responding to fatigue by resting reduces energy consumption.
Immobility	The greatest number of cases of immobility represent responses to pain and swelling. Immobilization promotes rest and, empirically, we believe that rest is important to healing. Many medical treatments, particularly after surgery or injury, include immobilizing a part or most of the body. Again, this protects against further injury by reducing energy demands, and promoting healing. In these kinds of situations, immobilization is protective and health promoting. Where there is loss of enervation, immobilization may become one of the most debilitating aspects of the disease.

Concept	*Explication of Protective Warning Function*
Chilling	Reflex responses to lowered ambient temperature include contraction of thousands of arrectores pilorum muscles that exert pressure on sebaceous glands to the extent that the skin around the glands becomes covered with an oily insulating secretion. Further body chilling causes shivering that is reported to start at the masseter muscles (Abbey et al. 1973).
Itching	The skin may itch because of irritants contacted in the external environment like poison ivy, soap, or insect bite. Skin may also become very sensitive as in allergy or when there is psychological stress. The itching may be perceived as a protective warning that the skin is in danger of being harmed by some noxious agent or it may possibly be a warning of psychological stress. Effective response at this point would prevent chronicity, ulceration of the skin, or infection of open, scratched surfaces.
Disorientation	This is probably the most difficult concept developed in this volume to define and, therefore, the most difficult to give functions for. It often occurs at the time of great stress when usual coping capacities and familiar orientating environment are not available. It may represent protection of the personality from intolerable stress. It often occurs after darkness falls and clears when daylight comes. Nurses have been heard to say that disorientation does not *start* when people are up and around. For affected people, disorientation may be a warning of sensory overload, sensory deprivation, or inability to cope with the problems at hand. Taken as a protective warning, the victims and nurses may act to

Concept	Explication of Protective Warning Function
	eliminate stresses before the patients' disorientation increases or becomes chronic. Disorientation here does not include chronic brain syndrome or other pathological conditions in which disorientation is part of the picture of confusion.
Bedsores	Bedsores represent the failure of a variety of physiological warnings to influence the behavior of the affected person toward protective strategies. Some of these warnings would be erythema due to pressure, pallor due to pressure, and loss of sensation due to pressure and ecchymoses due to pressure. Bedsores, then, are included to illustrate that when the body's protective mechanisms are not supported and are not successful within some time frame, the result is pathological resolution. Some bedsores represent lack of enervation and interference to normal circulation as well as interference to normal feedback mechanisms to the brain and spinal cord.

The following concepts, although not specifically covered in the text, also belong to nursing:

Concept	Explication of Protective Warning Function
Diarrhea	Frequent, loose stools represent an attempt by the gastrointestinal apparatus to rid itself of noxious materials so these materials will not be absorbed into the body proper. Irritation in the intestine creates an osmotic gradient that increases the amount of fluid in the intestine. This softens the stool, making it easy to expel and creates bulk in the sigmoid, which stimulates reflex activity experienced as the urge to defecate. In its primary function, diarrhea is protective.

Concept	Explication of Protective Warning Function
Constipation	Constipation conserves body water by absorption through the walls of the large intestine. The primary aim of this activity is protection but, associated with low activity level and diet lacking in bulk, becomes a source of concern and discomfort.
Flatulence	This function represents the major way pressure, created by gas formation during fermentation activity in the intestine, can be relieved. Its basic function is protection against buildup of pressure due to gas in the intestine and of the discomfort caused by unrelieved pressure.
Urinary frequency	Frequency occurs as the bladder attempts to rid itself of irritating substances in the urine as in a bladder infection. It may also occur in an attempt to relieve pressure on bladder walls as in distention. The bladder responds to protect by voiding the noxious agent.
Perspiration	When body temperature increases over the norm for a particular person at a particular time of day, reflex action mediated in the hypothalamus occurs. Peripheral vasodilatation permits the sweat glands to secrete an aqueous solution from extracellular fluids, which is poured forth from the glands on skin surfaces. The process of evaporation of this aqueous solution from the skin uses body heat, which cools the body. In its primary function, perspiration protects the body from overheating.

The synthesis resulting from the analysis of concepts allows the proposition that all the primitive physiological processes identified above, except pressure sores, have as a primary function *protection of the human organism.*

Time Limitations of Protective Mechanisms

Each basic physiological protective mechanism that attempts to remove threat has a specific time limit in which to accomplish its protective function. While time limitation is affected by many variables, if the protective function has not been completed within its time limit, the protective mechanism becomes an integral part of a pathological process.

All human phenomena have temporal relationships. We need to consider the relationships to instill meaning in the nature of the protection conceptualized in this chapter. Protective warning phenomena are not protective indefinitely. Each phenomenon probably has a range of time-limited effectiveness varied by age, state of health, ambient temperature, season of the year, environmental stress, and other factors. The temporal aspects of vomiting as protection, for example, would be affected by hydration at onset, health at onset, and age at onset. The protective function of vomiting would usually be much shorter for a healthy infant than for a healthy adult because of the varied rate at which dehydration would occur in the infant as compared to the adult. The protective function of immobility would be shorter in the aged healthy adult than in the young healthy adult—other factors being equal—because of the differences in amount of bone calcium and rate of decalcification as well as the differences in rates of soft-tissue replacement and repair. Insomnia taken to the limits of sleep deprivation has created considerable personality disorganization in healthy adults. More extensive information is required if temporal aspects of this kind of protection are to be assessed accurately and if the extent to which these aspects are useful in health promotion and disease prevention is to be determined.

Action Required by Protective Mechanisms

Some form of remedial action is required to damp protective mechanisms that occur.

1. Fatigue requires a person to rest and/or sleep.
2. Thirst requires a person to take fluids.
3. Hunger requires a person to eat.
4. Nausea requires a person to remain quiet, breathe deeply, apply ice to the left abdomen, or go with the demands of the body.
5. Vomiting requires going with the demands of the body while preventing aspiration.

Relief Associated with Protective Mechanisms

Intervention in existing protective mechanisms has a sequel called *relief*. Relief is alleviation, ease, or feeling of well-being following distress, discomfort, pain, or a return to some self-defined norm after intervention. At the personal level, the feeling experienced after responding to and dealing with these phenomena as warnings is taken for granted. It may be useful for the purposes of this discussion to make them explicit.

Phenomenon	Feeling after Responding to Protective Warning
Vomiting	After the event there are great relief and a return of sense of well-being.
Thirst	Enjoyment of the drink and a feeling of comfort and satisfaction after drinking are experienced.
Hunger	There is pleasure in anticipating, selecting, and eating food and a feeling of satiation and completeness after eating.
Insomnia	A feeling of sensual pleasure is related to being able to sleep and abandon cares.
Fatigue	Feelings of relief, comfort, or reward to rest, coupled with pleasurable sensations occur.
Immobility	Feelings of joy and power emerge as the return of function of muscles and joints occurs.
Chilling	Warmth brings comfort, joy, and relaxation.
Itching	Scratching, which tends to destroy small sections of nerve endings thus eliminating itching for 20 minutes or so, is pleasurable.
Disorientation	Feelings of relief follow lucidity, even though there is fear of return of symptoms.
Bedsores	Feelings of comfort and elimination of pain are experienced.
Diarrhea	Feelings of satisfaction and relief occur, even though diarrhea is accompanied by griping.
Constipation	Relief of anxiety and feeling of well-being result from defecation.
Flatulence	There is a feeling of power in the act and a feeling of relief and gladness after the act. Enjoyment, often humorous, is expressed about expelling flatus.
Urinary frequency	There is relief and a feeling of well-being on voiding. If there is infectious or other pathological process, relief is short or momentary.

Perspiration   On evaporation of perspiration, a feeling of
                               relief and comfort results.

To repeat, the sequelae of protective physiological responses and human intervention in protective warning responses includes a general theme of relief and
comfort.

Pleasure and Relaxation Associated with Relief

In addition to relief, as an outcome of successful action in response to the
occurrence of basic physiological protective mechanisms there are often feelings
of *pleasure* and *relaxation*. Pleasure is enjoyment, sensual gratification, experience of gladness, or feeling of energy revitalization. Relaxation is feeling at
ease, feeling muscle tension lessen, feeling at rest or able to rest, and/or feeling
mentally free and unworried.

Decision Making about Protective Mechanisms

People are involved in continuous decision making about basic physiological
protective mechanisms. There appear to be three types of decision making,
preventive, risk taking and uninformed. One purpose of the decision making is
to avoid instigating the protective mechanisms. Even though these protective
phenomena, as such, are welcome warning signals, a major thrust of human
behavior is preventing their occurrence. Most people know of ways to stay within
the margin of safety that deters, under normal conditions, activation of protection
responses. For example, one person may express this knowledge by saying, "If
I eat too many strawberries, I break out." Another will say, "If I drink too
much, I get sick," or, "Eating too much ice cream gives me diarrhea," or "I
don't drink gin; it makes me too thirsty." Most people discern relationships
between their behavior, emotional as well as physiological, and their feelings
of well-being. They use knowledge about these relationships to monitor their
lives, to restructure their behavior, to maintain their comfort, and to take health-
related risks. Much of this interaction between behavioral antecedents and physiological response goes on in a natural, matter-of-fact kind of way, in which
body control and responsiveness are taken for granted.

A great deal of continuous decision making appears to go into the maintenance
of dynamic physiological equilibrium, but not all of this decision making is
related to preventing the occurrence of protective or warning phenomena. Many
decisions are risk-taking decisions. Risk-taking decisions are judgments about
courses of action in which there is a chance of incurring a threat to the body
that will cause activation of one or more basic physiological protective mechanisms. These are decisions made while hoping against hope that dynamic equilibrium will not be affected. They are decisions like, "I really can't resist this

ice cream; I pray it doesn't show on the scales''; ''I really want this third martini, I hope I don't get sick (or drunk)''; ''I don't want to do my exercise today; one day won't really matter''; ''I should go to the bathroom, but I'm so busy that I guess I'll wait.'' These kinds of decisons are made by everyone. At what point does the number and kind of risk-taking decisions produce a life-style that is high-risk for frequent occurrence of protective warnings or even frank pathology? Knowing the range and frequency of risk-taking behaviors and their impact on various populations might be useful to nurses interested in protection as a component of life-style.

A third kind of decison making related to dynamic physiological equilibrium is the decison made in ignorance—whether through lack of self-monitoring and assessment or through lack of knowledge about health promotion and maintenance. Lack of motivation may also be related to uninformed decision making. This area is a challenge to all health care workers, but nurses could perceive it as a challenge to fulfill nursing's unique contribution to health.

Common Attributes of Protective Mechanisms

There are other attributes that some protective mechanisms share. The term *Common attributes* (i.e., attributes shared by two or more concepts) means that concepts are related to each other with an identified attribute or attributes.

Some of the protective mechanisms have type or method of protection in common—that is, they protect through the same general kinds of protective responses as illustrated in Table 23-1.

Relationships among Elements of Protection

In addition to the search for commonality in type of protection, associational relationships among some phenomena were identified. The search for relationships could be applied for all protective mechanisms, but is just illustrated here. Fatigue and restlessness appear to be the most commonly occurring concomitants. We could ask whether they are the most frequent protective mechanisms important to nurses along with responses considered psychological in origin like flight, freeze, startle, panic, and fight. If they do prove to be the most common physiological protective mechanisms, this would have implications for nursing priorities in health promotion. But this is speculative. The simple procedure of relating phenomena to each other is illustrated as follows:

Relationship of nausea to other behaviors.

Nausea often precedes vomiting.
Nausea warns of vomiting or the likelihood of it.

Table 23-1 Concepts Related by Type of Protection

Protective Mechanisms of the Human Organism—The Macrosystem

Increased drive or activity	Increased vigilance	Ejecting activity	Withdrawing activity	Withholding activity
Thirst	Restlessness	Diarrhea	Disorientation	Impaction
Hunger	Insomnia	Vomiting	Fatigue	Constipation
Chilling		Perspiration	Anorexia	Retention
Feeling hot		Incontinence	Tiredness	
Dyspnea		Coughing	Immobilization	
Itching		Frequency	Chilling and shiv-	
		Hiccoughs	ering	
			Nausea	

Protective Mechanisms of the Human Organism—The Microsystem

Healing
Immunity
Clotting
Stress response (fight/flight)—hypothalamic, pituitary, and adrenal systems
Integrative—nervous and endocrine systems

Nausea is accompanied by anorexia.

Nausea may be accompanied by fatigue.

Nausea may be accompanied by restlessness.

Nausea may be confused with hunger by those experiencing it.

Nausea damps hunger.

Nausea damps thirst.

Nausea often accompanies diarrhea.

Nausea may accompany constipation.

Nausea often accompanies pain and so may occur in immobilization and bedsores.

Nausea and a relationship to disorientation and itching (except where there is pain) was not found.

Relationship of vomiting to other behaviors.

Vomiting is preceded by anorexia.

Vomiting is often preceded by restlessness.

Vomiting often follows nausea.

Vomiting may accompany diarrhea.

Vomiting is often followed by thirst.

Vomiting damps hunger.

Vomiting may be followed by fatigue.

Vomiting is accompanied by considerable limitation of movement and function.

Vomiting may occur concurrent with or following pain.

Relationship of fatigue to other behaviors.

Fatigue may accompany nausea.

Fatigue may follow vomiting.

Fatigue may accompany diarrhea.

Fatigue may accompany constipation.

Fatigue may accompany or follow itching.

Fatigue may precede, accompany, or follow disorientation.

Fatigue may accompany or follow excessive perspiration.

Fatigue may accompany or follow anorexia.

Fatigue may accompany or follow weakness.

Fatigue may accompany or follow thirst.

Fatigue may accompany or follow hunger.

Fatigue may accompany or follow incontinence.

Fatigue may accompany or follow frequency.

Fatigue may accompany or precede the development of bedsores.

Relationship of insomnia to other behaviors.

Insomnia may accompany or be preceded by fatigue.

Insomnia may, in severe cases, be accompanied by nausea.

Insomnia may be accompanied by weakness.

Insomnia may be accompanied by anorexia.

Insomnia may occur concomitantly with frequency, dribbling, or incontinence.

Insomnia may occur concomitantly with diarrhea, constipation, or impaction.

Insomnia may occur concomitantly with urinary retention.

Insomnia often precedes or accompanies disorientation.

Insomnia may follow or be accompanied by weakness.

Insomnia may follow or be accompanied by thirst.

Insomnia may follow or be accompanied by hunger.

Insomnia often accompanies itching.

Insomnia often accompanies immobility.

Insomnia may precede or accompany bedsores.

Relationship of thirst to other behaviors.

Thirst often follows nausea.

Thirst often follows vomiting.

Thirst often follows diarrhea.

Thirst often follows frequency (i.e., due to diuresis).

Thirst may accompany or follow itching if the skin is broken.

Thirst often accompanies or follows perspiration.

Thirst may be part of hunger.

Thirst is damped in anorexia.

Thirst may occur in fatigue.

As already noted, fatigue is associated with many of the other phenomena. It may be that fatigue has a common denominator associational relationship to these protective phenomena as illustrated in Figure 23-1.

Figure 23-1 Fatigue in Common Denominator Association with Basic Human Physiological Protective Mechanisms

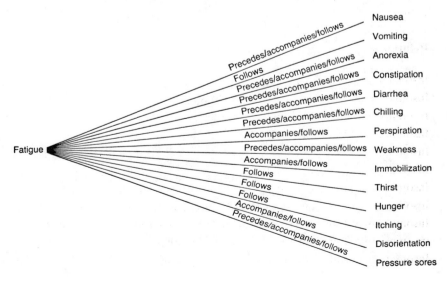

SYNTHESIS

It appeared that advance from the study of individual concepts and theoretical statements made about them as a whole required a formally constructed model that encompassed all the concepts.

So far, seven attributes that all named concepts have in common have been postulated. A variety of relationships between and among concepts have been identified. The next step is to advance the propositions emerging from the study of these concepts toward theory for nursing. The goal is to formulate a complex, organized whole that encompasses all propositions related to basic physiological protection mechanisms.

The results of one theory format used for this purpose are synthesized here as follows.

Scientific Assumptions about Protective Functions in Living Organisms

1. Living organisms maintain a dynamic homeostasis within the limits of which the organism exists in a state of well-being.
2. Living organisms are subject to attacks or forces that threaten this dynamic homeostasis.
3. These threats and attacks may be from forces in the environment but may also occur from autogenic forces.
4. The nature of these threats and attacks are varied and include
   a) Physical agents like heat, cold, friction, and pressure.
   b) Chemical agents like acids, alkalies, and toxins that may attack external or internal surfaces of living things.
   c) Pathogenic organisms.
   d) Lack of sensory input and sensory overload.
   e) Energy-depleting agents.
   f) Forced rapid physiological adjustments and adaptations.
   g) Loss of emotionally cathected objects.
   h) Change in life-style and routine.
   i) Loss of function and role.
5. Living organisms respond holistically to stress (e.g., threat), even though the stress may be expressed by one or two organ systems.
6. Living organisms, in order to conserve life, have developed protective functions or mechanisms.
7. Living organisms have built-in protective mechanisms at the levels of cells, organs, and systems and at the level of the total organism.
8. The more complex organisms become, the more complex and varied the protective mechanisms become. This is particularly true at the cellular level.

9. Humans have protective mechanisms typical of those of other complex living organisms.
10. Many protective phenomena in humans are observable as signs or reportable at the level of perceptions of experience.
11. Awareness of certain threats, whether innate or learned, allows living organisms to adjust in ways that maintain dynamic homeostasis.
12. Some protective mechanisms that evolved during earlier evolutionary phases still exist without function (e.g., motion sickness, the cuneiform appendix, scalp prickling in fear, and hair on neck stiffening when alarmed).
13. Protective mechanisms in humans operate in a variety of ways. They
    a) Warn of danger or need.
    b) Permit more rapid movement or withdrawal.
    c) Neutralize or destroy the threatening or attacking agent as in the development of immunity.
    d) Harden an area and make it impervious to attack, as in the formation of corns or in the clotting of blood.
    e) Reduce awareness as in emotional shock and syncope.
    f) Increase the rate or decrease the rate of functioning, as in physiological shock or production of epinephrine in fright.
    g) Draw upon hoarded energy supplies, as in glycogen and fat during the stress response.
    h) Promote return of function or wholeness, as in healing of wounds or fractures.
14. Protective mechanisms have a peak performance level. Maintaining peak performance is limited by many variables. When performance cannot be maintained, the protective function is inappropriate or fails. If the protective function has not been completed, it becomes part of whatever pathophysiological processes are operating.
15. Amount of noxious agent producing threat to the physiological response determines whether protective response will be initiated or whether the organism will go into physiological disequilibrium.
16. Strength or responsiveness of the organism in relation to threat determines whether the organism responds protectively or whether protection responses are overwhelmed.

Scientific Assumptions about Basic Human Physiological Protective Mechanisms

1. The identified physiological phenomena are, in their primary function, protective.
2. These phenomena protect by providing some kind of visually or sensibly observable warning.

3. The protective phenomena or mechanisms are experienced as bodily discomfort, need, or drive.
4. Resolution of the appearance of protective mechanisms is followed by relief.
5. Elimination of protective mechanisms is usually followed by feelings of ease and pleasure.
6. The identified protective mechanisms are operational for protection on a time-limited basis.
7. Each identified protective mechanism has its own specific time-limited effectiveness period.
8. People continually monitor and assess their bodily functioning to preclude the necessity of protective mechanisms.
9. People make decisions on a continuous basis that prevent the necessity of protective responses, or they make risk-taking decisions in which they take the chance of calling forth one or more protective responses.

Beliefs about Nursing and Basic Physiological Protective Mechanisms

1. Knowledge about basic human physiological protective phenomena is important to health maintenance and health promotion.
2. Knowledge about basic human physiological protective phenomena can contribute to self-care models for health and illness.
3. Nurses can enhance their contribution to health care by teaching self-care and healthy life-style maintenance in relation to basic human physiological protective phenomena.
4. Reinforcement and support of basic human physiological protective phenomena are necessary nursing activities.
5. Learning self-protection through self-care is a lifelong process.
6. Long-standing self-protective (self-care) practices become habitual and are then practiced at the level of the preconscious.
7. Habitual protective self-care practices are more likely to be carried on regularly than are newly learned practices.
8. Habitual nonprotective self-care practices are the hardest ones to break.
9. Self-care protective teaching and practice are a family function.

Values

1. Changing the perspective of the identified physiological phenomena from symptom to that of protective mechanism bodes well for people's health.
2. People will eventually use health knowledge to improve their life-styles in the direction of health.

3. When health professionals restructure their roles, people will take responsibility for individual and family health promotion.

Goals of action. Health professionals should work toward the following goals:

Effective response to protective mechanisms
Health promotion
Health maintenance
Illness prevention
Prevention of bodily discomfort

Actors' Roles. In the area of protective functions, nurses function as teachers, motivators, consultants, supporters, facilitators, debators, questioners, and collaborators.

Intervention. Nursing intervention involves awareness of both the foci and modes of health care. Foci include

1. Body listening and assessment skills
2. Decision-making skills
3. Knowledge of physiological protective phenomena
4. Relationship to one's body—rhythms, dynamic equilibrium, warnings, responses to warnings, and ease, relief, pleasures
5. Health-promoting life-styles

Modes include

1. Modeling
2. Motivating
3. Teaching by many methods
4. Supporting
5. Identifying resources
6. Consulting about problems and responsibilities
7. Consensual validation

Description of the Target Population

The target population of this beginning theory of physiological protective mechanisms includes all people who recognize and respond when dynamic physiological equilibrium threatens them. These are people who routinely and matter-of-factly monitor and assess their bodies in space and time. On a continuing basis, they make decisions that prevent occurrence of protective mechanisms.

They are people who promote and maintain wellness by responding to their body's warnings of threat to equilibrium. And once they have eliminated the warning, thus reinstituting unthreatened physiological equilibrium, they enjoy the resulting feelings of relief and pleasure. The adult target population also teaches its children to confidently listen to, assess, and make health-promoting decisions for themselves.

The target population make conscious, risk-taking decisions about disturbing dynamic physiological homeostasis that call forth warning protective mechanisms.

Discussion

The identified phenomena. In the final analysis, all of the phenomena specified in this volume are related. Taken as a whole, they reflect a comprehensive mechanism for survival—cellular adjustment and cellular repair—in terms of threat to an organism's total integrity. These protective mechanisms originate at precortical or subcortical levels as reflex actions or, in some cases (e.g., hunger and thirst) as drives. This ability of an organism to protect itself ultimately depends on the endogenous biological capability of the organism to

1. Eject the threatening agent or repair the damage done by the agent.
2. Neutralize the invasive agent if not ejected, as in the case of the inflammatory response or the antigen–antibody reaction. During the total period of threat, endogenous mechanisms are working to neutralize toxins (e.g., endogenous antibodies).
3. Withdraw from the threatening agent.
4. Maintain appropriate metabolic response to stress (e.g., while stressed organism is insulin antagonized, glycogen reserves are mobilized; gluconeogenesis occurs to maintain an adequate supply of carbohydrate for brain function and fatty acid oxidation provides high energy yield to other cells). Anorexia in this phase is an appropriate and protective response. Eating at this point to provide energy substrate might lead to a more energy-demanding disequilibrium for the organism in that eating could lead to nausea and vomiting.
5. In the case of prolonged or overwhelming threat, protective functions may exceed their optimum functional capacity and no longer function to protect (e.g., toxin production exceeds neutralization; energy production does not meet demands; pain outstrips psychological tolerance or the threatening agent cannot be ejected). These inappropriate responses culminate in widely deranged metabolic activity with accompanying cell necrosis, which the organism experiences as illness. And the protective function is terminated as its effective time period expires.

Nursing. In this chapter, an attempt was made to synthesize and thus provide greater meaning to the work of this volume. While this is a useful activity in theory building, explanation of phenomena is not all the information nurses need to practice. As indicated earlier, another kind of knowledge—theory or scientific knowledge—is needed in deciding how to use explanation provided by theory and scientific knowledge. Nurses also need *practice theory* and knowledge that they use to draw upon substantive knowledge of the discipline (e.g., content related to basic physiological protection mechanisms).

Theory. The umbrella concept of protection as developed in this text incorporates a broader range of variables and permits more sophisticated prediction than nurses have conceptualized about basic physiological protection of the human organism in previous studies. As more clinicians, theoreticians, and researchers study and critique the concept, its application potential in nursing practice will be realized.

REFERENCE

Abbey, J., Andrews, C., Avigliano, K., Blossom, R., Bunke, B., Engberg, N., Halliburton, P., and Peterson, J. A pilot study: The control of shivering during hypothermia by a clinical nursing measure. *J. Neurosurg. Nurs.* 5:78–88, 1973.

Chapter 24

The Relationship of the Protective Phenomena to Nursing

Catherine M. Norris

By definition . . . a discipline is not global; it is characterized by a unique perspective, a distinct way of viewing all phenomena (Donaldson and Crowley 1978).

Nursing knowledge, because of nurses' close alliance with medicine, has been traditionally oriented to symptoms. Symptoms represent processes whose end-products are failure of bodily systems unless there is medical intervention. It follows that much of nursing assessment has arisen out of identifying a problem and tracing it back into the medical model where it is considered from the point of view of failure of the human organism. Much of nursing intervention has emerged from attempts to assist in or complement medical intervention and to provide measures that reduce the discomfort caused by the pathology or medical treatment of it.

NAMING FOR NURSING

In this volume, some basic physiological protective phenomena for nursing have been named. So many of my colleagues and students questioned the importance of "naming" that it seems necessary to explain the significance here. In concrete terms, a few symptoms commonly associated with medicine have been analyzed and certain components of these symptoms have been named *basic physiological protective mechanisms*. What is so significant about this change? To return to the work of Donaldson and Crowley (1978), some nursing concepts have been separated from medical phenomena; this separation provides a unique nursing perspective for viewing the concepts. This naming makes nursing concepts visible; it gives the concepts a quality and value they previously lacked. Naming is an early step in the search for meaning (i.e., bringing inarticulate knowledge to a level where it is possible to proceed to study it). Naming provides a springboard for study, research, and ultimately, practice. Naming is a beginning step in defining nature. Only within a system of names can we experience reality. Failing to name phenomena is to mystify, devalue, and make them invisible. Naming for nursing requires action. Nurses must determine whether basic physiological protective phenomena represent reality and whether they are meaningful for nursing. If the phenomena do not represent reality, the nursing action is to reject them; if they do represent reality, nurses can then initiate the search for meaning.

EVALUATING CONCEPTS FOR NURSING

Concept clarification is a recognized initial step in theory building. An initial step in evaluating concept work, however, is deciding whether the concepts are basic or important to the discipline. Nurses will have made, by this point in their reading of the text, some decisions about whether the concepts clarified and the construct of protection have potential for useful theory building in nursing.

Each concept clarified may be examined under a guideline of what is possible now, using the criteria of meaning that includes things like theoretical and operational definitions, specification of the limits of inclusion, a typology with mutually exclusive categories, and descriptions of empirical referents. Besides meeting the criteria of degree of generality, level of abstractness and degree of complexity may be used in evaluating concepts.

Nursing concepts are also evaluated in terms of their usefulness in understanding the meaning of the phenomena that confront nurses. Concepts are judged in terms of whether they advance the knowledge of the discipline. This includes evaluating the scope of the work and whether the hypotheses stated are testable and predictive. Ideally, concepts are stated in ways that make them easily testable and have high predictive value. If hypotheses are not stated, the concepts need to be related to theory or theoretical principles. Concept clarification cannot be isolated from theory construction.

Concepts need to be evaluated in terms of their precision. If the vernacular of the particular society is the language used, it is bound to have limited communication value. The common sense language of the laity is usually too imprecise and too vague for professional practice.

The ultimate clarity is represented in an operational definition, a structural model, and the facility with which we can move from one level of abstraction to another—from the multiple concrete to levels of generality and back again to observed specifics. If new terms are invented, they must also be operationally defined to meet the criteria of clarity and precision.

Concepts can also be evaluated by the kind of reasoning that appears at all levels of the work. Contradictions, overgeneralizations (i.e., going beyond the information at hand), ambiguity, equivocation, and excursions into unrelated matters are all traps.

Concepts are not true or false, right or wrong, good or bad. They cannot be verified (by relying on tradition, authority, or past experience). Some scholars have relied on their reputations, on getting the work published, on inventing new terms for concepts, or on simply asserting that their work was important in the development of the science of the discipline. But concept work can only be verified by research.

LOOKING TO THE FUTURE

If the named concepts are accepted in the profession, one unique perspective of nursing might be its priorities in assessing health, facilitating health-producing behaviors, conceptualizing health-producing life-styles, and supporting behaviors that reduce health risks. These priorities require a substantive body of knowledge about health.

A major component in a program of health promotion and reduction of risks to health is protective. All of the concepts dealt with in this volume except pressure sores have one or more aspects that can be subsumed in the category of protection—physiological protection that forms the foundation of any hierarchy of needs. These are low-level (primitive) human protective functions in an evolutionary sense. That is, they emerged phylogenetically before higher level intellectual and social needs. They represent the body's first line of defense, or warning system, against attack. They are behavioral phenomena that can be described in their primary roles as healthy coping activities. Pressure sores represent a kind of secondary coping because they represent failure of the protective functions of the skin in coping with a variety of stressors. Pressure sores are related to the other phenomena discussed in that they are all coping mechanisms that protect up to a point. The failure of protection is represented by pathological processes. The approach to pressure sores in this volume is in considerable contrast to the search for meaning in some other chapters and provides an excellent contrast to the search for meaning in physiological failure as opposed to physiological protection. The chapters on chronic itching, thirst, nausea in MI patients, and immobility were approached from the standpoint of pathology with the recognition that these phenomena have protective phases.

A CHANGING PERSPECTIVE FOR NURSES

Once phenomena, identified in a pathophysiological framework as symptoms, are identified as protective (i.e., representing healthy coping activity), questions arise related to what extent should they be encouraged and supported.

What are the criteria that identify each of these behaviors as protective?

To what extent would we initiate any of these protective phenomena and under what circumstances?

What are the criteria for terminating supporting activities (i.e., for assessing protective behavior)?

What are the criteria for intervening in the various protective behaviors?

Are there situations in which the behaviors would be supported but where other dimensions of the situation indicate tamping?

What are the criteria for making the diagnosis of failure or inappropriateness of each of these protective behaviors?

What is the total range of human (physiological and psychological) phenomena that compose the body's first line of defense?

What are the ways that basic physiological protective mechanisms fail and cause disequilibrium?

Are there nursing interventions that support protective behavior and discourage or delay the loss of physiological equilibrium?

For example, if thirst and hunger do not accomplish their function, levels of consciousness are changed and autistic thinking occurs. These changes cause the individual to lie, cheat, steal, fight, or gorge on food and fluid even though the possible complications—including death—are known to the individual. Ultimately, fluid and electrolyte imbalance, weight loss, and other serious physiological imbalances occur. The questions raised above need to be answered by practicing nurses who identify the criterion attributes of these phenomena and raise critical questions. Clinicians then articulate their work with nurse researchers who have methodologies and some of the instrumentation needed for studying the questions.

Primary Protection

As noted in Chapter 23, each person knows to some extent how to prevent the occurrence of basic physiological protective mechanisms in the self. Each person knows of measures to prevent nausea, chilling, overheating, thirst, hunger, and the like. Each person also monitors and assesses his or her behavior and relationship to the environment as a way of maintaining dynamic equilibrium. Further, each person carries on considerable risk-taking behavior when there is conflict between the priority to prevent the occurrence of protective mechanisms and some other priority. Some people are able to listen less in self-monitoring and others are more frequent risk-takers. If nurses sought baseline data about the health of risk-takers as compared to the sensitive listeners and less frequent risk-takers, the risk-takers might demonstrate need for a new kind of primary protection.

Secondary Protection

Once a protective mechanism occurs, nurses need to respond in damping, rather than preventive, ways. Then they need to consider prevention of future incidents by assessing the basis of decision making, past experience with the protective mechanism, self-monitoring, level of risk-taking, and advice of others. While some nursing assessment could be carried on at the present time, now, much of this level of protection depends on what questions will be asked, how they will be studied, and what kinds of findings evolve.

Protective responses may demand or be assigned priority according to some hierarchy or other criterion. Degree of discomfort or need for relief might function as a criterion. Nausea, thirst, and itching might all produce demands for immediate relief. Cause and effect might function as criteria in terms of consequences if the protective behavior fails, as in dehydration or pressure sores. Duration might be another temporal component used in viewing priority for nursing. If diarrhea, vomiting, or profuse perspiration occurs over a period of time there is danger that these protective functions will have reached their limits; they then become part of an illness process. Frequency of occurrence, as in morning sickness, may be a criterion indicating a high priority for nursing. Threat to integrity might also function as a criterion in determining priority since it is known that incontinence, for example, is a last-ditch failure of human integrity. Groups of protective responses, occurring simultaneously or in sequence, might be important in setting priorities for nursing as in the sequence of constipation, diarrhea, and impaction. Of all the protective phenomena that fall within the context of nursing, we wonder which is the most protective.

When we view the variety of protective mechanisms of the human organism, the questions of which responses are more important and what criteria should be used in determining priorities for nursing attention arise. The most obvious criterion would be to relate the protective response to some hierarchy of needs to give priority to responses originating in lower-level needs (e.g., dyspnea). Another criterion might give priority in terms of general response versus specific organ response. For example, elevated temperature, being a general response, would receive more attention than flatulence. Temporal criteria might determine nursing priorities. Sleep disturbance, restlessness, and fatigue have been identified as early protective responses and it may be that intervention at this point would promote rapid reinstatement of dynamic homeostasis.

It is obvious to clinicians that many people are out of touch with healthy homeostasis and protective functions with resulting dissynchrony between their behavior and their bodies' responses to their behavior. We can all name people who consistently overwork or abuse the body's first line of protective defenses. We can speculate about whether people who frequently abuse their first-line defense system are more prone or more vulnerable to health breakdown and disease. There is some evidence for some protective functions (e.g, coughing from cigarette smoking) that this may be so. It is interesting to contemplate whether the majority of people in healthy dynamic equilibrium consciously structure this state of existence or whether it is encultured ritualistic practice that requires no conscious thought or little awareness.

NURSES AND SELF-CARE

It appears that both primary and secondary prevention in relation to the protective warning phenomena must be the responsibility of each person or each family for obvious reasons. If self-care is the modus operandi, what then is the role of nursing? When physicians have relied on the role of exhorter, nurses have explored roles as participant observers, facilitators, supporters, teachers, and motivators. While these roles require much more study and testing, nurses have made a beginning and may be ready to move effectively in this area as knowledge about basic human protective mechanisms is developed. Nurses also have the contexts with large captive audiences in which to function—especially schools, industry, and well-baby clinics.

CONCLUSION

This book constitutes a beginning attempt to develop knowledge of the discipline of nursing using an inductive approach. It represents a transitional phase between nonsystematic concept clarification and concept clarification using sophisticated exploratory and descriptive methodologies. The text represents solid advances for concept clarification for nurses. Responsibility for continuing to build and hone theory for the discipline rests with concerned nursing professionals.

> The major area needing nursing research is the identification of the specialized concepts which constitute nursing practice. This relatively untouched domain is fraught with risks, but one in which we must risk "significant failures" rather than settle for "trivial successes" (Kramer, 1970).

In the future, whole scholarly books will be written about a single nursing phenomenon. No nurse could possibly study a concept in all its contexts or in all its meanings, but as more nurses study phenomena from both general and specific perspectives, nursing will be able to articulate the findings of their research and other scholarly activities to create, ultimately, the body of knowledge called nursing.

REFERENCES

Donaldson, S.K., and Crowley, D.M. The discipline of nursing. *Nurs. Outlook* 26:113–120, Feb. 1978.

Kramer, M. Concept Formation. In M.V. Batey, *Communicating Nursing Research*. Boulder, Col.: Western Interstate Commission for Higher Education, 1970.

Index

A

Abortion, and morning sickness, 151
Acetaminophen, for shivering control, 237
Adaptation
  avoidance of fatigue and, 254
  as behavior concept, 14
  to disorientation, 317–21
  Roy's model, 188–89
  as theory, 5
  thirst process as, 192
Advances in Nursing Science, 37
Affect
  data on hunger, *202*
  in description, *73*
Analysis
  See also Methods
  knowledge and, 12
Anesthesia, stress and, 282–83
Anorexia
  hunger and, 212
  nausea and, 87
  underlying malfunctions in, 200
Anorexia nervosa, 103
  vomiting and, 92
Antibiotics. *See* Drugs

Anxiety
  as behavior concept, 4, 14
  in disorientation, 310, 315
  immobilization and, 336, 337, 348
  infant, 326
  insomnia and, 305
  maternal, 326, 331, 332
Appetite, defined, *209*
Arthritis, as cause of immobility, 334, 347
Ascites, defined, *177*
Associations, as relationships, 56
Atherosclerotic plaques, in heart disease, *111*
Automatic behavior syndrome, 311
Awareness of Dying, 31

B

Basic physiological protective mechanisms
  biological capability and, 402
  common attributes, 394, 395
  decision making and, 393
    avoiding protection mechanism, 393
    in ignorance, 394
    risk-taking, 393–94

Note: Italicized page numbers include references to defined or "clarified" nursing terms and concepts.